www.harcourt-international.com

Bringing you products from all Harcourt Health Sciences companies including Baillière Tindall, Churchill Livingstone, Mosby and W.B. Saunders

▸ **Browse** for latest information on new books, journals and electronic products

▸ **Search** for information on over 20 000 published titles with full product information including tables of contents and sample chapters

▸ **Keep up to date** with our extensive publishing programme in your field by registering with **eAlert** or requesting postal updates

▸ **Secure online ordering** with prompt delivery, as well as full contact details to order by phone, fax or post

▸ **News** of special features and promotions

If you are based in the following countries, please visit the country-specific site to receive full details of product availability and local ordering information

USA: www.harcourthealth.com

Canada: www.harcourtcanada.com

Australia: www.harcourt.com.au

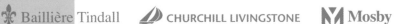 Baillière Tindall CHURCHILL LIVINGSTONE Mosby 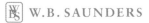 W.B. SAUNDERS

Physical Signs
of Child Abuse

Commissioning Editor: Deborah Russell
Project Development Manager: Tim Kimber
Project Manager: Rolla Couchman/Scott Millar
Designer: Jayne Jones
Page Layout: Jim Hope

Physical Signs of Child Abuse

Second Edition

Christopher J. Hobbs BSc FRCP FRCPCH

Consultant Paediatrician
Department of Community Paediatrics
St James University Hospital
Leeds UK

Jane M Wynne FRCP FRCPCH

Senior Clinical Lecturer
Department of Community Paediatrics
St James University Hospital
Leeds UK

W.B. SAUNDERS

London • Edinburgh • New York • Philadelphia • St Louis • Sydney • Toronto 2001

WB SAUNDERS

An imprint of Harcourt Publishers Limited

© Harcourt Publishers Limited 2001

 is a registered trademark of Harcourt Publishers Limited

First published 1996

ISBN 0-7020-2582-8

British Library Cataloguing in Publication Data
A catalogue record for this book is available from the British Library

Library of Congress Cataloging in Publication Data
A catalog record for this book is available from the Library of Congress

Note
Medical knowledge is constantly changing. As new information becomes available, changes in treatment, procedures, equipment and the use of drugs become necessary. The editors/authors/contributors and the publishers have taken care to ensure that the information given in this text is accurate and up to date. However, readers are strongly advised to confirm that the information, especially with regard to drug usage, complies with the latest legislation and standards of practice.

Existing UK nomenclature is changing to the system of Recommended International Non-proprietary Names (rINNs). Until the UK names are no longer in use, these more familiar names are used in this book in preference to rINNs, details of which may be obtained from the British National Formulary.

The publisher's policy is to use paper manufactured from sustainable forests

Printed in Spain

Contents

Preface

The first edition of our colour Atlas was well received and has been widely used in teaching. We are to develop a teaching pack of selected slides/CD set to sell with the Atlas to enhance the teaching opportunities for colleagues.

We continue to talk about Jigsaws and would urge colleagues to advise against instant, snap diagnoses: there is no substitute for clinical method.

The Atlas has grown.

Certain abuses are increasingly recognized – for example, emotional abuse and neglect and this is recognized in the Atlas. Paediatricians, in common with most adults, find the notion of child sexual abuse difficult. The standards of proof required in the courts have risen and levels of denial are high as professionals in the field are "attacked" professionally but also in the media.

Additionally there are very real worries as to the management of sexual abuse. If the mother believes the child the outlook immediately improves.

The best that is achieved for children is early recognition and thereby damage limitation. Prevention of abuse remains the long term aim: but it's a long haul...

We hope that this Atlas will help children and thank all our colleagues who have supported us.

Many slides have been sent to us by fellow paediatricians and particularly those attending the monthly "colposcope meeting" where slides are discussed (and donated!)

SECTION 1

INTRODUCTION

Chapter 1

Methods of Examination

The medical examination of the child who may have been abused or neglected

The paediatrician's role in the evaluation of possible child abuse or neglect extends beyond the physical examination and has been described in some detail (Hobbs *et al.* 1999; Royal College of Physicians 1997; Bamford and Roberts 1998).

The findings of the examination are seen in the context of the 'whole child examination' to include a view of the child's current and past medical history, his growth and development, in addition to any signs of trauma and infection. These findings may become part of a multi-agency assessment (which includes social services, the police and other health professionals) as to the probability of abuse.

The completed 'jigsaw' (Figs. 1.1, 1.2) attempts to clarify the clinical method and emphasizes the need to build up the diagnosis from the relevant pieces of information; this approach should minimize misdiagnosis. The diagnosis of child abuse may be straightforward but on occasion it is extremely difficult, for example 'fictitious illness'.

The physical injuries sustained by the child may be recognized as a pattern of typical assault but on other occasions the signs are non-specific and interpretation is difficult.

Healing of injuries may be rapid and early examination is usual to record injury, treat, for example, fractures or a sexually transmitted disease and collect 'forensic swabs'.

The main reasons for examining a child who may have been sexually abused have been described (Bamford and Roberts 1996):

- to detect any traumatic or infective disorder which needs treatment;
- to evaluate the nature of any abuse;
- to provide forensic evidence which may be helpful in the future protection of children;
- to reassure the child;
- to begin the process of recovery.

These criteria for examination of children are valid when evaluating other abuses and, in any event, the children are frequently abused in several ways.

The timing of injuries is difficult and imprecise and recent research into bruising, for example, confirms that yellowing occurs after 18 hours but all other colours are variable in ageing.

Consent for examination:

- If uncertain take legal advice.
- The co-operation of the child is needed and older teenagers may give their own consent if 'Gillick competent' – on occasion a general anaesthetic is required.
- Consent is usually given by the adult who has parental responsibility (Children Act 1989) – oral consent is equally valid as written, there should be no coercion and the implications of consent are understood.
- Additional consent is required for photography, radiography and other investigations.
- Once legal proceedings have been started the Court's permission is required for medical investigations or examination.

History from parent	History from child	Any disclosure
Physical symptoms	Child's behaviour	Bruises/injuries
Physical examination	Sexually transmitted infection	'Forensic' investigation
Police inquiry	Social work assessment	Siblings

◀ **Fig. 1.1 The 'jigsaw' in the diagnosis of child sexual abuse**

◀ **Fig. 1.2 The 'jigsaw' in the diagnosis of physical abuse**

History from parent	History from child	History from third party
Physical symptoms	Bruises/other soft tissue injuries	Fractures/head injury/abdominal injury
Physical examination	Blood tests, e.g. clotting disorder	Skeletal survey/ brain scan/ other radiology
Police inquiry	Social work assessment	Siblings

Method of examination

Children should be examined by trained paediatricians in child-friendly but appropriately equipped clinics.

The gender of the doctor is less important than the manner of the examiner, but older children often have a preference which should be respected.

There should always be a chaperone (General Medical Council Guidance 1999).

The initial examination follows usual clinical methods, including measurement of growth and use of standardized growth charts.

Increasingly paediatricians are using colposcopes when examining the ano-genital area which provides:

- good illumination;
- magnification;
- an integral camera, i.e. improves recording;
- an important 'distance' from the child which is appreciated by the child and the examiner.

It is important to record the method of examination

For example:

- when examining the anus 'left lateral buttocks parted for 30 seconds';
- when examining the genitalia 'supine, frog-legged with labial separation or labial traction' or, 'knee-chest position'.

Inspection is adequate for the examination of pre-pubertal girls but from puberty a vaginal examination is needed. A case has not been made to justify rectal examinations. The stage of puberty must be recorded using Tanner stages.

Description of the child and his injuries

At the beginning of each chapter there is a more detailed description of the physical findings seen in association with the category of abuse.

- Physical state: describe any signs of neglect including dental caries as part of usual paediatric examination (Chapter 16).

- Growth: signs of malnutrition, stunting (Chapter 17).
- Behaviour seen during the examination.
- Developmental screen.
- Physical injuries: bruises, burns, bites.
- Genito-anal examination for signs of trauma and infection.

Organizing the paediatric assessment

- Referrals may be via the general practitioner, social services department, health visitor, police, paediatrician, family – child protection requires a flexible, positive approach from the doctor. Undue delay may allow healing and renders the examination less useful. Some forensic and microbiological swabs must be taken urgently.
- What are the indications for the assessment? Do you have adequate information? Is there any urgency? Are siblings at risk? Has the child been prepared?
- Is the paediatrician adequately trained/supervised?
- Is the gender of the doctor important? Older children may have a preference but the manner of examination is more important for most children.
- Is the clinical accommodation appropriately child friendly, with staff trained to treat children (including a chaperone)? Remember the need for security, i.e. for the family and the professionals.
- Is there the necessary equipment for the examination and any investigations – a colposcope, camera (record the number of photos), bright light source, microbiological swabs, 'forensic' swabs, access for blood tests and X-rays.
- Facilities to conduct an examination under general anaesthetic – this is rarely necessary; the exceptions are a distressed child who may require surgery (usually child sexual abuse), the child may have a sexually transmitted disease and is unable to co-operate, an examination is felt to be necessary to protect the child.

Notes on conducting the examination

- Children should be prepared by the carer before arriving at the clinic and understand why the appointment has been arranged and the extent of the examination. Children should never be physically restrained, the exception being pre-verbal infants. Talk to the child before and during the examination and explain the process; maintain as much privacy as possible and build up the child's confidence. Draw the injuries, examine the genitalia and anus at the end of the examination, taking colposcope pictures during the examination.

◆ If the child is very young or apprehensive use usual strategies, e.g. examine with the help of the mother, on the mother's knee; teenagers may need a further appointment.

◆ Recording: notes should be dated, signed, legible and contemporaneous. Often a proforma is available and is useful as an aide-memoire (swabs to do, results to file, etc.).

◆ Reports and police statements should ideally be written the day of the examination, but do not give an opinion under pressure before you have had time to think/consult.

The structure of paediatric assessment is based on usual practice and includes:

◆ A history (presenting, past history, general health, family and social history).

◆ A full physical examination – the child may choose who is to be with him during his examination: carer, social worker, friend. Do not examine any child alone; if in doubt ask the clinic nurse to be present.

◆ An assessment of the child's growth (height, weight, mid-upper arm circumference, head circumference and stage of sexual development).

◆ A brief assessment of the child's development.

◆ An assessment of any maltreatment – neglect, physical injury, sexual abuse and an indication as to the child's emotional wellbeing.

◆ Further history, previous medical records (school, hospital and general practitioner) may only be available later.

◆ If social services department have requested the examination the social worker should accompany the family and be informed. (Note: avoid asking the child a detailed history if this is likely to cause distress, talk to the carer, social worker, etc., but if necessary ask for history of pain, bleeding and a detailed urinary and bowel history, last period, tampon use.)

Recording of the examination should be careful – a proforma with line figures, details of specimens taken and later results of any medical investigations should be available.

◆ The child's demeanour, response to carer, play, attention, behaviour during the examination. (Note: record any comments made by the child verbatim.)

◆ Usual examination: mouth (teeth, petechiae, palate), ENT, eyes, cardiovascular and respiratory system, abdomen and genitalia/anus.

◆ Signs of neglect, e.g. dirty.

◆ Physical injuries:
  – bruises (site, size, colour) and soft tissue swelling
  – lacerations, abrasions (site, depth, width, length, healing?);
  – burns (contact, scald) and (site, dimensions, healing?);
  – swelling, deformity, disuse of limb ± bruising and pain on examination? fracture;

  – bites (site, shape, colour, laceration, dimensions) – consider swab for saliva, orthodontist opinion.

◆ Sexual abuse: note stage of puberty and position of child (supine, frog-legged, knee-chest, left lateral), method of examination (labial separation or traction), length of time (less than 30 seconds), buttock separation. Note if hymenal opening remains closed.

◆ Erythema, bruises, burn, laceration, etc., to external genitalia/perianally.

◆ Labial fusion (length and thickness of fusion)

◆ Injury to perineum (scars, thickened ± shiny skin, bruises, laceration).

◆ Hymenal opening gaping before labial separation

◆ Vulvitis or vulvovaginitis-erythema ± discharge (colour, amount, odour).

◆ Abrasion, scar at posterior fourchette

◆ Hymen configuration (i.e. annular, crescentic, fleshy, obliterated), infantile/prepubertal, pubertal (oestrogenized), erythema, swelling, dimensions, notches, deficits, bumps, tags, dimensions of opening, thickened rolled margin, attenuated hymen, rarely scars. Notes:
  – hymen is thickened under the influence of oestrogen in infancy or puberty and is thickened/'redundant', prepubertally the hymen is thinner with increased erythema and visible vascular pattern and continuous fine margin.
  – vaginal ridges are normal and may give an irregular appearance to the hymenal margin.
  – there is no indication for a digital examination prepubertally; however it is mandatory postpubertally as the redundant, petal-like hymen may obscure a dilated vagina. Record, e.g. fifth finger (1.5 cm) with ease, index finger (2.5 cm) caused discomfort. Terms such as 'roomy vagina' are more difficult to classify.

◆ Anus: examine in left lateral position, gently part buttocks and inspect anus. After 30 seconds let buttocks come together and repeat examination. (Note: erythema, swelling, bruising, scratches perianally, anal laxity, reflex anal dilation, veins (halo, act, swollen), scars, fissure(s), skin tags.)

◆ Infection: erythema, vesicles, warts, discharge (urethral, vaginal, rectal, oral) – screen for a sexually transmitted disease (STD).

◆ Forensic: swabs for semen, sperm, saliva, blood stain, blood sample of DNA, etc. (see later).

Differential diagnosis

◆ skin disorder, e.g. lichen sclerosis;

◆ blood dyscrasia, e.g. ITP;

◆ fractures, e.g. osteogenesis imperfecta, osteoporosis;

◆ failure to thrive, e.g. coeliac disease.

Diagnosis

◆ Do you need advice? Is another opinion needed?

◆ Are you able to make a diagnosis?

◆ Do not be pushed into a quick diagnosis, say if you need more time.

References

Hobbs CJ Hanks HIG Wynne JM 1999 *Child Abuse and Neglect. A Clinician's Handbook* Churchill Livingstone

The Royal College of Physicians 1997 *The physical signs of sexual abuse in prepubertal children.* London

Bamford F Roberts R 1989 Child Sexual Abuse Chapter in *ABC of Child Abuse* ed. SR Meadow BMJ publication London

General Medical Council guidance on Chaperones 1999; Consent 2000, London

Additional Reading

A Physician's Guide to Clinical Forensic Medicine 2000 ed. MM Stark Humana Press New Jersey US

Chapter 2

The Use of the Colposcope

The colposcope is an instrument widely used in gynecology for the examination of the cervix uteri. Interest in the process of diagnosis has encouraged the adoption of new methods of physical examination including the use of the colposcope.

The essential requirements for examining the genital tract in female children include illumination and magnification. The colposcope fulfils those requirements better than any of the other methods which have been tried.

The colposcope is a binocular system of lenses of varying strength coupled to an integral light source and mounted on a rigid structure, usually a stand or cantilevered arm. Cameras (35mm, Polaroid, digital and video) can be attached.

It has been estimated that an additional 10 per cent of suspected cases were corroborated than would have been using conventional examination techniques. The colposcope is important in difficult or subtle cases. Others have concluded that examination with the unaided eye is adequate for most children. Despite these contradictory views, the popularity of the colposcope continues to increase.

Applications

The colposcope can be used in the examination of the anus in both boys and girls, and both prepubertal and pubertal genitalia in the female. Its use is non-invasive and 'creates an environment in which the examination is done with care and attention to detail' (Woodling and Heger 1986).

The colposcope combines an integral photographic facility. Photography of all visible findings in abuse is increasingly expected as the standard of good practice. Images produced by colposcopy can be recorded by:

◆ 35mm standard photography using a single lens reflex (SLR) camera; (to date 35mm photography provides the highest quality images);
◆ Polaroid photography producing instant photographs;
◆ digital image;
◆ videotaped recording.

When combined with a one-way screen which overlooks the consulting or examination area, physicians in training may obtain the benefit of being able to observe the examination findings within the context of the clinical consultation whilst preserving minimal intrusiveness for the child. Full permission is required from the child and carers.

An additional advantage of the colposcope is the capability, in some models with integral eyepiece measuring devices, for direct measurement of examination parameters, for example the hymenal opening diameter. The colposcope can also facilitate the taking of fine 'ENT'-sized swabs for microbiological investigation by means of trans-hymenal insertion under close visual control.

Good quality photographs enable findings to be discussed with colleagues and studied with more time and attention than can usually be achieved in the emotionally charged atmosphere of the consulting room. Nowadays there is a tendency for examiners to undertake this work in teams. Each doctor has an on-call commitment and support is obtained by regular peer review meetings. The case file and photographs form the basis for discussions of cases and diagnostic evaluations can be shared with colleagues. Video-conferencing extended to trusted colleagues has allowed for greater consultation in other hospitals and centres geographically distant and for difficult cases.

Acceptability for patient and parent

In the modern health care system, the use of medical technology is accepted and expected as an adjunct to competent and professional clinical practice. The alternative, that of attempting to peer between a child's legs with an otoscope held a few centimetres from the child's genitalia is less appealing to examiner and patient. The colposcope places the examiner about 20–40 cm away from the child and allows a more relaxed examination. Verbal consent is usually adequate for the examination and is sought from parent and child. Additional consent is required for photographs. Information is given that photographs are used to document the medical record and may be seen by other doctors who are asked to provide opinions. If there are legal proceedings and the court permits other doctors to become involved then this information will be made available to them and may avoid the need for further examination of the child. They may also be used for teaching and research.

Technique

The instrument can be introduced to the child so as to gain co-operation. Some children enjoy looking down it, whilst others find interest in the green light. The child lies in the supine position at the end of an examination couch with perineum about 10 inches from the end of the couch. Examination of the anus is usually undertaken with the child in the left lateral position. Ideally the colposcope should be at 90 degrees to the plane of the genitalia and anus. Our experience with the current versions of the Olympus colposcope is that the couch may need slight elevation to achieve this with anal inspection. Measurements can be obtained using standard measuring devices held close to and in front of the anatomical structure to be measured and photographed. Parallax error should be avoided by close apposition.

The shutter release and film wind on are operated by a simple foot-operated switch connected via a remote cable to the camera winder. Photographing patient details using standard information cards at the beginning of the examination enables identification of photographs. A camera data back is used to automatically imprint the date onto the photographic slide as a further check.

Some units now routinely use video-colposcopy with images stored on videotape. The full examination is then recorded.

Advantages

◆ Non-invasive technique.
◆ Good light and magnification allow detailed and careful examination.
◆ Facilities for non-intrusive photography (requires no flash illumination). Photographs can be used for second opinions, legal work, teaching and peer review.
◆ Acceptable to child, parents and doctor.

Disadvantages

◆ Expensive.
◆ Relatively non-portable.
◆ May discourage unaided examination and be seen as essential.
◆ Danger of over-interpretation of minor signs.

References

Woodling BA and Heger A. (1986) The use of the colposcope in the diagnosis of sexual abuse in the pediatric age group. *Child Abuse and Neglect* 10: 111–114.

Further Reading

De San Lazaro (1985) Making Paediatric assesment in suspected sexual abuse a therapeutic experience. *Archives of Disease in Childhood* 73: 174–176.
Hobbs CJ, Wynne JM. (1996) Use of the colposcope in examination for sexual abuse. *Archives of Disease in Childhood* 75: 539–542

Chapter 3

Photography in Child Abuse

This can be undertaken by a medical photographer, a police photographer, a doctor who is seeing the child or other designated professionals working as part of the investigative team.

Photography may be used to record:

◆ injuries, e.g. bruises, burns;
◆ genital and anal signs (usually injury or infection);
◆ growth and development;
◆ appearance, including demeanour, emotional signs and signs of neglect.

The uses of photographs in child abuse work are:

◆ to document any visible findings;
◆ to share findings with others who may need to know;
◆ for peer review;
◆ for teaching and research.

Good medico-legal practice

◆ In child abuse cases the standard is that all visible lesions should be photographed.
◆ Consent is required − from child and parent (verbal is adequate).
◆ Photographs must not be copied without consent of the doctor responsible for the child's care.
◆ Photographs must be made available for second opinions on a doctor-to-doctor basis

Showing photographs in court

◆ Prior warning must be given − notice for experts and to ensure that projection facilities are available.
◆ Prints − give copies to each party; slides can be projected for all parties to see.
◆ Slides should always be returned after use (property of health authorities/police).
◆ The doctor confirms the identity of photographs.

Photographic technique and quality

Taking adequate photographs requires:

◆ equipment: camera, including lens;
◆ light source;
◆ film (colour, reproducible quality, e.g. Agfa asa 100 professional slide film);
◆ basic knowledge of photographic composition;
◆ patience;
◆ professional laboratory services.

Types of camera

1. single lens reflex (usually 35mm) − recommended;
2. point and shoot, compact − simple to use, but results less predictable;
3. instant or self-developing camera − not advised for this work.

Lenses

◆ telephoto (85−105mm) for faces;
◆ macro facility for close ups;
◆ aperture (f−number) determines depth of field.

Lighting

◆ affects colour, texture, depth and contour;
◆ studio lighting ideal (send child to medical photography department);
◆ electronic flash is generally most practical;
◆ ring flash (e.g. for anus/genitalia to avoid shadows but not usually necessary).

> **Useful tip:**
> Always keep to hand fresh spare batteries for flash unit.

Film − slides or prints taken according to preference

◆ 35mm colour transparency/reversal;
◆ transparency − projection or prints;
◆ print film − has more latitude of exposure, forgiving of mistakes;
◆ speed: 100 ISO daylight/tungsten, e.g. 160T for colposcope photography.

Storage of film and photographs

◆ store unused film in fridge;
◆ slides − unmounted in case notes or glass mounted in cabinets;
◆ prints − in case notes or separately according to local policy;
◆ photographs should carry name and date as minimum information.

Identification of photographs (doctor responsible for identifying photographs)

◆ identifier on film (photograph names of child and examiner, hospital no. date)
◆ use one film per child;
◆ data back imprint − use date or other identifier automatically printed onto film;
◆ frame counter reference and log book.

Photographic composition
- show scale and location of lesion (vary distance from camera to child);
- show injury realistically;
- serial photographs for change;
- incorporate landmarks and close up;
- >1 frame per lesion (take plenty);
- vary angle and perspective;
- non-reflective, matt, uncluttered background (e.g. green surgical towels).

Common pitfalls and problems
- no film, camera not switched on, film not properly loaded/wound on;
- too light/dark exposure: check exposure compensation and film speed settings;
- film dark/orange cast: flash failed to fire − not switched on, dead batteries;
- blurred image − child/photographer moved, out of focus.

Tips for photographing children
- explain what is going to happen;
- provide comfort for child;
- flexibility, use trusted supporter;
- use automated techniques/film advancer to avoid delays;
- use photographs sensitively.

Useful tip:
The doctor must show the photographer what to photograph.

Digital photography
New technology is enabling photographs to be taken without the use of photographic film. The digital revolution has spread to photography and some doctors are adopting this technology to record their clinical findings. There are advantages and disadvantages.

- The new cameras are only just now producing images of comparable quality to conventional photography.
- There is no processing of films required and hence no delay.
- Trainees may be able to obtain opinions from colleagues with greater ease and rapidity.
- The possibility of manipulating the image is greater with digital photography. This could pose a problem in the legal arena.
- Storage of images may be facilitated on computers but data protection issues will need addressing.
- There may be a saving in cost.
- It is possible to send images for second opinions via the internet without time-consuming scanning.
- Security will, however, be a consideration.

It is likely, however, with the passage of time and developments in technology that digital photography will replace conventional photography.

Reference
Ricci L.R. 1991 *Photographing the physically abused child: principles and practice.* Am J Dis. Child. **145: 275−281**

SECTION 2

PHYSICAL ABUSE

Chapter 4

Bruises and Soft Tissue Injuries

General characteristics of physical abuse
◆ Repetitive pattern of injury.
◆ Injuries not consistent with the history − i.e. too many, too severe, wrong kind, wrong distribution, wrong age.
◆ Presence of other signs of abuse − e.g. neglect, failure to thrive and sexual abuse.
◆ Unusual behaviour in the parents − e.g. delay in seeking medical advice, refusal to allow proper treatment or admission to hospital, unprovoked aggression towards staff.
◆ Incidental discovery of injury: child allowed to go to school, to nursery or to another person's care where injuries found and reported. Parents may deny knowledge of the injury and provide no satisfactory explanation.
◆ Patterns of injury which strongly suggest abuse:

   ◆ bruising to a young baby;
   ◆ multiple injuries following a moderate fall;
   ◆ severe head injuries in babies or toddlers;
   ◆ rib fractures; subdural haematoma and retinal haemorrhage from violent shaking;
   ◆ multiple cigarette burns;
   ◆ fractures in infants and toddlers.

Documentation of injuries
Diagnosis involves the assessment of lesions visible to the unaided eye and accurate documentation by means of words, drawings and photographs.

Descriptions should be brief but detailed and include:

a. Probable nature of the lesion and approximate age (colour for bruises).
b. Site.
c. Shape.
d. Size (in cm).
e. Any unusual distinguishing features.
f. Where possible, an estimate of its likely causation.

Injuries should be listed one by one and related to body drawings, which give the best indication of patterns. Drawings should be outline with sizes (e.g. of bruises) marked.

Patterns of inflicted bruises
◆ Hand marks.
◆ Marks of implements − e.g. straps, sticks, buckles.
◆ Bruises from throwing, swinging or pushing the child onto a hard object.
◆ Bites.
◆ Bizarre marks (including petechiae).
◆ Kicks.

Hand marks
1. Grab mark or fingertip bruises, for example on limbs, face, chest wall.
2. Hand print or linear finger mark.
3. Slap mark − often vaguely two or three finger-sized linear marks are seen with stripe effect. Rings may leave a telltale mark.
4. Pinch marks − a pair of crescent-shaped bruises, facing one another.
5. Poking marks − fingernail may cut the skin.
6. Fist − diffuse often severe bruising to face, penetrating recesses, e.g. eye socket.

Ageing of bruises
◆ If there is doubt that a lesion is a bruise − serial examination.
◆ Studies emphasize the difficulties of ageing bruises.
◆ Yellow bruises are older than 18 hours.
◆ Other colours − red, blue, purple or black can occur from any time from 1 hour to resolution.
◆ Bruises of identical age and cause on the same person may not appear as the same colour and may not change at the same rate.
◆ Multiple bruises have often been inflicted on a number of occasions and there will be different ages as well as size and shape.
◆ After a single accident, bruises will be of the same age and few in number.
◆ Falls downstairs are not associated with multiple bruises in many sites and of different ages.

Sites of bruises
◆ Buttocks, lower back and outer thighs − often related to punishment.
◆ Inner thigh and genital area − sexual abuse or punishment for perceived toiletting misdemeanours.
◆ Head and neck − slap marks on the sides of the face and ears, extending onto the scalp.
◆ External ear − unusual following accidents (protective effect of the triangle created by the shoulder, skull and base of neck).
◆ Bruises on the lower jaw and the mastoid − strongly with associated with abuse.
◆ Neck, suggests choking or suffocation.
◆ Black eyes can occur in normal school children (direct injury).
◆ Very hard blow to forehead for blood to track down around one or both eyes.
◆ Distal to elbow and knees less significance than thighs and upper arms.
◆ Trunk (chest and abdomen) − suspicious of abuse and lower abdomen should suggest sexual abuse.

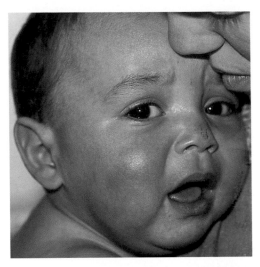

◀ **4.1** ▽ **4.2 Male aged 5 months**
Well-nourished infant with a history of rolling off a bed causing bruising to the right cheek, an irregular bruise to the outer aspect of the right thigh. Injuries not consistent with history.

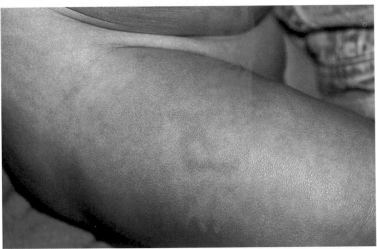

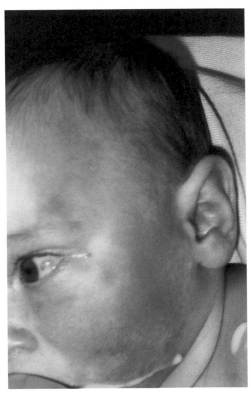

▶ **4.4 Male aged 10 months**
He was failing to thrive, with multiple bruising on head. No history offered to account for injury.

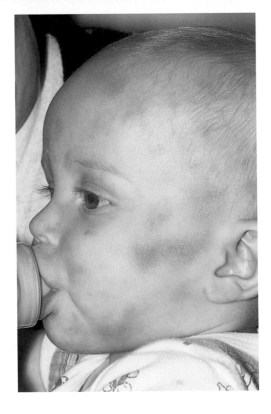

▲ **4.3 Male aged 9 months**
Presented with subconjunctival haemorrhage, irregular bruising to outer aspect of left orbit of different colours and shapes. No history given. This child had previously been shaken by his mother who denied hurting him and went home for further injury.

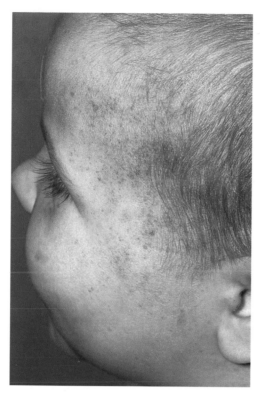

▲ **4.5 Male aged 3 years**
Presented with extensive petechial bruising over left side of head, likely to have been caused by blow with a flat hand.

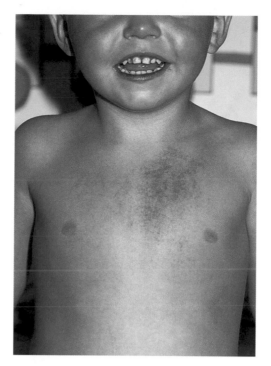

▲ **4.6 Male aged 4 years**
The same child as in Fig 4.5 but 1 year later, with ill-defined petechial bruising on the left side of upper chest and carious teeth. Injury likely to have been caused by blunt force through clothing.

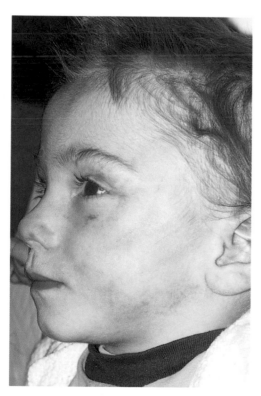

▲ **4.7 Male aged 10 months**
Child with cerebral palsy aged 10 months, failing to thrive and fading hand mark on left side of face. Children with disability are more likely to be injured by carers.

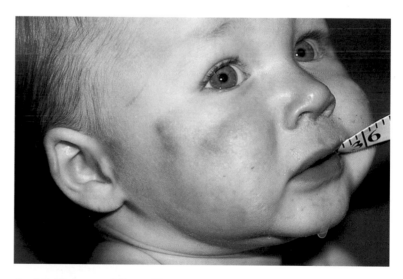

▲ **4.8 Male aged 5 months**
Presented as having 'hit himself with a bottle'. Old, paired, irregular shaped bruises on the cheek, consistent with a pinch mark made by an adult, are shown.

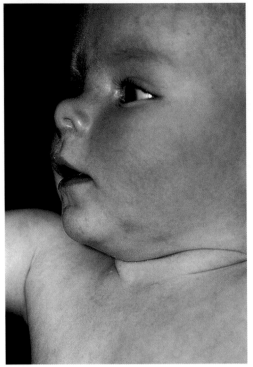

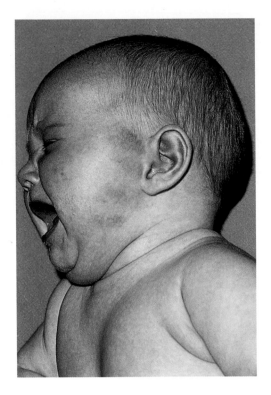

△ 4.9 Female aged 3 months
Presented as having 'rolled over in her cot against the bars'. Different coloured bruises on the cheek and lower jaw can be seen, due to fingertip bruising.

◁ 4.10 Male aged 5 months
His mother admitted to slapping him. Four linear bruises can be seen in front of and extending across the ear and cheek, consistent with an adult hand slap.

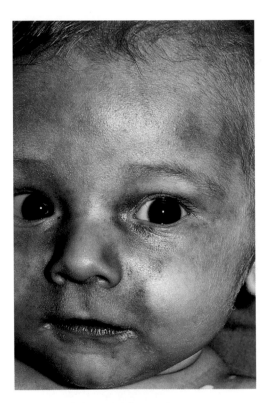

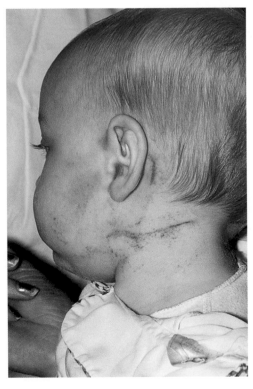

◁ 4.12 Female aged 8 months
She was claimed to have been 'choking on feeds'. Recent extensive bruising to the left side of the face is seen, with a characteristic hand mark seen as linear petechial bruises.

△ 4.11 Male aged 9 months
He was supposed to have 'fallen off the settee'. Recent extensive bruising to the forehead, nose and left orbit is evident. This was caused by multiple adult hand slaps, with fingertips discernible on the left forehead.

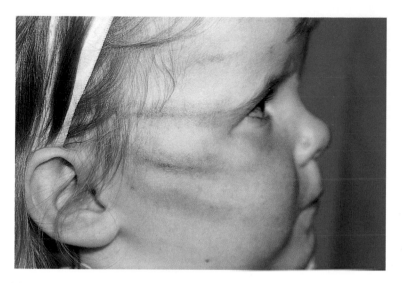

▲ **4.13 Female aged 3 years**
She presented as having 'fallen downstairs'. Recent horizontal linear bruises extending across the cheek are consistent with an adult hand slap.

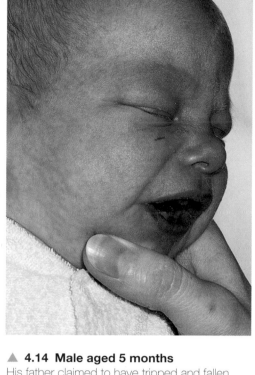

▲ **4.14 Male aged 5 months**
His father claimed to have tripped and fallen against a door jamb whilst holding him. Swelling of the orbit with bruising below the eye and a short abrasion can be seen. This was caused by being hit in the face with a clenched fist; the scratch is possibly due to a ring.

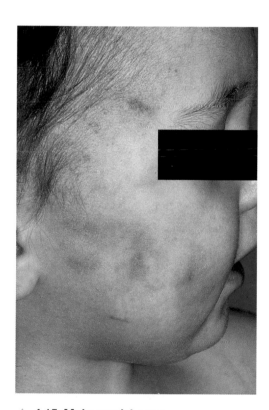

▲ **4.15 Male aged 4 years**
No history available. Two generations of bruises can be seen: scattered petechial bruising in rough lines over the temple extending back into the hairline, and patchy old yellowing bruises over the cheek. These were due to two separate assaults. Probably hand marks are also evident.

▶ **4.16 Male aged 2 years**
He was left in the care of a babysitter. The babysitter, who was known to the social services having murdered her own child, claimed the child fell off the settee onto a carpeted floor. Extensive petechial bruising over the forehead, eyelids and cheek are seen, caused by repeated adult hand slaps.

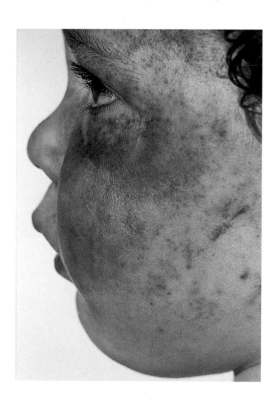

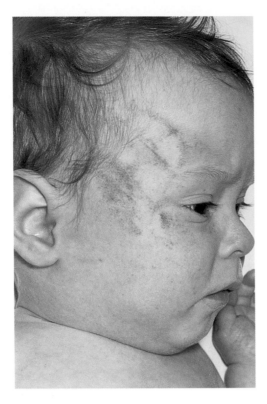

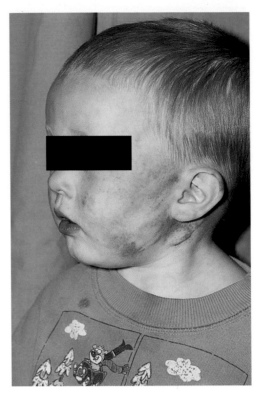

▲ **4.17 Female aged 4 months**
She presented as having 'rolled over on toys on the floor'. Four linear red marks with scattered petechiae are seen on the right side of the face, consistent with an adult hand slap. Note also the anxious expression.

▲ **4.18 Male aged 3 years**
He was assaulted by his mother's male partner. There is extensive recent diffuse and petechial bruising with swelling across the cheek, ear and behind the ear, caused by an adult hand slap.

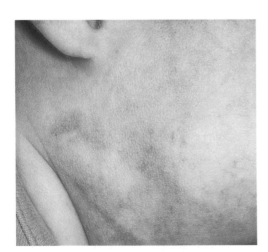

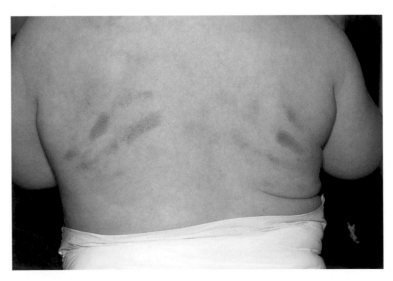

▲ **4.19 Male aged 3 months**
Presented with thumb mark across the lower jaw. The child had feeding problems and the parents were force-feeding. Note: the child was not underweight.

▲ **4.20 Female aged 2 years**
She had unusual bilateral linear parallel marks on her back. The cause of these marks was not clear; she did however have other injuries which suggested that these were all inflicted injuries, possibly hand marks.

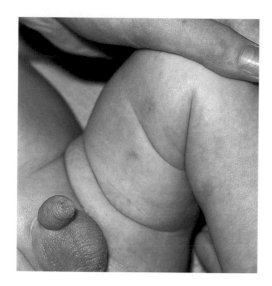
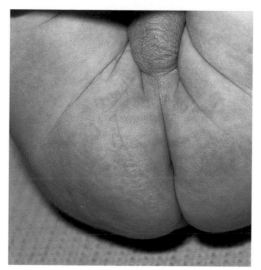

▲ **4.21,** ▲ **4.22 Male aged 3 months**
He presented with what might appear initially to be insignificant bruising on the inner aspect of the left thigh, the left lower leg and also a larger bruise on the left buttock. However, further investigation showed fractures of the ribs and femur.

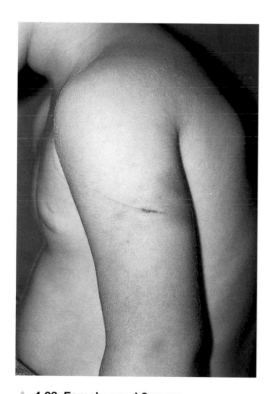
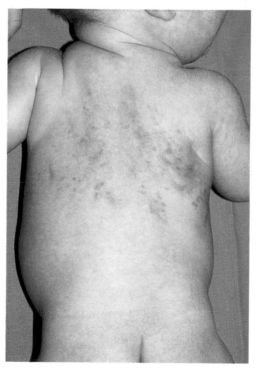

▲ **4.23 Female aged 2 years**
This photograph shows an area of diffuse old bruising with an overlying linear scratch. The injuries are unexplained.

▲ **4.24 Female aged 4 months**
Her doctor was called for a night visit because she was crying. Diffuse petechial bruising is seen over the entire upper back, caused by adult hand slaps through clothing.

▶ **4.25 Female aged 4 years**
She had a previous 'accidental' laceration of the liver when she fell on a vegetable knife. At paediatric follow-up bruising was found. The photograph shows two circular old brown bruises, which are unexplained, and in an unusual site for accidental bruising. They are probably fingertip bruising.

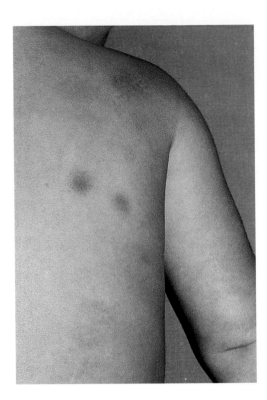

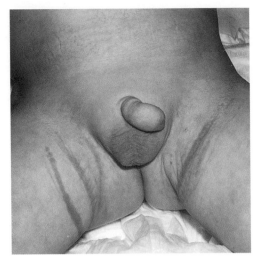

▲ **4.26 Male aged 2 years**
He was referred by his nursery because of unexplained marks in the groin. The linear red marks encircling inner thighs were caused by the child being sealed into his nappy at night with parcel tape. This was done to prevent the child removing his nappy in the morning.

▶ **4.27 Male aged 12 years**
He complained at school that his older brother had hit him. Recent extensive bruising over the upper half of the back can be seen, the configuration of bruising suggesting finger marks. This was due to multiple blows from an outstretched hand.

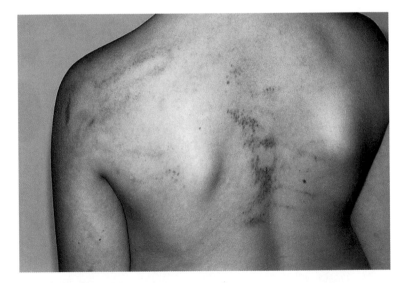

▶ **4.28 Female aged 3 weeks**
The midwife noticed bruising at a routine follow-up. Recent, complex bruising of the buttocks can be seen, due to unexplained serious non-accidental injury.

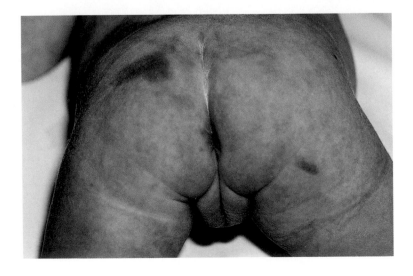

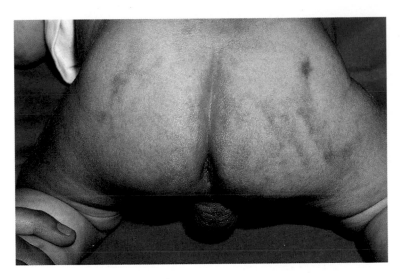

4.29 Male aged 2 weeks

He was taken to the clinic by his mother because of his 'crying'. Recent linear bruising of both buttocks can be seen, probably caused by repeated blows from an outstretched hand.

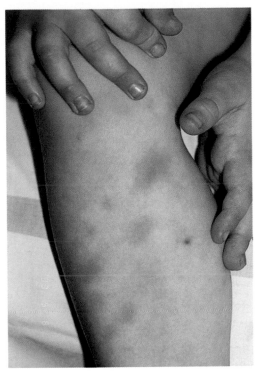

4.30 Male aged 4 years

He was referred to the paediatrician by his doctor because of behaviour problems. The photograph shows a cluster of roughly circular bruises of similar age on the inner aspect of the lower leg. These are probably grip marks. The child later disclosed anal abuse.

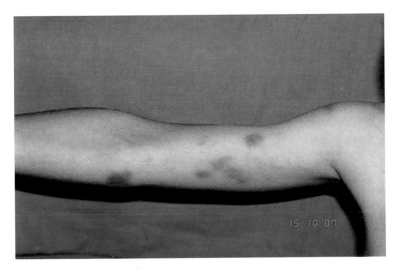

4.31 Male aged 6 years

He was seen as a routine after his younger sister presented with neglected burns. Multiple bruising can be seen, of similar age but differing in size, over the shoulder and inner aspect of the upper arm and elbow. These are unexplained bruises in an unusual site, probably grip marks.

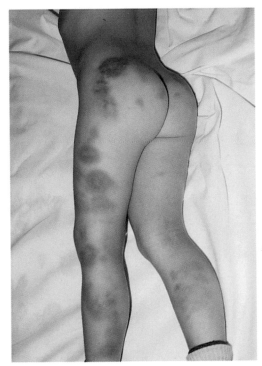

4.32 Male aged 5 years

He had recently come to the UK from Hong Kong. His mother admitted disciplining her son by kicking him. The photograph shows multiple large irregular bruising, mainly on the outer aspect of the legs, of varying ages, consistent with kick marks.

▶ **4.33 Male foster child aged 2 years**
When seen to have bruising at his nursery, he said 'Daddy hit me'. There is diffuse complex ageing bruising on the outer aspect of the left upper thigh, consistent with being hit with a hard object, or kicked.

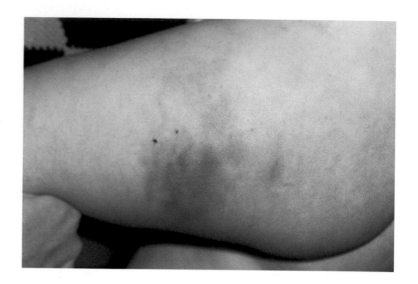

▶ **4.34 Male aged 6 months**
He presented with facial bruising and the examining doctor noted a reluctance to move the left arm. A swollen left elbow can be seen, diagnosed as a pulled elbow in association with other non-accidental injury.

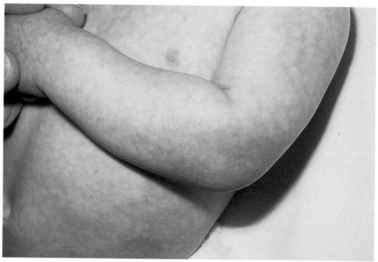

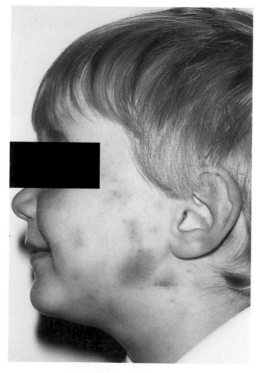

▶ **4.36 Female aged 5 years**
She presented with bruise caused by thumb mark over inner aspect left clavicle. There is also fingertip bruising over the left upper back (not shown).

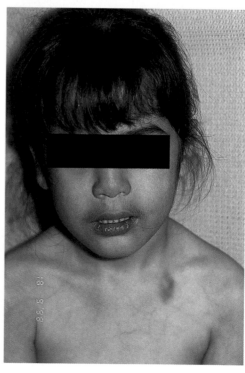

▲ **4.35 Male aged 4 years**
He presented with multiple bruising of the left side of face and over angle of the jaw. The exact cause of these bruises is not known but they have not been caused by any ordinary accident.

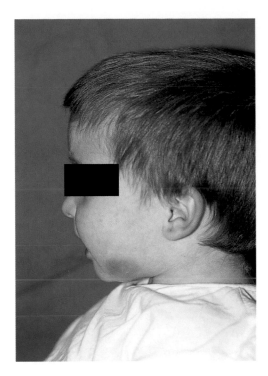

▲ **4.37 Male aged 3 years**
Presented with bleeding from laceration on penis and found also to have large irregular bruise over the left mandible and cuts in mouth. The injuries to the mouth are likely to have been caused by the blow to the lower jaw (see Chapter 7 and Chapter 20).

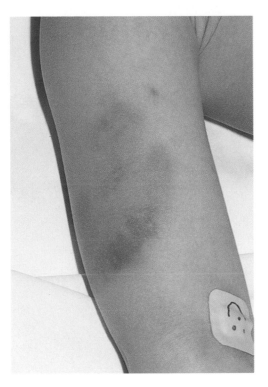

▲ **4.38 Male aged 5 years**
He had irregular bruising on the outer aspect of the arm, which might have been caused by a twist or a kick.

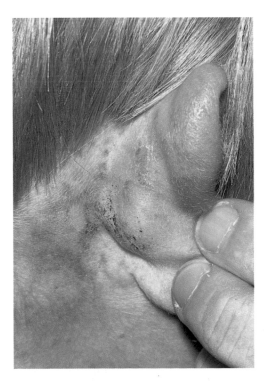

▲ **4.39 Male aged 6 years**
He presented with extensive bruising behind the ear. It is necessary to look behind the ear when injuries are seen anteriorly on the pinna.

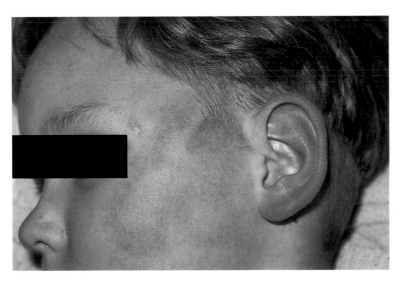

▲ **4.40 Male aged 7 years**
Th`e extensive swelling and bruising of the left cheek and left ear was said to have been caused when roller skating. The injury is too extensive for the history given. The ear is usually protected in accidental falls by the parietal area of the skull and the shoulder, giving a protective triangle.

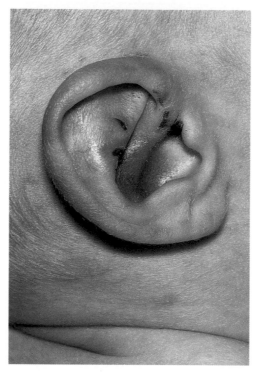

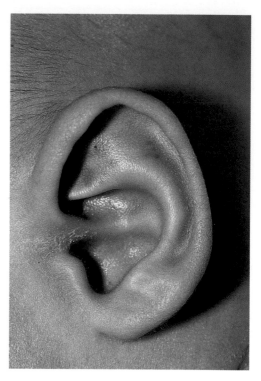

▲ **4.41 Male aged 2 years**
Presented with extensive bruising and laceration of the right ear. The site of this injury is typical of non-accidental injury.

▲ **4.42 Male aged 3 months**
He was taken to see his GP because of minimal bruising on the inner aspect of the left upper ear. This child had also had a shaking/impact injury and was admitted to hospital later the same day, fitting.

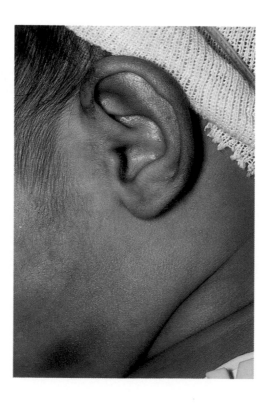

◄ **4.43 Female aged 3 months**
She was admitted seriously ill to hospital following a shaking/impact injury with bruising across the left mandible and skin loss and injury to the left ear. The ear has the appearance of increased pigmentation, raising the question of earlier severe injury.

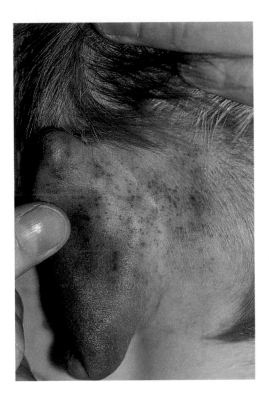
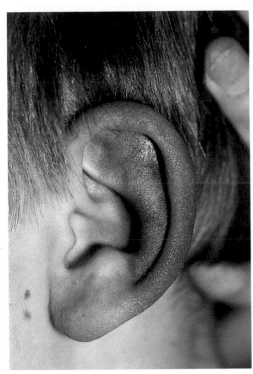

▲ **4.44**, ▲ **4.45 Male aged 6 years**
His school teacher noticed a 'rash' when the child complained
of earache. Multiple petechial bruises of pinna and temporal
area of skull are consistent with a hand slap by an adult.

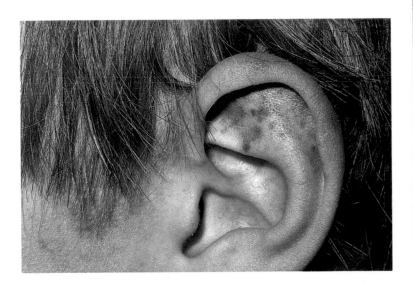

▲ **4.46 Male aged 8 years**
He was beaten up by his mother's male partner. In addition to multiple
bruises elsewhere, there is bruising of the upper rim and helix of the
pinna, caused by a blow to the ear.

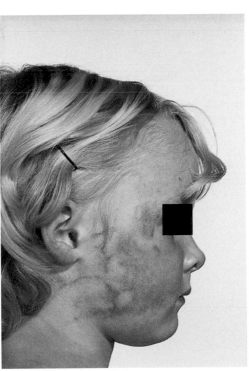

▲ **4.47 Female aged 6 years**
Her mother had called the social services and
told them that she had hit her daughter to
punish her for wandering around the streets.
There is extensive recent petechial bruising and
swelling, with a prominent vertical and several
horizontal lines extending across the cheek.
These were caused by a hand slap, the vertical
line representing the metacarpophalangeal joint.

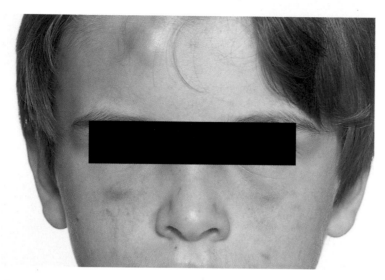

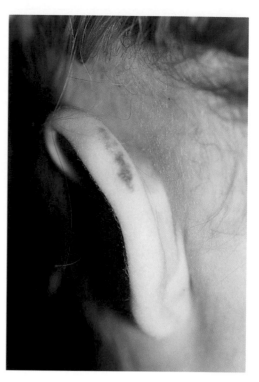

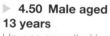

▲ **4.48 Male aged 8 years**
He was claimed to have been 'fighting with his brothers'. There is a swollen ageing bruise on the mid-forehead and recent bruising of both orbits inferiorly, which are unexplained.

▲ **4.49 Male aged 5 years**
He was admitted to hospital because of gastroenteritis, and found to have unexplained scalds in both groins and signs of anal abuse. The photograph shows bruising of the upper rim of the pinna, which is probably a pinch mark.

▶ **4.50 Male aged 13 years**
He was assaulted by his father. There is petechial bruising above the left orbit and extending below the eye, and a swollen lower lip with a scratch mark. The injuries were caused by fist blows to the eye and mouth.

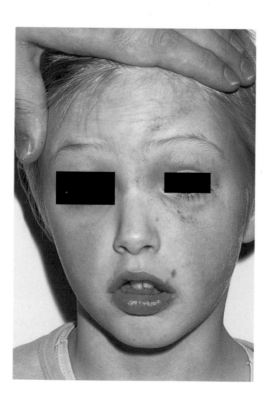

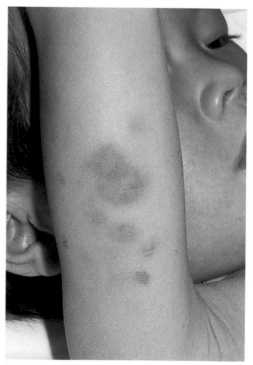

▲ **4.51 Male aged 5 years**
He presented with bruising on the outer aspect of the left upper arm. The bruises are circular and probably represent a punch and possible knuckle marks from a fist.

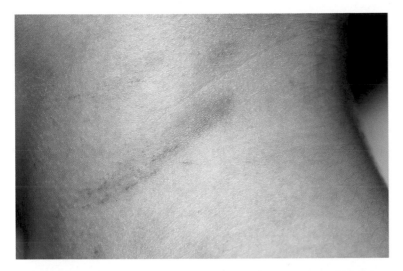

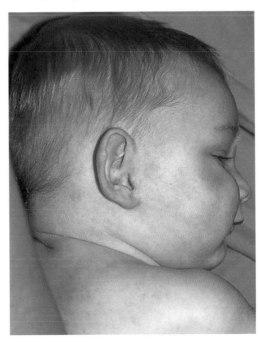

◀ **4.52 Male aged 14 years**

He was in a fight with his father. The linear mark round his neck was caused by his shirt collar. Teenagers are involved in fights with their carers but tend not to be recognized as the victims of abuse. Fighting with carers may be a prelude to running away from home.

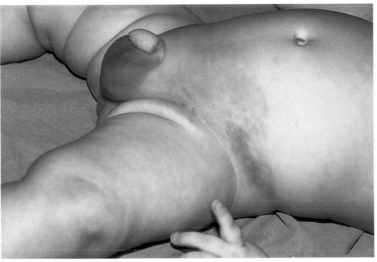

▲ **4.53,** ▶ **4.54 Male aged 6 months**

Presented with diffuse bruising of the lower abdomen with tracking down to scrotum and the base of penis. Injury caused by blunt force applied to lower abdomen, probably a kick. Unexplained bruise over right maxilla. NB This child had von Willebrand's disease which is not associated with an increased frequency of bruising but characteristically after operation the wound continues to ooze. This child had no bruising in foster care.

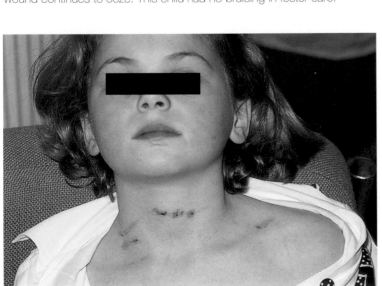

◀ **4.55 Female aged 10 years**

The irregular lacerations round her neck are likely to have been caused by an adult with long nails grasping her from behind. This is a physical assault.

▶ **4.56 Female aged 14 years**
Presented at A&E with linear mark around her neck. She had a history of self-harming and had previously taken an overdose. This mark is compatible with attempted strangulation.

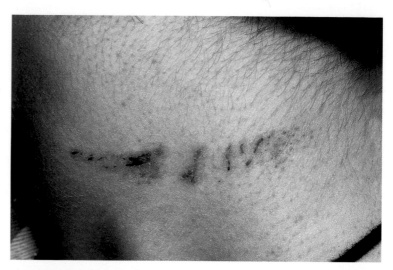

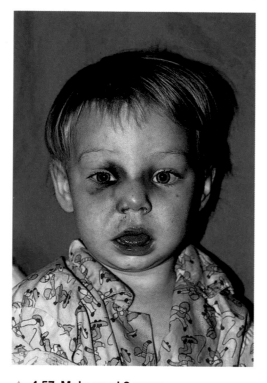

▲ **4.57 Male aged 2 years**
He presented with a history of having fallen downstairs but note bruising of the orbit, swollen nose, swollen upper lip with bruising. This injury is consistent with a penetrating blow to the right orbit, i.e. a punch, not a simple fall.

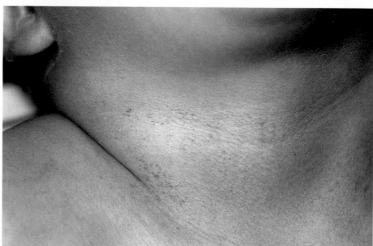

▲ **4.58 Male**
Young child with scattered petechiae round the neck. Marks like these are seen in attempted strangulation; also look for petechiae in the orbit, especially upper eyelids.

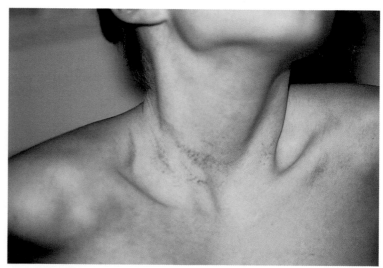

▲ **4.59 Male**
Presented with linear petechial bands round the root of his neck. Marks like these are seen in attempted strangulation.

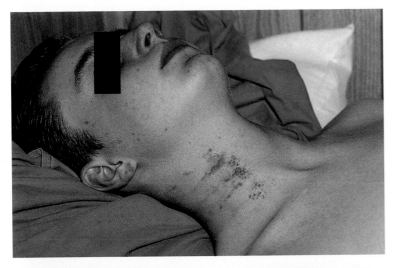

◀ **4.60 Male aged 14 years**

He was assaulted by his father after he and a friend drank a bottle of his father's whisky. Scattered petechiae and linear marks round neck anteriorly are seen, caused by attempted strangulation with a hand around the neck.

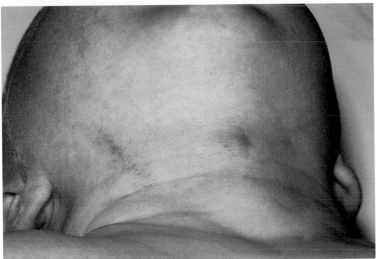

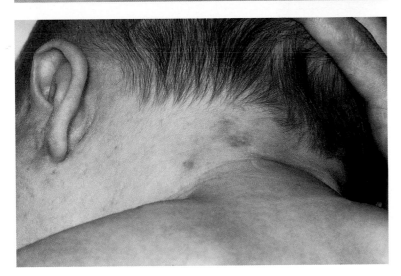

▲ **4.61,** ▲ **4.62 Female aged 6 months**

Her older brother was seen to have multiple bruising on his face, arms and back in the day nursery, and therefore she was seen in the clinic as well. Petechial bruising seen round neck, caused by strangulation. (Note: strangulation may cause petechiae round the neck, upper eyelids and behind the ears, but it should be remembered that in many cases of strangulation there are no abnormalities seen on the neck.)

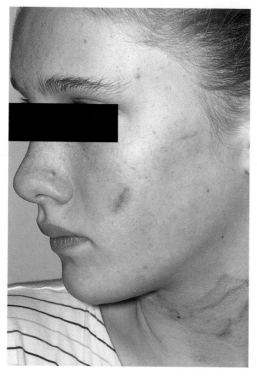

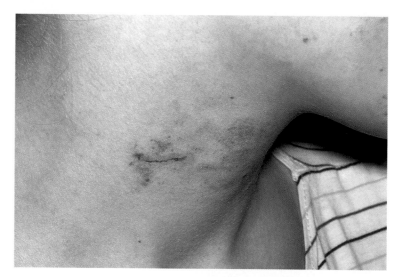

▲ 4.63, ▲ 4.64 Female aged 14 years

She told her teacher that her mother had attacked her the previous evening. The photograph shows fingernail scratches to the side of the face and extensive lacerations with petechial bruising around the neck, caused by serious physical assault. (Note: lacerations were caused by long fingernails, an extremely scaring assault for this child.)

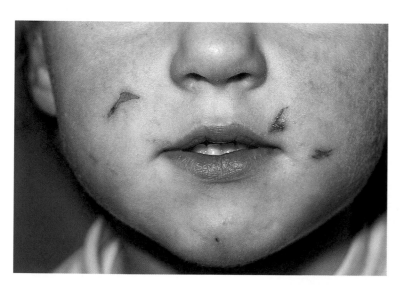

▲ 4.65 Female aged 2 years

This photograph shows irregularly shaped superficial lesions of the face showing early healing. They are probably finger scratch marks.

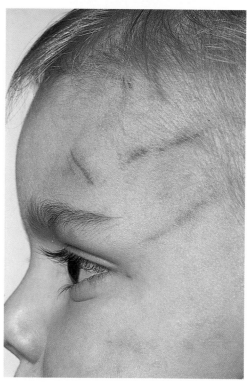

▲ 4.66 Male aged 3 years

Father said that he had hit the child across the face as he was choking on baked beans, thereby saving his life. Two parallel linear bruises, and two shorter red linear marks at right angles to the upper mark are seen, consistent with being hit across the face with a hand, and the shorter marks due to impact from a ring.

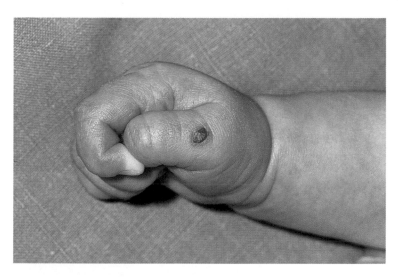

▲ **4.67 Female aged 4 weeks**
She was born pre-term. The midwife on a home visit noticed unusual lesions on the hands and feet 1 day after discharge from the neonatal unit. The photograph shows a superficial abrasion on the outer aspect of the thumb. This is an inflicted nail injury by an adult.

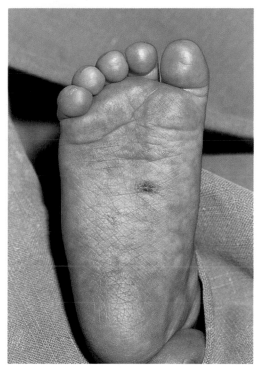

▲ **4.68 Female aged 4 weeks**
The same child as in Fig. 4.67. This photograph shows an abrasion to the sole of foot, a nail injury inflicted by an adult.

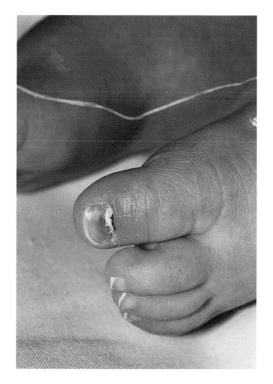

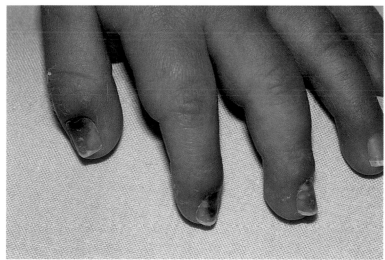

▲ **4.69,** ▲ **4.70 Male aged 6 months**
His father took him to hospital because of vomiting. Bruises can be seen under the nails of the hand and foot. The child was very ill with intestinal obstruction, but also had, on skeletal survey, unexplained fractures, an old subdural haematoma, and these inflicted injuries on the hands and feet.

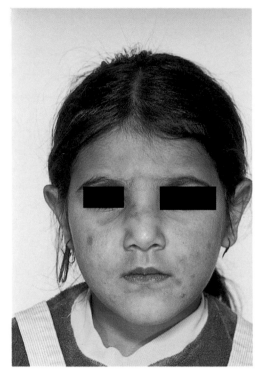

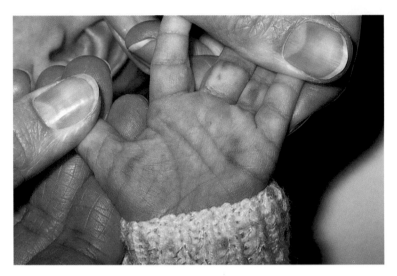

▲ **4.71 Female aged 7 years**
She was referred to social services by her
school, because of concern that the child was
withdrawn and had repeated scratch marks on
her face. There is bruising over the bridge of
the nose and infra-orbitally on the right, and
scattered scratch marks in various stages of
healing across the face and chin. These were
due to unexplained injury: the parents explained
that the children kept fighting. (Note: further
investigation was unsatisfactory and the child
was not protected.)

▲ **4.72 Female aged 4 weeks**
Her mother asked the health visitor about a bruise on the palm of the
hand. The photograph shows multiple abrasions and a bruise with
superficial abrasion on the palm of the left hand. This is an unexplained
injury in a very young baby.

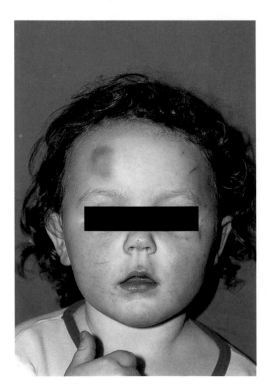

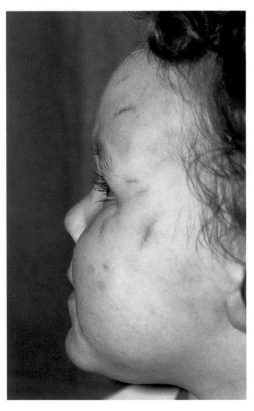

◀ **4.73, ◀ 4.74
Female aged
3 years**
Her parents had a
fight one evening,
the police were
called and observed
injuries to the
children. The child
said her mother had
banged her head on
the cupboard door.
An old circular bruise
is seen on the right
frontal area, and
multiple fingernail
marks in various
states of healing on
the forehead and
cheeks. The bruise
is consistent with a
bang against a hard
surface as
described; the
scratches were
inflicted by
fingernails.

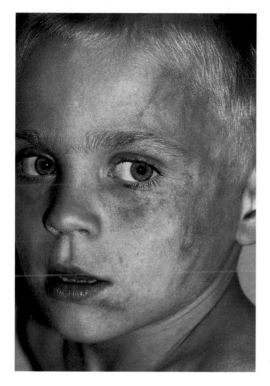 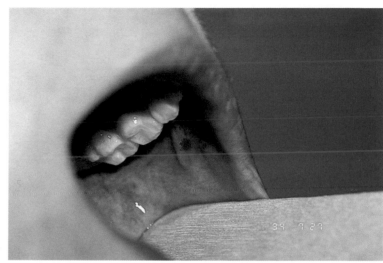

▲ **4.75,** ▲ **4.76 Male aged 5 years**

He claimed that his mother had hit him. The photographs show a slap mark on the left side of the face and bruising on the buccal surface on the left cheek due to the cheek impacting on the teeth. This was diagnosed as a non-accidental injury. (Note: When bruising of lips or cheeks is seen then remember to look inside the mouth.)

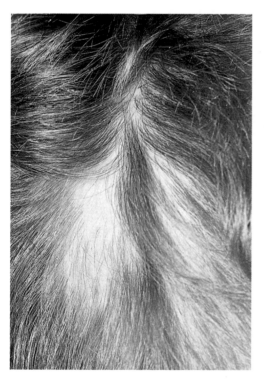 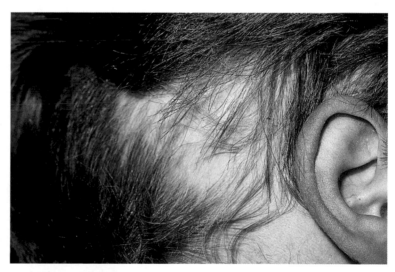

▲ **4.78 Female aged 3 years**

She was referred because of multiple bruises. Examination revealed an area of hair loss (as shown in photograph) resulting from the child's hair being pulled; there were also signs of physical and sexual abuse.

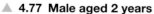

▲ **4.77 Male aged 2 years**

He presented with facial bruising, fracture and signs of sexual abuse. Examination revealed hair loss that had been caused by the child's hair being pulled.

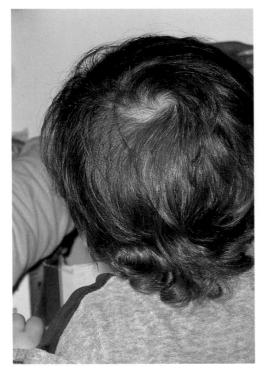

▲ **4.79 Male aged 4 years**
He attended school with a bald patch and said his father had 'done it'.

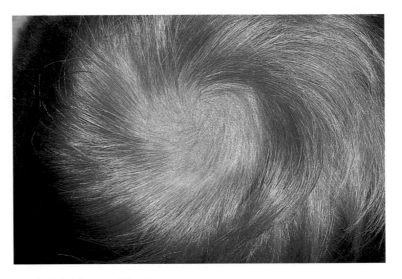

▲ **4.80 Male aged 2 years**
He presented with unexplained bald patch, probable trauma. Bruises to ears and failure to thrive also present.

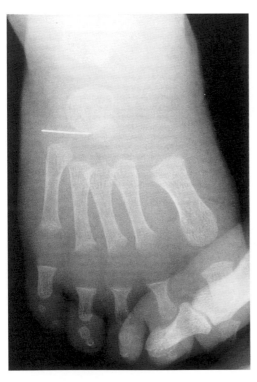

▲ **4.81 Female aged 9 months**
Presented with broken hypodermic needle embedded in top of foot. No history. Signs consistent with sexual abuse in brother.

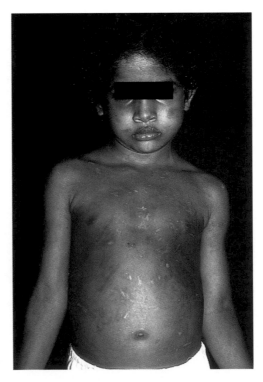

▲ **4.82 Female aged 12 years**
Child servant showing multiple scars from injuries. She also had a calcified haematoma in the thigh. (With permission of Professor H. de Silva.)

Chapter 5

Injuries Caused by Implements

Marks from implements

In a community sample of 700 children, by 7 years of age, 26% of boys and 18% of girls had been hit with an implement.

Commonly used implements include:
1. strap or belt;
2. cane or stick;
3. slipper or shoe;
4. miscellaneous objects, e.g. riding crop, golf club, baseball bat.

Characteristics of marks from implements

◆ Belts or straps − parallel-sided marks which tend to curve with the contours of the body.
◆ Stick or canes − less clearly defined linear marks over prominent areas, usually thinner than strap marks.
◆ Loops of flex − circular closed-end thin lines.

> **Practice point:**
> **Photograph both the injury and the implement**

◆ Slipper or shoes − large confluent areas of bruising, commonly on buttocks, tops of thighs.
◆ Ties or ligatures − circumferential bands around limbs and penis.
◆ Gags − abrasions from the corner of the mouth.
◆ Strangulation − petechiae on the upper eyelids and face as well as bruising to the neck.

Implements may also be used to burn a child, e.g. clothes iron, hair curler, soldering iron.

Identification of implements requires co-operation between doctor and police officer, who may be able to identify the object during a search at the child's home.

▶ **5.1,** ▶ **5.2 Male aged 5 years**
Presented with unusual marks on the outer aspect of the right buttock. The injuries were caused by a blow from this construction toy as shown.

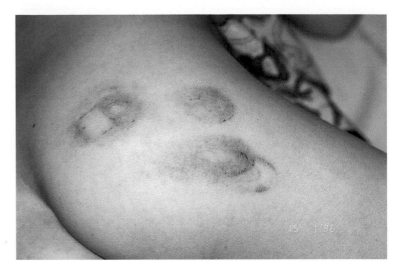

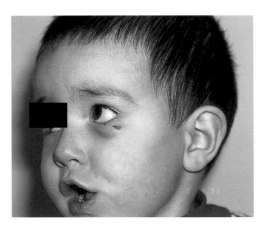

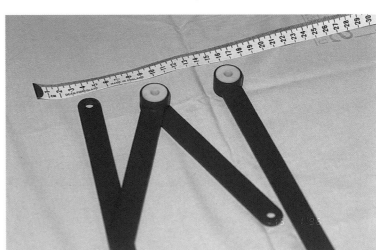

▲ **5.3 Male aged 3 years**
He presented with a black eye and laceration to outer aspect of orbit: caused by baseball bat, but no further details given. This is not an 'ordinary injury'.

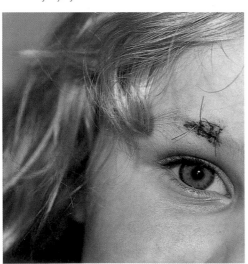

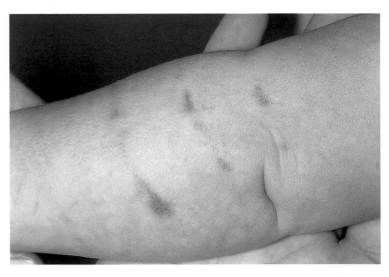

▲ **5.4 Female aged 4 years**
Her stepfather hit her with a plastic sword, causing a laceration to the outer aspect of the right eyebrow.

▲ **5.5 Female**
Unexplained parallel marks round left arm. Clearly an explanation must be sought in such a young child.

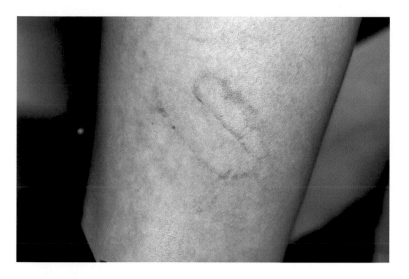

◀ 5.6 Female
Presented with unusual marking on outer aspect of thigh: caused by an undisclosed implement.

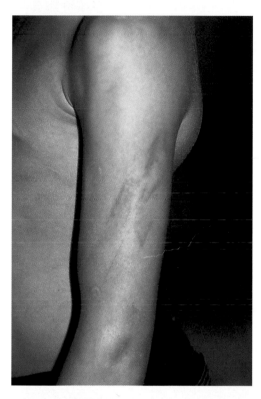

◀ 5.7 Male aged 7 years
He presented with weals on the outer aspect of left upper arm, likely to have been caused with a stick.

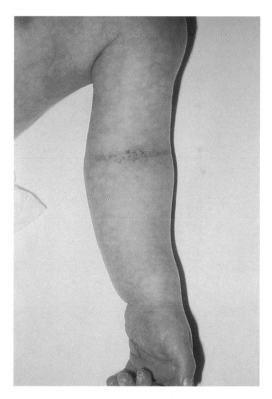

▲ 5.8 Male aged 3 months
There is a ring of petechial bruising round left upper arm, presumably constriction band. This infant warrants urgent investigation for other injuries.

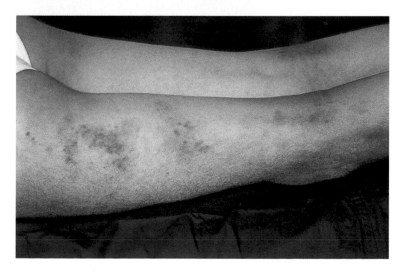

◀ 5.9 Male aged 9 years
He was beaten with a cane by his mother because of poor school performance. His younger sister initially claimed she had caused the marks. The child was underweight.

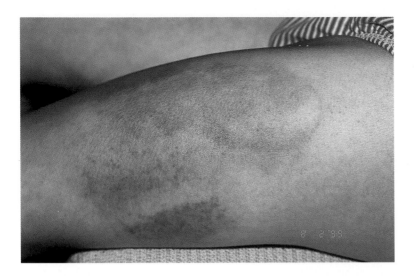

◀ **5.10 Male aged 5 years**
Presented with this injury having allegedly fallen downstairs carrying his toys. The injury on the upper thigh has the shape of a shoe and the lower injury may have been caused similarly.

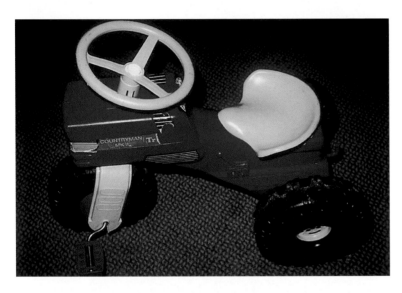

◀ **5.11,** ◀ **5.12**
It is always important to see the alleged implement, the wheels on the toy tractor and baby buggy do not fit the shape and size of the injury shown in Fig. 5.10.

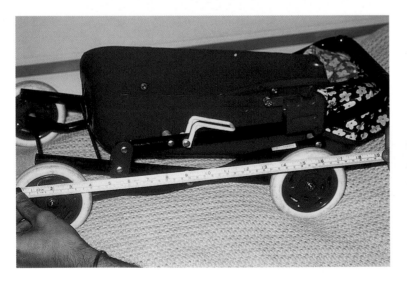

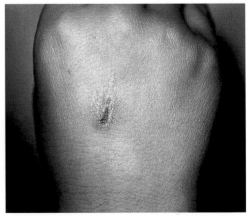

▲ **5.13**
An unexplained laceration was also found on the dorsum of his hand.

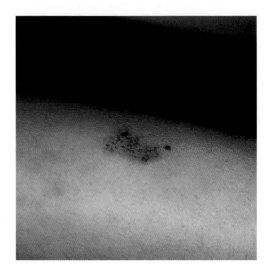

▲ **5.14**

Also, an unexplained lesion on the outer aspect of the left arm was said by his carers to have been a carpet burn, but this is uncertain. Further examination showed signs compatible with anal abuse. Later the child disclosed that he was hit with a shoe and sexually abused.

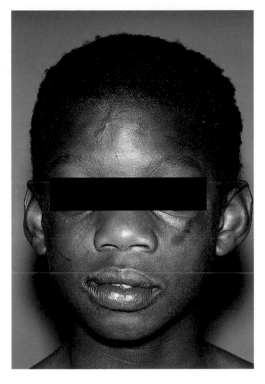

◀ **5.15–5.17**
Male aged 9 years
Presented with recent bruising below the left orbit and old keloid scarring on the forehead.

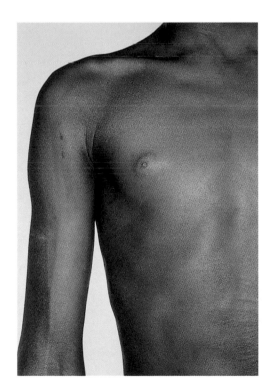

▲ **5.16**
Linear marks on the forearm compatible with blows from a stick.

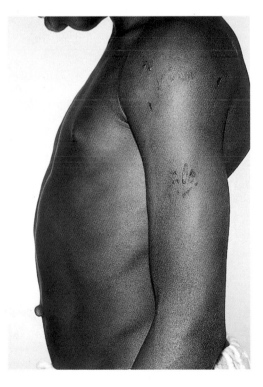

◀ **5.17**
Scarring on outer aspect of left upper arm. Whilst examination of children with darkly pigmented skins may be difficult, scars are sometimes clearly evident.

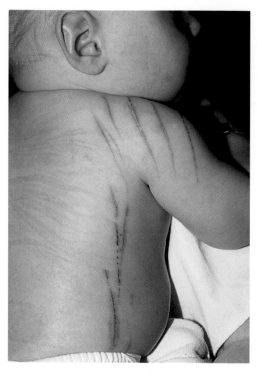

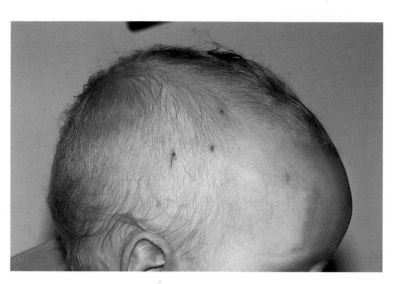

▲ **5.19 Male aged 9 months**
The same child as in Fig. 5.18. This photograph shows small puncture marks in the scalp and a linear vertical bruise above the right eye. The marks fitted a carpet gripper rod. The bruise on the forehead is unexplained but consistent with a fall against a hard object.

▲ **5.18 Male aged 9 months**
It was claimed that he had fallen down uncarpeted stairs, and scratched himself on carpet tacks. The photograph shows parallel scratches over the shoulder and side. These are inflicted scratches, probably caused by a metal dog grooming comb.

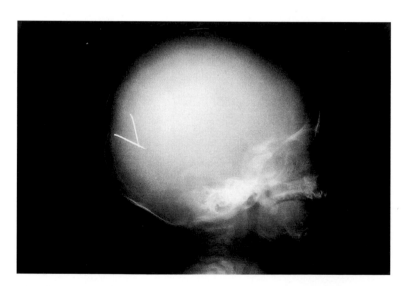

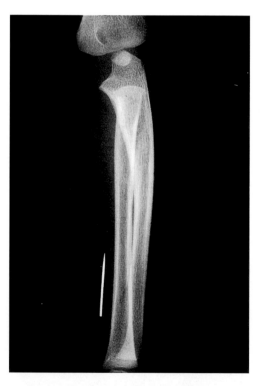

▲ **5.20 Female aged 4 weeks**
She died suddenly due to pneumonia. A skeletal survey was performed because of abuse in an elder sibling. The lateral skull X-ray shows fragments of three sewing needles, two posteriorly within the skull and one lying subcutaneously over the vertex. The needles were deliberately inserted by an adult. (Photograph supplied by Dr A. Habel.)

▲ **5.21 Female aged 18 months**
A sibling of the child in Fig. 5.20. There was a previous history of failure to thrive and non-accidental injury, and she was examined following the death of her sibling. A needle is seen to be present intramuscularly in the forearm, inserted by an adult. (Photograph supplied by Dr A. Habel.)

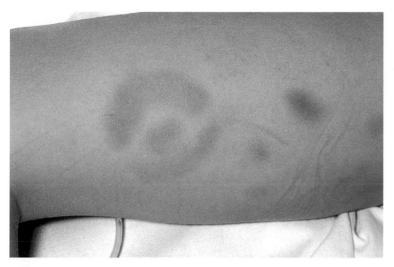

◀ **5.22 Male aged 2 years**
He presented in the hospital emergency department with a severe head injury. The photograph shows a circular ring bruise with central bruising, and a cluster of adjacent bruising. The ring bruise was shown to fit precisely the shape of the base of a torch; the cluster of bruises is consistent with fingertips, i.e. grip marks.

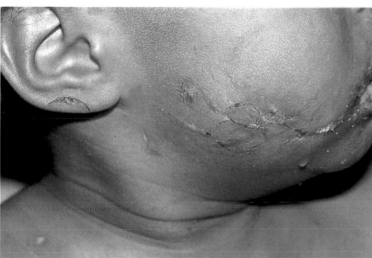

◀ **5.23 Male aged 2 years**
He presented to the hospital emergency department with burns to his hands, feet, mouth and trunk and injury to both sides of his face. There are multiple superficial excoriations/lacerations, which extend from the angle of the mouth symmetrically on each side of the face towards the ear, and are at various stages of healing. The injury is consistent with some form of gag.

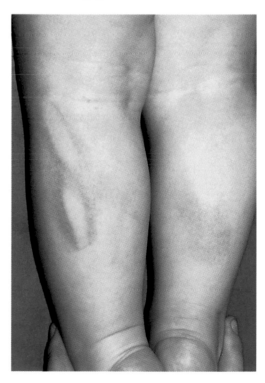

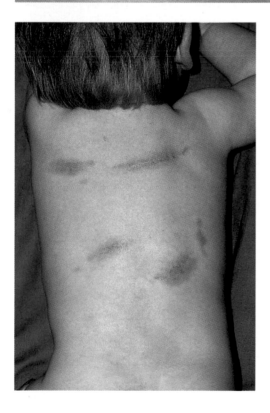

◀ **5.24 Male aged 18 months**
Social worker was shown marks on a routine home visit. (The child had suffered previous neglect.) The mother claimed he had been hit with a fire engine by his 6-year-old sibling. There are several linear bruises with a central line of petechiae, horizontal, oblique and vertical, caused by repeated blows from an unidentified object.

▲ **5.25 Male aged 15 months**
He had repeated unexplained marks noticed in day nursery. The parents were both full-time students and complained that the child cried. Two similar-shaped parallel red marks can be seen on the back of the lower leg, inflicted by an adult with some implement; it was later found to be a riding crop.

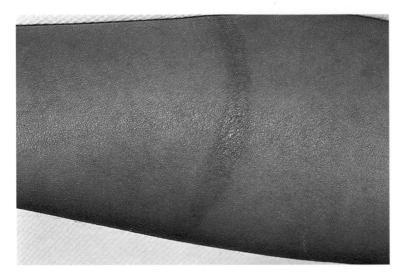

▲ **5.26 Female aged 3 years**
She had unexplained marks noted at nursery school. There is a healed ligature mark around the leg.

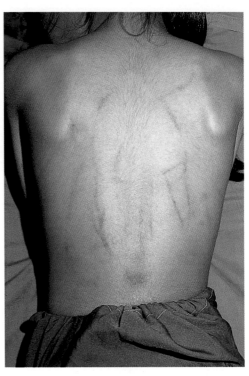

▲ **5.27 Female aged 7 years**
The child complained to her teacher that her mother had beaten her. She said that this was a punishment for losing her little brother in the park. Multiple linear petechial bruising can be seen. These are inflicted marks, consistent with beating with a stick.

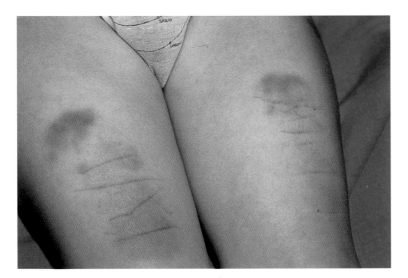

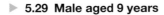

▲ **5.28 Female aged 8 years**
Her school noted unusual marks. Her parents said she was injured while playing. The photograph shows old, symmetrical bruising and linear scratches to both anterior thighs, due to unexplained but non-accidental injury.

▶ **5.29 Male aged 9 years**
His teacher noted extensive bruising during a sports lesson. There is extensive bruising on the outer aspect of the upper thigh and buttock, comprising loops, linear marks, and diffuse bruising of recent origin. This is inflicted bruising due to blows with a looped skipping rope.

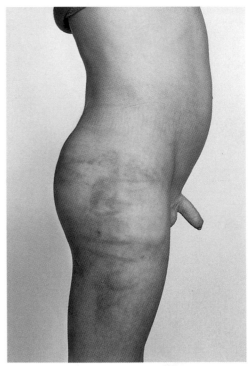

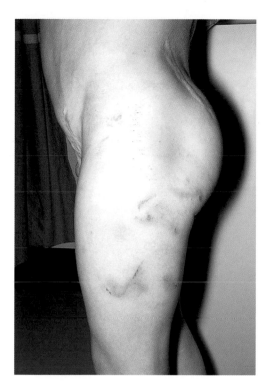

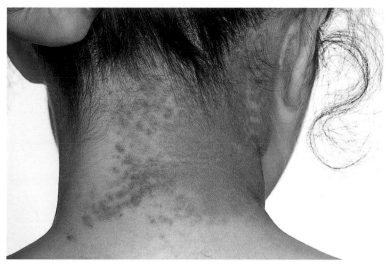

▲ 5.31 Female aged 11 years

She complained of a sore neck at school. Later she said she had been hit by her mother with a slipper. There is an extensive confluent and textured bruise extending on the back and side of the neck extending into the hairline and ear consistent with multiple blows.

▲ 5.30 Male aged 6 years

Mother found him lighting a fire in the middle of the sitting room floor and hit him with a belt. Multiple linear marks and abrasions to the outer aspect of the upper thigh are seen. These are not typical belt marks, but consistent with the history given. (Note: scarring due to surgery for ectopic vesicae.)

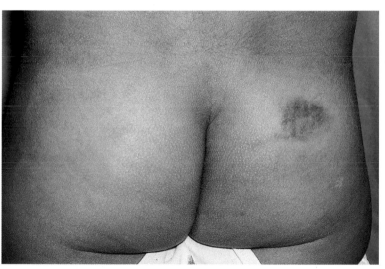

▲ 5.32 Male aged 4 years

He presented because of bruises seen at day nursery. The child had previous behaviour problems. The photograph shows one of several identical roughly circular bruises with linear marking – this one on the right buttock. The mother later admitted to hitting him with a golf club.

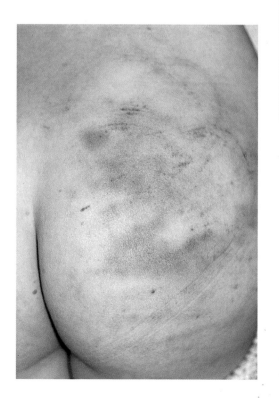

◀ 5.33 Male aged 8 years

He had run away from home several times previously, and was punished by being put in a dog kennel. On this occasion when he was returned by the police he complained he had been beaten. An extensive complex area of recent and old bruising is evident over the right buttock. Loops and linear marks can be seen within the bruising. The injuries are consistent with repeated beatings, including the use of a belt.

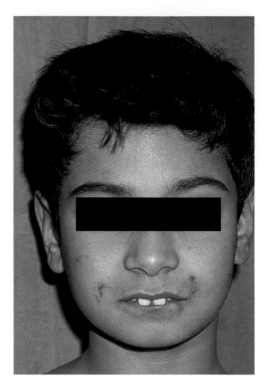

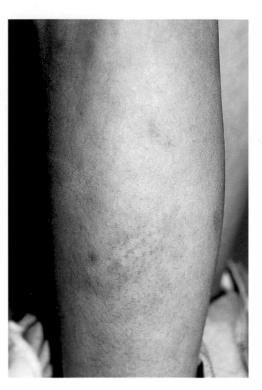

▲ **5.34 Male aged 12 years**
He had stolen money from a doctor's surgery where his mother was a cleaner. The mother admitted hitting him with a shoe, but had shared the money. There are multiple irregular lacerations on the face, and a similar lesion was seen on the scalp, caused by repeated blows from the heel of a shoe.

▲ **5.35 Male aged 13 years**
His parents admitted the injury as punishment for the boy spending housekeeping money on gambling machines in an amusement arcade. The photograph shows one of several identical marks on the body – linear bruise marks separated by a linear reddened mark. They are consistent with the history of beating with a stick.

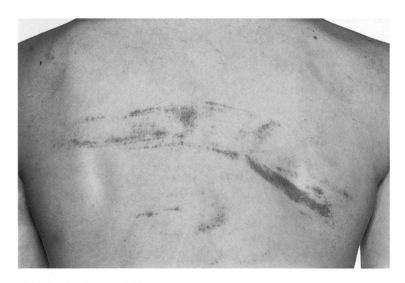

▲ **5.36 Male aged 13 years**
He was belted by his father for playing truant. Parallel linear red marks across the upper back are consistent with belt marks.

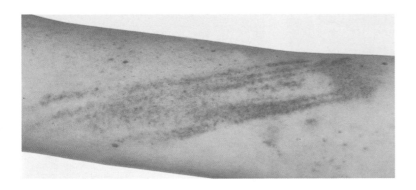

◀ **5.37 Male aged 13 years**
The same child as in Fig. 5.36. This photograph shows a similar lesion on the forearm, i.e. a belt mark.

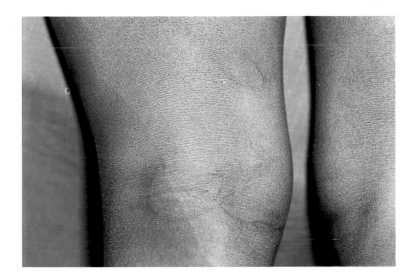

◀ **5.38 Male aged 6 years**
Presented because of a history of bed-wetting, when unusual marks were noted on the backs of the legs. Fine pigmented open-ended semicircular marks are seen on the back of the thigh and knee. These are healed loop marks – the mother admitted to previously hitting the boy with a looped electrical flex.

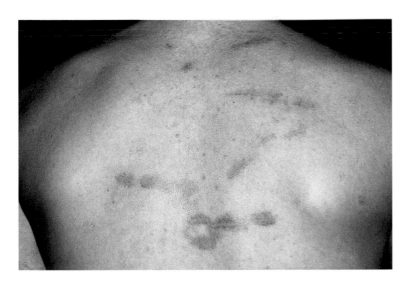

◀ **5.39 Male aged 17 years**
He was resident in hospital because of severe learning difficulties. Day staff found unexplained marks on his back. The photograph shows extensive bruising over the back, of characteristic linear shape and 'key shape'. This was an inflicted injury, although the actual weapon used was not discovered. (Note: people with disability of any sort are more vulnerable to all forms of abuse.)

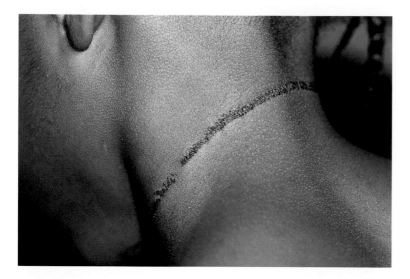

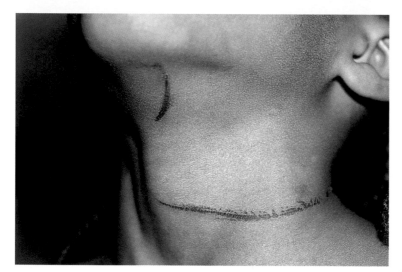

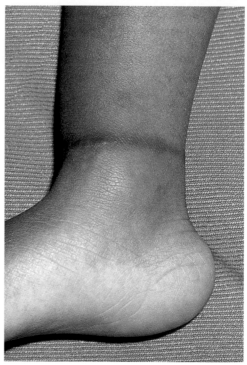

▲ 5.42 **Male aged 4 years**
He was referred because the neighbours had heard a child screaming at night. He had a pigmented circumferential band round lower leg with keloid scarring anteriorly. The ligature mark was caused when the child was tied to his bed.

▲ 5.40, ▲ 5.41 **Male aged 5 years**
He was referred by a psychologist during a therapy session because of marks around the neck. The child had a history of emotional, physical and sexual abuse. The photograph shows an incomplete circumferential abrasion around the neck (Fig. 5.40) with a similar lesion under the chin (Fig. 5.41). The lesions had the appearance of a cord burn but the exact nature of the 'accident' was unknown.

Chapter 6

Bites

Bites

- Resulting marks − paired crescent-shaped bruises with or without breaks in the skin.
- Always non-accidental in origin.
- Can be animal or human, adult or child.
- Identification of perpetrator possible if mark is recent and clear.
- Individual tooth marks may be identified if the injury is recent.
- Animal bites, e.g. dog or cat, result in puncturing, cutting and tearing of skin by the carnivorous dentition.
- Intercanine distance (measurement across the mouth between the third tooth on each side) is greater than 3.0 cm in the adult or older child and less than 3.0 cm in a young child with primary teeth.

Is it a bite?
- Human or animal?
- Adult or child?
- Photograph with rule, daily ×7.
- Washing for saliva (ABO group).
- Perpetrator identification − forensic odontologist.

Suspect identification

- Can be attempted with the help of a forensic dentist or odontologist.
- Series of photographs, starting as soon as the injury is identified, are taken at intervals of 24 hours with a millimetre rule incorporated.
- Suspected perpetrators are asked to provide a dental impression to compare with the photographs.
- ABO blood grouping can be determined from saliva washings of the skin surrounding a bite. Approximately 0.3 ml of saliva are deposited and it can be difficult to obtain sufficient by swabbing.

▶ **6.1 Male aged 5 months**
Presented with probable bite on the right shoulder. This was an adult bite – see notes on further investigation of bites.

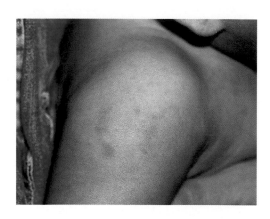

▶ **6.2 Female aged 6 weeks**
A bite on her cheek was noticed by staff at a mother and baby home. The photograph shows a typical bite mark on the cheek, and a deep healing laceration in the pinna. Diagnosis is an adult bite on cheek, and the laceration in the ear is consistent with nail injury.

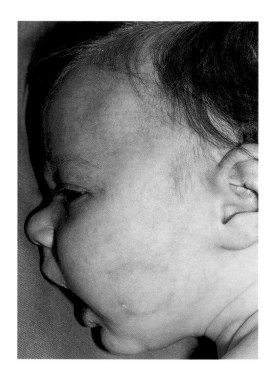

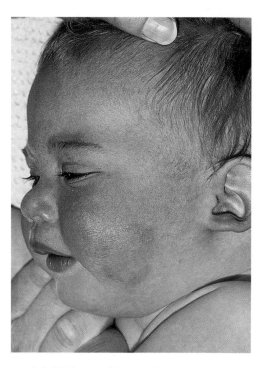

▲ **6.3 Male aged 9 months**
Bruising was noted by staff at a child health clinic. A double elliptical yellowing bruise can be seen on the cheek, probably due to an adult bite.

▶ **6.4 Male aged 6 years**
He presented having fallen off a gate. The photograph shows an incomplete bite with individual tooth marks visible. This is probably an adult bite. The boy had also been sexually abused.

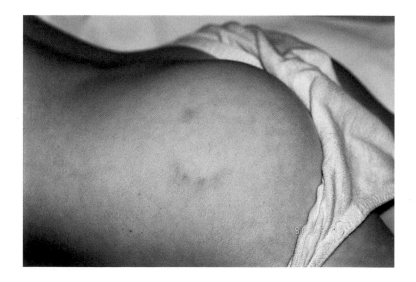

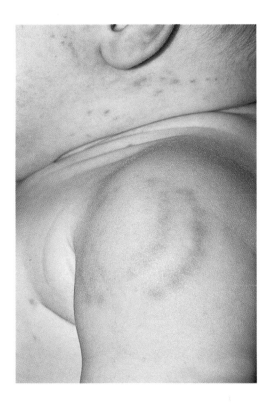

◀ **6.5 Female aged 11 months**

Mother showed marks on the baby's shoulder to a health visitor. A double bite mark can be seen on the outer aspect of the upper arm/shoulder. When approached by a forensic odontologist, the father admitted biting the child.

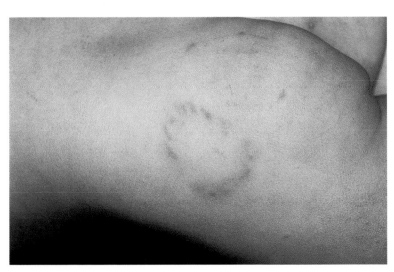

▲ **6.6 Male aged 3 years**

He presented as a neglected child with a healing burn on the chest and a mark on the bottom. A bite mark is seen with individual tooth marks visible, caused by an unidentified perpetrator.

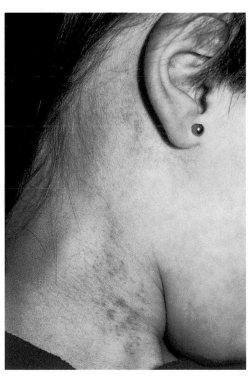

▲ **6.7 Female aged 4 years**

She was said to have fallen out of bed. The child had been repeatedly sexually abused at home where her mother lived with a female partner. There is multiple petechial bruising over a circumscribed area of the neck, due to a 'love bite'.

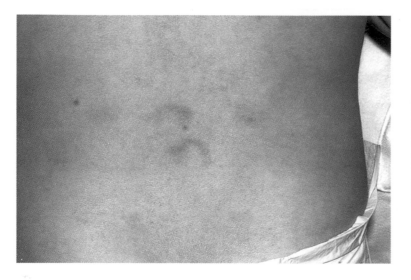

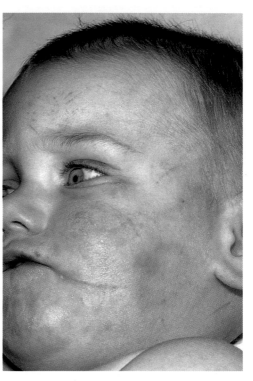

▲ 6.8, ▶ 6.9, ▶ 6.10 Male aged 14 months

His grandmother noticed bruises and scratches when caring for the child. The mother was known to be abusing drugs. There are multiple healing, semilunar facial scratches; an old yellowing bite on the left cheek; a linear, purple/blue bruise on the right cheek, and semicircular bruises on the back. These are due to fingernail scratches and an old bite (probably adult); in addition, there are unexplained old injuries to the back.

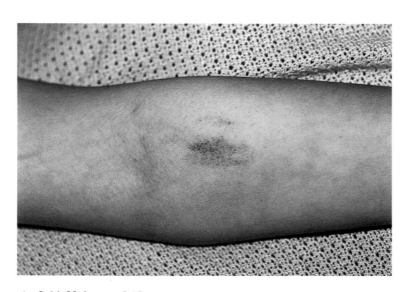

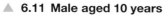

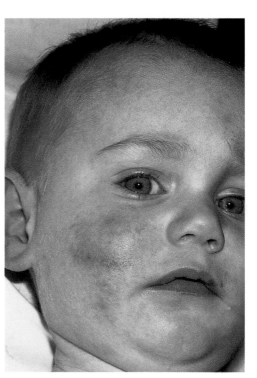

▲ 6.11 Male aged 10 years

Self-inflicted 'love bite' on the arm of this boy. Note petechiae. There was a long history of sexual abuse.

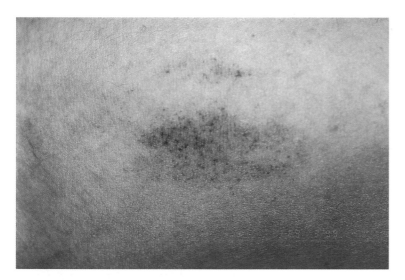

▲ **6.12 Male aged 10 years**
Same injury as Fig. 6.11, but with greater detail due to higher magnification.

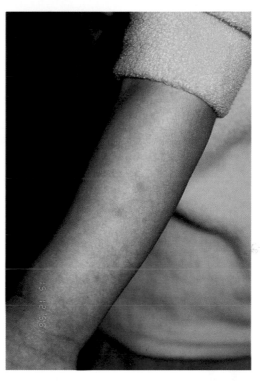

▲ **6.13 Female aged 3 years**
She presented with self-inflicted bite; she had been sexually abused and this amounts to self-mutilation. Note: children as young as 2 years have been seen with injuries due to self-mutilation.

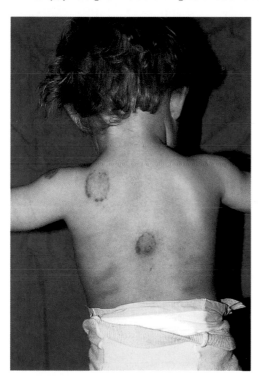

◀ **6.14 Female aged 1 year**
Child with multiple bites and other non-accidental injury to back.

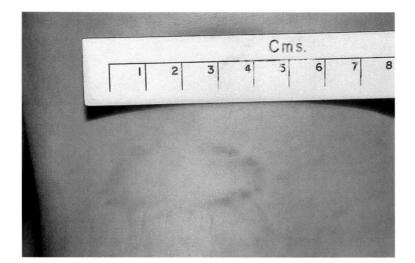

◀ **6.15–6.19 Male aged 2 years**
Presented at his day nursery with bites of differing ages. There was a 5-year-old sister and parents in the household. By taking dental impressions it was shown that the 5-year-old girl was biting her younger brother. The bites were seen in day nursery over several days and advice was sought when the third bite appeared and was unexplained. (With permission of Dr. S. Fayle.)

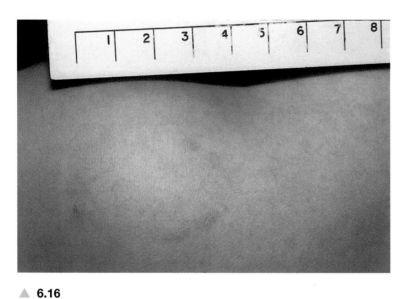

▲ **6.16**
The most recent bite.

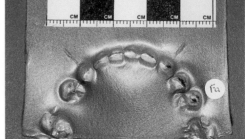

▲ **6.18**
The dental impression of the 5-year-old child, which fitted the bites very closely.

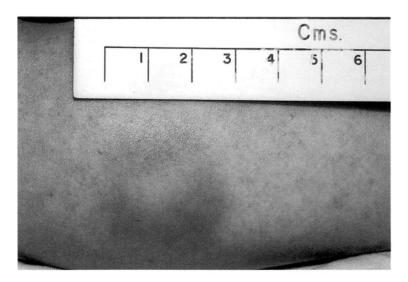

▲ **6.17**
The oldest bite.

▲ **6.19**
Dental impression of father, which excluded him as the biter.

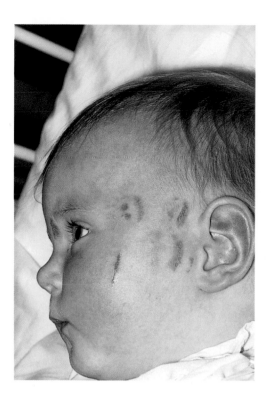

◀ 6.20 Female aged 12 months

Taken to see a doctor because she was 'irritable'. She was also reported to have been 'assaulted' by her disturbed, abused 4-year-old cousin. The photograph shows a bruised pinna, a graze to the nose, a superficial scratch to the cheek and three paired, elliptical lesions with surface abrasion. They are possibly caused by bites.

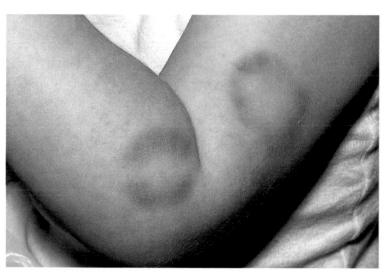

◀ 6.21 Female aged 4 years

She had been previously sexually abused. Two bite marks are seen on her arm, probably child bites obtained in the day nursery.

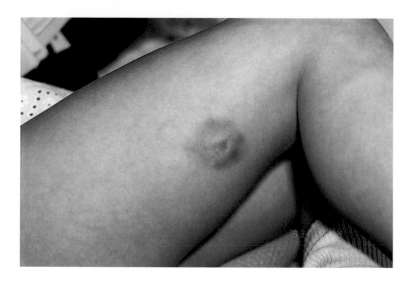

◀ 6.22 Female aged 3 years

A small radius bite with a central suction mark, on the back of the thigh, was a chance finding at a routine follow-up appointment following sexual abuse. This is a worrying unexplained bite because of the type of bite and position.

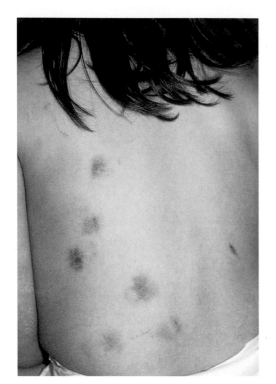

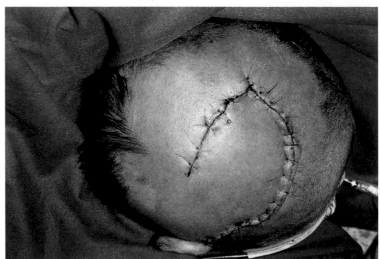

◀ 6.23 Female aged 3 years

She presented with unusual marks at day nursery. The marks have the appearance of 'love bites' although we were not able to confirm the diagnosis.

▲ 6.24 Male

This infant suffered bites from the family's Rotweiler on day 2 of life. An extensive neurosurgical flap with repair of depressed skull fractures is shown. At 15 months the child has a marked left hemiplegia but is otherwise developing well. The family unwillingly parted with the two 'guard dogs'.

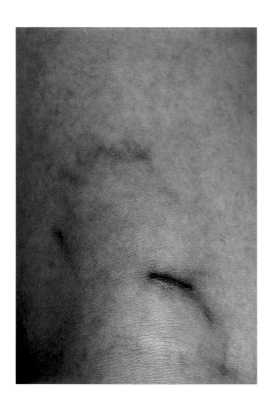

◀ 6.25 Male aged 8 years

He was bitten by a neighbour's Rottweiler. A faint healing semicircular mark with scarring is seen on the knee, and an inferiorly deeper laceration not yet healed.

Chapter 7

Injuries to Mouth

How common are dental injuries in abuse?

If examined by a skilled dentist, up to 1 in 4 physically abused and 1 in 6 sexually abused children have evidence of mouth injury.

Findings which could indicate abuse in the mouth include:

- oral lacerations;
- jaw and teeth injuries;
- frenulum tear;
- signs due to neglect.

Facts about the tear of upper lip frenulum

- association with abuse;
- examine carefully for recent and healed tears;
- usual history of falling;
- in pre-mobile infant is usually abuse;
- direct blow or force feeding;
- alone or with other injuries;
- toddler fall may be accidental.

Lip injuries

- common in abuse;
- contusions, lacerations, abrasions, burns;
- blunt force traps lip between teeth and object e.g. fist;
- injury often mainly visible on under side;
- burns: hot food, utensils, cigarettes.

Injuries to deciduous teeth

- very common injury 50% under 5 years;
- luxation, intrusion, avulsion, fractures;
- does the history fit?
- are there other injuries consistent with abuse?
- could there be a facial/jaw fracture?

Dental neglect

- How severe is the condition?
- Has treatment been sought?
- What is the parent's understanding?
- What is the child's general state?
- What is the child's diet?
- Has the child failed to thrive?
- Is he underweight for his age?

▶ **7.1 Male aged 3 years**

He has healing lacerations to either side of his tongue caused when his jaw was hit from below. See Chapter 4, Fig. 4.14.

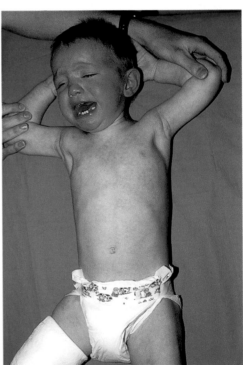

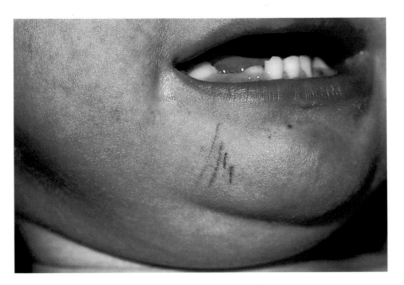

▲ **7.2 and** ▶ **7.3 Male aged 15 months**

He was found by his carers at night standing by his bed. His mother noticed he had a swollen, painful leg and took him to the A&E Department. X-ray showed a fractured tibia. Further examination showed chipped teeth, caused by trauma. No history was forthcoming to explain the fracture – it is unexplained and warrants urgent investigation.

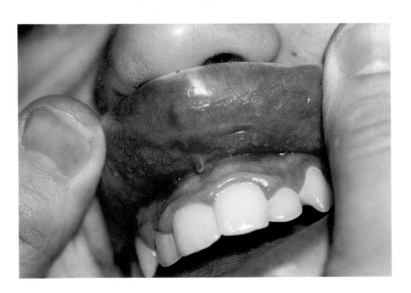

▲ **7.4 Male aged 6 years**

He lived in a residential home where he was bullied. This escalated and led to the injury to the upper lip, showing marked swelling, bruising and torn frenulum. The likely mechanism is a blow to the mouth.

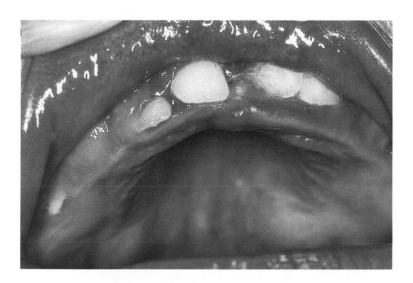

◀ **7.5 Male aged 18 months**
He was seen initially following a fall from his buggy but later seen again in hospital with injury to the mouth causing displacement of the teeth and gum margin. Full investigation showed he also had a fractured forearm and signs consistent with sexual abuse.

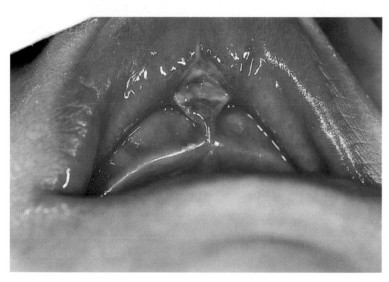

◀ **7.6 Male aged 3 months**
He was referred with recently torn frenulum. Further investigation showed fractured ribs.

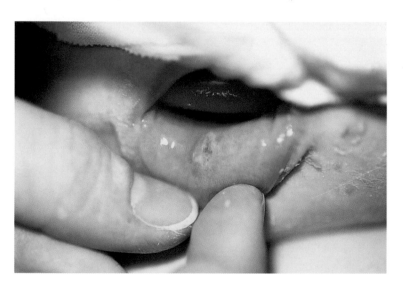

◀ **7.7 Female aged 15 months**
She has healing laceration on inner aspect of lower lip. This child also had a lacerated liver following a blow to the abdomen.
Note: intra-abdominal injuries may be difficult to diagnose. Late diagnosis accounts for the high mortality of up to 50% where there is a rupture. There were also three limb fractures.

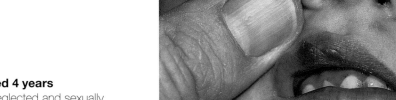

▶ **7.8 Female aged 4 years**
She presented as neglected and sexually abused with an unexplained mouth injury. The photograph shows a swollen, bruised, abraided upper lip caused by an unexplained injury, probably a blow to the mouth.

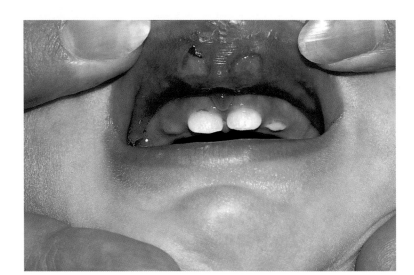

▶ **7.9 Male aged 10 months**
His mother mentioned bleeding from the mouth at a routine follow-up appointment in the neonatal clinic. There is a torn frenulum and swollen upper lip with tooth mark imprints, ulcerating and fresh bleeding. These were due to two mouth injuries: one probably inflicted by a bottle, causing the torn frenulum, and the second by a blow to the mouth.

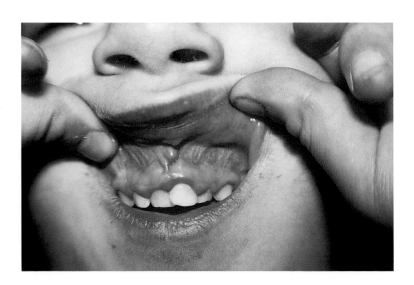

▶ **7.10 Male aged 5 years**
Presented with unexplained bruising (not described). An old, healed tear of the frenulum is seen, and the right central incisor is misaligned. This is an old mouth injury.

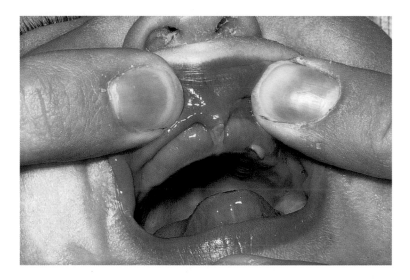

◀ 7.11 Male aged 7 months

He presented with a fractured humerus. The photograph shows a healing tear of the frenulum. This is an old mouth injury, in conjunction with recent further injury.

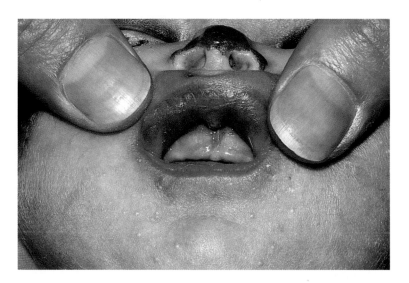

◀ 7.12 Female aged 3 months

She presented unconscious in the hospital emergency department. A grossly swollen upper lip with recently torn frenulum is seen. There were also other serious injuries. These injuries were caused by a blow to the mouth, and other trauma.

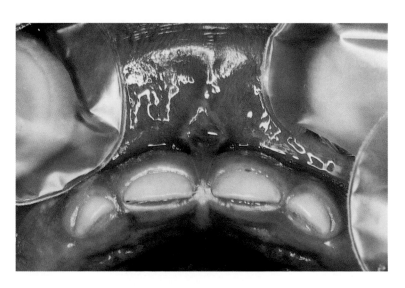

◀ 7.13 Female aged 18 months

She attended at her doctor's surgery with a history of not using her right arm for 3 days. The photograph shows an old healed complete tear of the frenulum, caused by a blow to the mouth. In addition, failure to thrive and other multiple injuries including supracondylar fracture were seen.

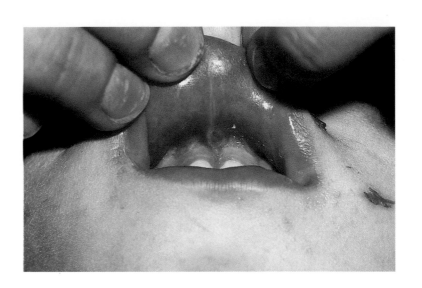

▶ **7.14 Female aged 2 years**
She presented as having 'fallen off a climbing frame in the park'. Recent bruising at the margin of the upper lip and gum, and a recently torn frenulum are seen. These constituted unexplained mouth injuries in a child who had been physically and sexually abused. The child had other multiple injuries.

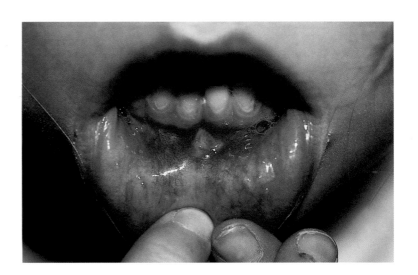

▶ **7.15 Female aged 5 years**
The torn, ulcerated frenulum of the lower lip was an incidental finding at a paediatric follow-up clinic following previous sexual abuse by the mother's partner. The mother said the doctor had diagnosed an aphthous ulcer. This indicated physical abuse.

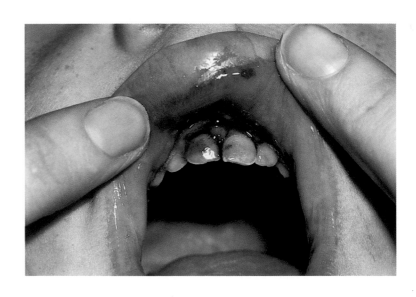

▶ **7.16 Male aged 4 years**
He was taken to hospital's emergency department by his parents with a history of having fallen against the toilet. Examination showed a swollen upper lip with abrasions, bleeding from the gum, and also chipped incisor teeth. The injury was compatible with a fall against a hard surface or a blow to the mouth. But there were numerous other bruises not typical of accidents.

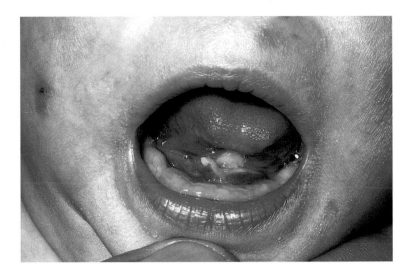

◀ **7.17 Male aged 5 months**

He was described as a miserable baby who would not take feeds properly. Extensive ulceration of the frenulum below the tongue can be seen. This is a healing injury; the mother later admitted to forcing a spoon into the infant's mouth.

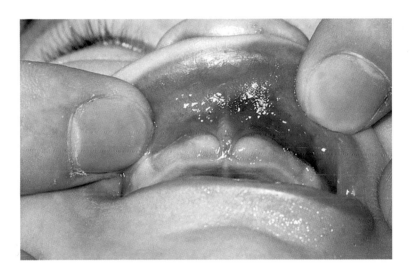

◀ **7.18 Male aged 2 months**

Presented at the hospital emergency department with unexplained bleeding from the mouth. Recent extensive injury to the inner aspect of the upper lip and frenulum is seen with bruising and bleeding. This is a feeding bottle injury.

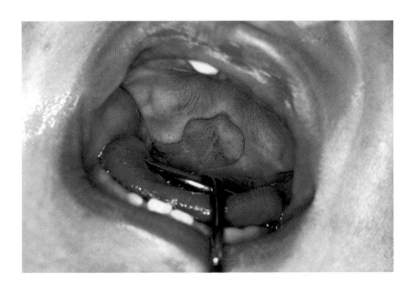

◀ **7.19 Male aged 12 months**

The child had a history of feeding problems. A traumatic ulcer of the hard palate is shown in the photograph; it was probably caused by a spoon. There were also three limb fractures.

Chapter 8

Injuries to the Eye

Ophthalmic injuries in abuse
Structure

◆ Eyelids, periorbital tissue
— arise from blunt trauma, e.g. fist.
— bruising 'black eye' recovers.

◆ Cornea, conjunctiva
— blunt/penetrating trauma, haemorrhage, laceration.
— burns, chemicals, abrasion, ulceration, scarring — visual loss if in visual axis.

◆ Lens, anterior structures
— blunt or penetrating trauma, iris sphincter rupture, vossius ring glaucoma.
— dislocated lens, intraocular scar formation, cataract.

◆ Posterior structures, vitreous
— anterior injury transmitted to vitreous haemorrhage, retinal scarring, papilloedema.

◆ Retina
— whiplash, shaking. Haemorrhage, retinal detachment, optic atroply.

◆ Fractures of orbit
— optic nerve injuries. Resolution and visual loss variable.

◆ Visual cortex
— head injury contrecoup — cerebral contusion
— cortical blindness.

Examination of the eye requires ophthalmological assistance.

Causes of retinal haemorrhages
◆ 60−95% of shaken infants have retinal haemorrhages;
◆ vaginal birth (30%);
◆ blood dyscrasias;
◆ not high impact head injuries from RTA;
◆ CPR unlikely to cause retinal haemorrhages;
◆ No association with epileptic fits.

▶ **8.1 Girl aged 14 months**
Presented with bruising to upper orbit associated with fracture of the frontal bone (Battle sign). This child was neglected and had had a fall from around 20 feet, fracturing a forearm bone.

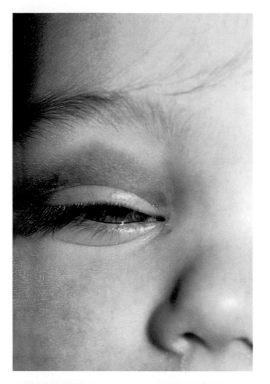

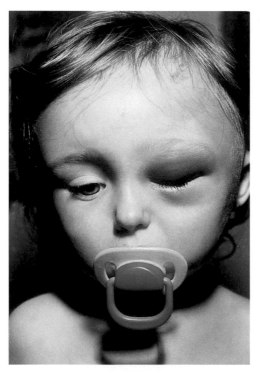

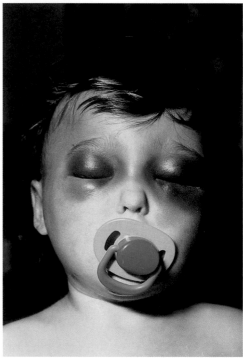

▲ **8.2,** ▲ **8.3 Female aged 2 years**
Admitted to hospital because of a swollen eye. Over the next 24 hours both eyes became very swollen and closed. The history was that she had fallen from an ordinary divan bed. The severe injury is not compatible with the history given. The photographs show the evolution of the bruise.

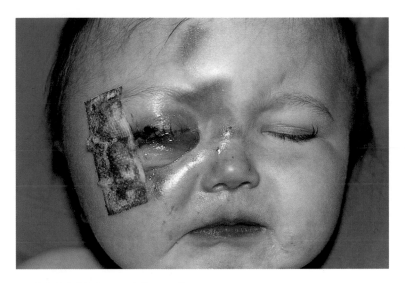

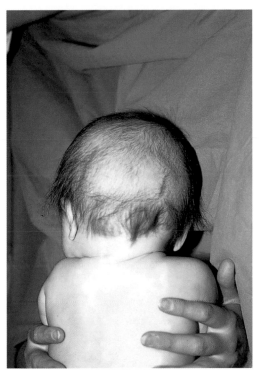

▲ **8.4-8.8 Male aged 6 months**
Presented at the A&E Department with signs of severe swelling to the right eye which initially was thought to be cellulitis. There was bruising on the forehead and blood was seen within the orbit and within the eye. The ophthalmologist confirmed a diagnosis of trauma. Surgical decompression of the orbit was necessary in an attempt to preserve the vision. The mother gave a history that the infant had put his head through the bars of the cot, causing this injury. The child's mother was also a victim of severe physical abuse, having suffered a hammer blow to her head resulting in a hemiplegia. She was wheelchair-bound.

▲ **8.5**
Shows unexplained linear marks to either side of the occiput. There was also an unexplained red mark to the inferior aspect of the occiput to the left.

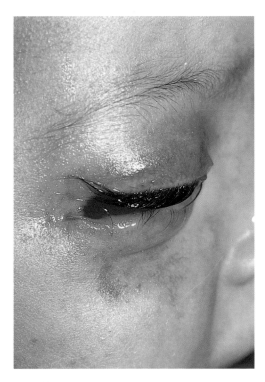

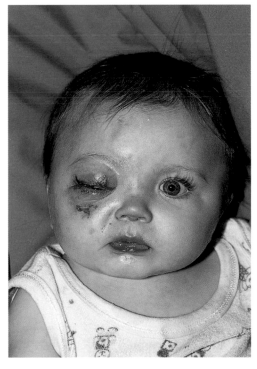

▲ **8.6**
Shows marked swelling of the orbit with erythema. This photograph was taken after orbital decompression.

▲ **8.7**
This photograph was taken 3 weeks later, showing how long the eye took to heal.

▶ **8.8**
On follow-up, the child had an amblyopic right eye with squint.

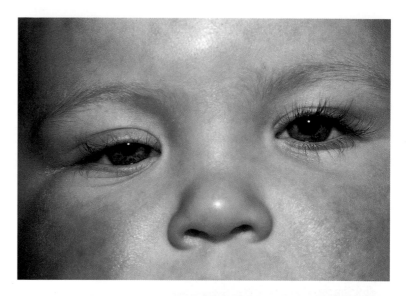

▶ **8.9 Female aged 3**
She was brought to the A&E Department with a history that the bedroom door had fallen on top of her. The injuries seen were two black eyes, a swollen nose with bleeding, a graze on the chin and bruising on the lower cheek. The two black eyes and swollen nose may be due to one or more punches to the face. The graze on the chin is unexplained. The history was clearly erroneous because these are penetrating eye injuries.

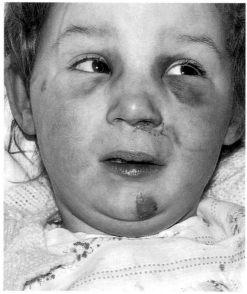

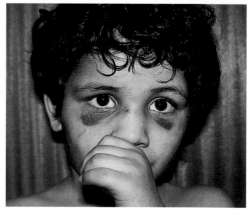

▲ **8.10 Male aged 3 years**
The health visitor observed injuries when visiting the house to see a new baby. The photograph shows bilateral infra-orbital haematoma with a small laceration to the bridge of the nose. Old linear scarring of face is also noted, and he was also failing to thrive. The injuries suggest a blow to the frontal area with blood tracking downwards. There was a history of previous physical abuse in this family and also failure to thrive.

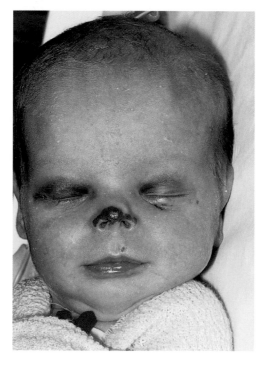

◀ **8.11 Female aged 3 months**
The child was found fitting when her parents awoke in the morning. The photograph shows a deeply unconscious infant with peri-orbital haematoma and an extensive carpet burn to the nose. This infant had suffered a severe head injury with skull fracture and intracerebral haemorrhage. She survived but now has severe cerebral palsy and significant learning difficulties.

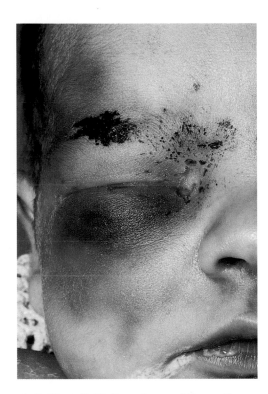

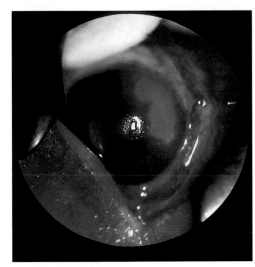

▲ **8.12,** ▲ **8.13 Female aged 2 months**

The mother's male partner accidentally dropped her on the stairs. A laceration above the right eye is seen, showing signs of healing, with marked oedema to the right side of the face, infra-orbital and cheek bruising. There is dried blood about the nose, and an injury to the lip (not shown on this photograph). Further examination showed a burn of the right cornea, demonstrated using fluorescein (Fig. 8.13). Further investigation showed a complex parietal skull fracture, caused by impact with a firm object. The other injuries are consistent with blows to the face and head. The cause of the corneal burn is unknown, but the presumption was that it was a cigarette burn. She subsequently suffered a detached retina to the right eye and is now blind in this eye.

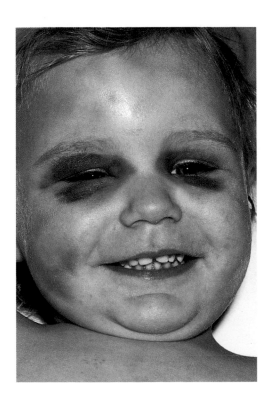

◄ **8.14 Female aged 2½ years**

The child presented with unexplained bruising, which had been noted by a social worker on a routine visit. There is marked swelling across the forehead with bruising and tracking of blood giving bilateral peri-orbital haematoma. The eyes are not injured. (Note: fading bruise around the angle of the right jaw; bruises were also seen on the upper arms, abdomen, back and thighs.) This child had been punished for not using her potty by having her head banged against the floor. She was thus the victim of physical assault, emotional abuse and subsequent investigation showed she had also been sexually abused.

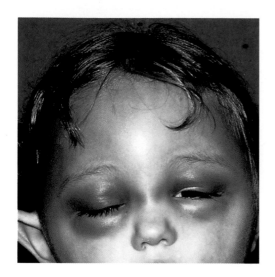

▶ **8.16,** ▶ **8.17 Male aged 13 years**
The child told his teacher at school that he had been 'beaten up' by his father. Bilateral subconjunctival haemorrhage can be seen with a small area of skin loss over the bridge of the nose, and extensive diffuse bruising over the back. Subconjunctival haemorrhage may be caused by blunt trauma, e.g. a fist causing direct damage to the orbit, or a similar injury may be seen due to strangulation, where there may or may not be associated petechiae of the upper eyelids. Subconjunctival haemorrhage may also be caused by bouts of paroxysmal coughing, e.g. whooping cough. The combination of injuries here is consistent with the boy's history, i.e. he has been beaten up.

◀ **8.15 Male aged 4 years**
The boy returned from an access visit to his father with unexplained black eyes and multiple burns. There is swelling of the forehead and bilateral peri-orbital haematoma, with no injury to the eyes. He also had burns to the genitalia, buttocks and lower legs, and he gave a history of attempted buggery. (Note: there is an association between sadistic burns and sexual abuse.)

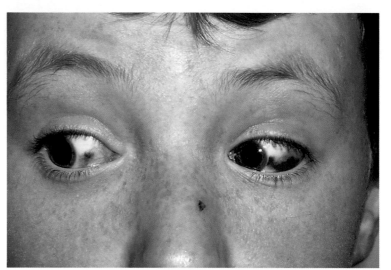

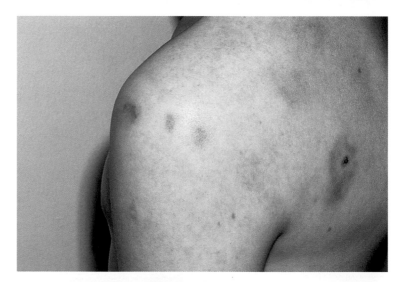

▶ **8.18 Male aged 3 years**
The child was taken to the hospital emergency department by his parents because of bleeding from his mouth. He was said to have fallen off the settee. There is subconjunctival haemorrhage, but also bruising around the orbit. This eye injury is consistent with a blunt injury, e.g. a fist. The child also had a markedly swollen upper lip, also consistent with blunt trauma. (Note: this pattern of injury is not caused by a simple fall as described.)

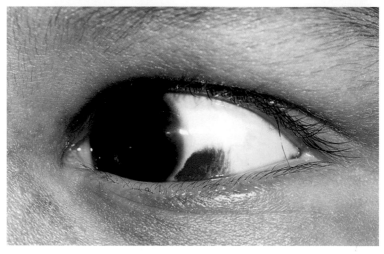

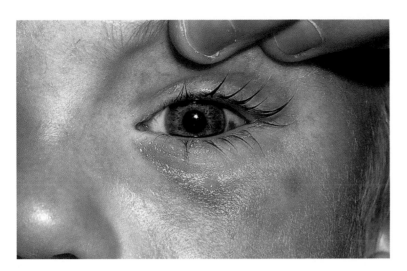

▲ 8.19 Male aged 4 years

The child returned home crying saying he had been hit by older boys. The photograph shows subconjunctival haemorrhage, with peri-orbital swelling and bruising. The injury is consistent with a blunt impact, e.g. a fist in the orbit. (Note: the changing colour of the bruising, suggesting this bruise may have been more than 1 day old, i.e. at variance with the history.)

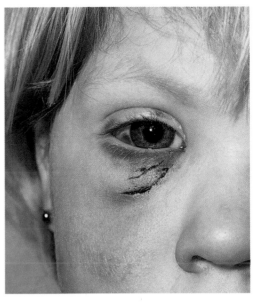

▲ 8.20 Female aged 4 years

The history given was that her mother's male partner was putting her to bed when he accidentally poked her in the eye. There is peri-orbital haematoma with two parallel lacerations below the eye and a subconjunctival haemorrhage. The injury is not compatible with the history given but likely to have been caused by a clenched fist, and the lacerations due to rings on the fingers of the assailant. (Note: this child was later found to have been sexually abused; in any child where there has been a physical injury sexual abuse should also be considered.)

▶ 8.21 Female aged 12 years

The parents took the child to the doctor complaining of an allergic reaction to bath cleaner which had accidentally fallen into the bath. The doctor confirmed this diagnosis. The photograph shows bilateral peri-orbital haematoma, which is consistent with a blunt injury to the forehead. (Note: the father, who was a convicted child abuser, had 2 years earlier admitted to banging the girl's head against a wall causing a similar injury. The girl was also self-mutilating, and was thought to have been sexually abused although this was not confirmed.)

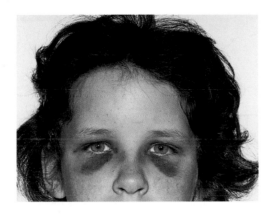

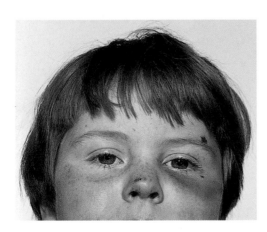

▲ 8.22 Male aged 7 years

The child told his class teacher that his father had hit him when he had wet the bed. There is bilateral old infra-orbital bruising with minor abrasions with skin loss about the orbit at the left and on the nose. The injuries are consistent with multiple blows to the face.

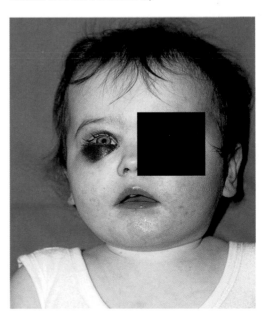

▲ 8.23 Female aged 2 years

The injury to the eye was noticed by a health visitor. A recent right peri-orbital haematoma with swelling is seen. This is a serious unexplained injury in a very young child. There were other bruises on examination of the child but none were diagnostic of physical abuse.

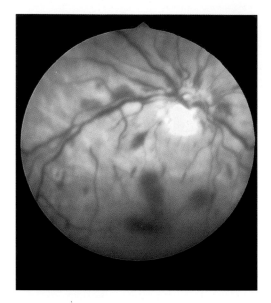

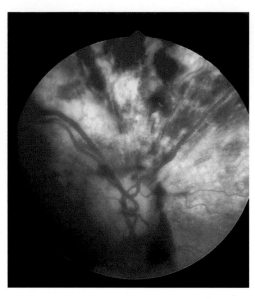

▲ **8.24 Male aged 4 years**
The mother returned from a shopping trip to find the child in her male partner's arms and was unable to rouse the child. He was deeply unconscious with bruising of the face, bleeding from the nose and bruising to the back. The bruising is of different ages. Further investigation revealed recent retinal haemorrhages. There were also signs of anal abuse. The boy died of his head injury.

▲ **8.25 Male aged 4 months**
Mixed retinal haemorrhages in a baby who had been shaken violently.

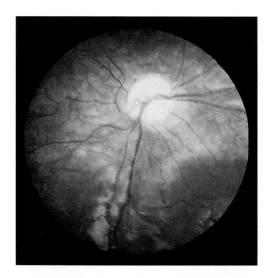

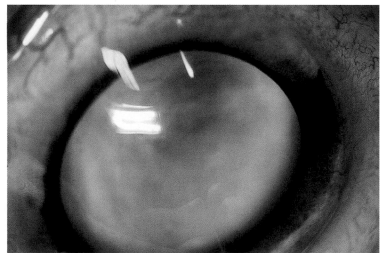

▲ **8.26,** ▲ **8.27 Male aged 2 years**
Figure 8.26 shows optic atrophy resulting from a severe shaking injury in a child who survived. (Photograph provided by Mr R.M.L. Doran.) Another complication of non-accidental injury is cataract, as shown in Fig. 8.27.

Chapter 9

Head and Abdominal Injuries

Types of head injury

1. Scalp injury – bruises, traumatic subgaleal haematoma.
2. Skull fracture.
3. Subdural, subarachnoid and intraventricular haemorrhage.
4. Cerebral contusion, haemorrhage and oedema.
5. Eye and other associated injury.

Skull fractures are common in the severely battered child.

Diagnosis

- Plain X-ray examination (also seen on bone windows of CT).
- Depressed or wide ('growing') fractures can be palpated.
- Presence of bleeding or cerebrospinal fluid (CSF) from an ear or nose.
- Swelling over the scalp.
- Cannot readily be aged.
- Difficulties in diagnosis arise in infancy because of the presence of aberrant suture lines.

Fractures should be accurately described and measured, either on the radiograph or at post mortem.

Patterns

- Single linear.
- Multiple or complex.
- Depressed.
- Growing fractures.

Reports of skull fractures should include

- site – which bone(s);
- whether suture lines crossed;
- configuration – e.g. linear, crazy paving, stellate, branching;
- orientation – horizontal, vertical, oblique;
- length (cm) of each component, maximum width (mm);
- other features – e.g. depression, growing;
- presence of soft tissue swelling (use bright light source).

Skull fracture – differentiating abuse from accident

- Does the injury fit the explanation?
- Most histories in young children usually involve relatively minor falls or impacts.
- Every skull fracture will need to be evaluated carefully.
- Differentiation on the basis of fracture characteristics on radiology findings alone is not possible.

Findings associated with greater severity of impact:

- complex;
- multiple;
- large depressed areas;
- wide, involving more than one bone;
- basal, occipital (in general non-parietal in site);
- associated with intra-cranial injury;
- uncomplicated linear parietal fractures are the most frequently encountered fractures following both abuse and accident.

Intracranial injury arises from:

- shaking;
- impact;
- both.

Findings include

- diffuse or focal cerebral oedema;
- subarachnoid haemorrhage;
- subdural haemorrhage (interhemispheric, convexity – acute or chronic);
- intraventricular haemorrhage;
- contusional haemorrhage;
- post-traumatic hydrocephalus and cerebral atrophy;
- eye injury.

Shaken baby syndrome (SBS)

Minor injuries such as falls from low height, infant swings, bumpy roads, or routine play do not cause this syndrome. The relatively large head and weaker neck musculature and poor head control increase the whiplash effect.

Clinical presentation

- SBS is characterized by 'much obscure and subtle rather than immediately clinically identifiable' (American Academy of Pediatrics).
- Subdural haemorrhage and retinal haemorrhage provide strong evidence of shaking.
- Many cases are missed.

Retinal haemorrhages

- thought to arise in shaking from vitreous traction.
- provide strong evidence of abuse outside the newborn period.
- 60–95% of shaken infants have retinal haemorrhages, sometimes unilateral.
- vaginal birth (30%);
- blood dyscrasias;
- high impact head injuries from RTA – possible, uncommon;
- CPR and epilepsy – very rarely.

Diagnosis – investigations

- Ultrasound, CT or magnetic resonance imaging (MRI) confirms the presence of intra-cranial injury.
- Fractures are best identified by plain films and a full skeletal survey incorporating individual films and not babygrams is essential.
- Full social investigation is needed if head trauma suspected without adequate history.
- Other conditions which occasionally lead to intracranial bleeding should be considered.

Abdominal injury – features

- Less common than limb fractures or cranio-cerebral injuries.
- Threat to life.
- Delay in diagnosis is common.
- Usually results from a kick, stamp or punch.
- Hollow gastrointestinal as well as solid organs may be injured.
- There may be no signs of external injury, e.g. bruising.

Types of abdominal injury

1　Perforation of the gut – stomach, duodenum and duodeno-jejunal flexure, jejunum, ileum.
2　Haemorrhage – major vessel.
3　Laceration, contusion, haematoma – liver, spleen, duodenum, pancreas, mesentery, kidney.
4　Other, e.g. bladder injury, rectal perforation from abusive anal penetration in young child.

Clinical presentation

- Seriously injured child, presumed head injury, poor response.
- Acute abdomen.
- Sudden unexplained collapse.
- Unexplained peritonitis.
- Abdominal bruising.
- Persistent abdominal pain, vomiting.
- Other, e.g. haematuria, inferior vena cava thrombosis.

Investigations

Clinical abdominal examination

- Is there distention?
- Insert nasogastric tube, empty stomach. Is blood, food or bile obtained? Does distention remain?
- Is rectal examination required?
- Are there signs of injury (sexual abuse can perforate the rectum in infancy), blood, anterior tenderness?

Laboratory investigations

- Serial haematocrit for blood loss.
- Serum amylase (raised in pancreatic and in some cases of splenic injury because the spleen lies close to the pancreas).
- Serum aspartate aminotransferase, alanine aminotransferase, lactate dehydrogenase (raised in liver laceration).
- Urine: gross or microscopic haematuria (>20 RBCs per high power field suggests damage to the kidney or urinary tract).

Radiology

- Chest X-ray – rib fracture, pneumothorax, pleural fluid/haemothorax.
- Posteroanterior abdominal and chest radiographs, taken in supine and erect positions, allow visualisation of free air and fluid levels following perforation of a hollow viscus.
- Plain X-rays of abdomen may reveal ground-glass appearance of intraperitoneal haemorrhage (or fluid from other cause).
- CT scanning is the most sensitive method of identifying injuries of the lungs, pleura and solid abdominal organs, including pancreatic injury and duodenal haematoma.

Note:
Urgent laparotomy is the most appropriate way to confirm the presence and site of a perforation.

▶ 9.1 Female aged 3 months

This child was taken ill whilst out with her parents shopping. She was in the baby buggy when her mother noticed she was gasping for breath so she took her to the GP who organized an immediate ambulance to hospital. She was resuscitated in hospital and ventilated. Investigation showed extensive subdural haematoma. Her clinical recovery was stormy and she had many fits. She was discharged to foster care and has severe learning difficulties and associated cerebral palsy. The family gave a history that a poltergeist injured the baby.

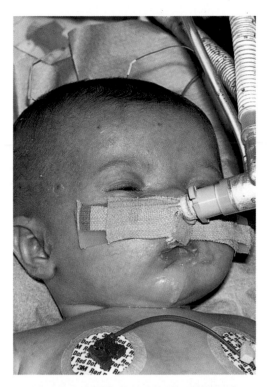

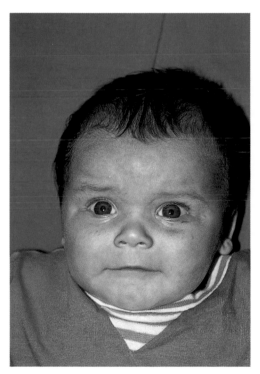

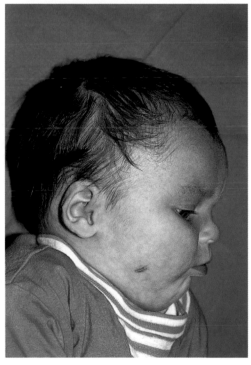

▲ 9.2–9.4 Male aged 4 months

He was admitted after an apnoeic spell at home. His mother gave a history that she was winding him over her shoulder when his head inadvertently was banged on the wall behind her. He had an old burn on his calf that was said to be from the car seat and bruising below the left eye.

▲ 9.3

He also had an abrasion on the right cheek, which was said to have been caused by his mother's ring.

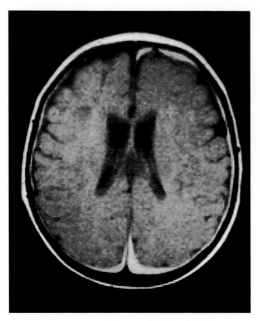

▲ 9.4

MRI scan showed an acute subdural haematoma and there were also retinal haemorrhages. He has made a good recovery.

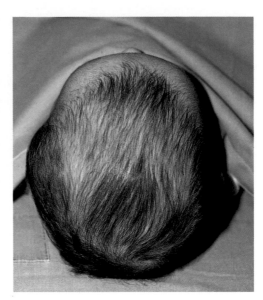

The mother noticed a large bump on the side of his head. She later gave a history of the television falling on his head 3 days previously, a fall against a coffee table, and a relative then said that the child's head had been kicked. There is a large fluctuant swelling over the parietal eminence. Further investigation showed a long parietal fracture with overlying haematoma. This injury would be consistent with a kick from a boot. Young infants seen with a swelling on the side of the head and no history of trauma are likely to have been abused.

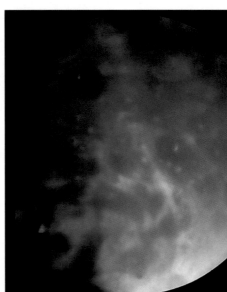

▲ 9.6 Male aged 3 months

The child was seen in an infant welfare clinic with rapid head growth. This is a classic picture of abuse 20 years ago, showing sites where diagnostic and therapeutic subdural taps have been performed. (From 1974: Dr M.F.G. Buchanan.)

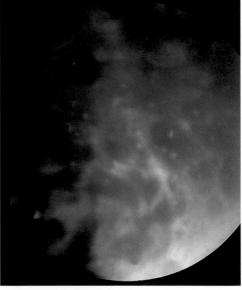

▲ 9.7 Female aged 6 weeks

This child was admitted to hospital unconscious and in need of urgent resuscitation. The mother said she had fallen with the baby in her arms over a sweeping brush but the baby's head had not been damaged in the fall. Investigation showed she had got an acute subdural haematoma which was evacuated immediately. She had unilateral retinal haemorrhages.

▶ 9.8 Female aged 6 weeks

The same child from Fig. 9.7. After making a good recovery from the head injury the mother and daughter were admitted to a residential unit. Within 2 weeks of discharge back home alone with her mother the child twice had bruising on the face. She has now been adopted and developmentally appears to be doing very well with no signs of persisting neurological damage.

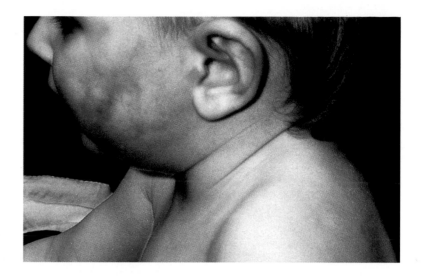

▶ 9.9 Female aged 5 months

The child was brought to the hospital emergency department by parents because she was 'unrousable'. She was deeply unconscious with multiple injuries to the face, scratches and early bruising with oedema of the face. Further investigation revealed retinal haemorrhages and subdural haematoma on CT scan. This baby had been physically assaulted, causing the injuries to her face, and she had also been shaken.

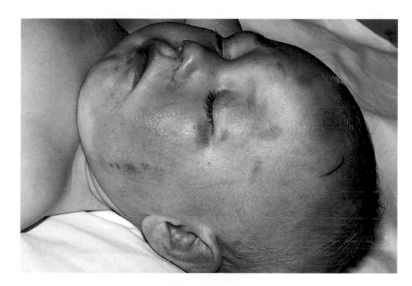

▶ 9.10 Male aged 2 days

He was admitted following bite from the family guard dog. Skull X-ray showed three discrete portions of bone embedded deeply in the brain substance. Apart from fitting initially he made a good post-operation recovery. On longer-term follow-up the infant has developed a left hemiparesis but is a bright, alert little boy.

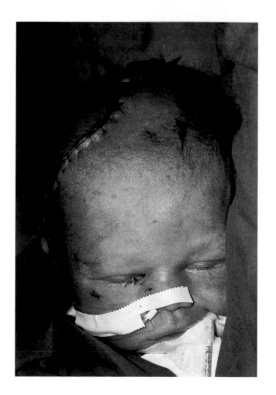

▶ **9.11 Female aged 5 weeks**

Admitted because of respiratory arrest at home. The father gave a history that the child had been restless in the evening and he had given her a little shake. The abrasion on the nares were said to be due to a dummy rubbing. This seems an unlikely explanation. There were three small round bruises on the left side of the face. Skeletal survey showed a fracture of the lower end of the left tibia. The infant did very badly and fitted continuously over the next 2 or 3 days and at follow-up has severe cerebral palsy and microcephaly. At 6 months she shows signs of hydrocephalus. At 18 months she is severely handicapped with uncontrolled epilepsy.

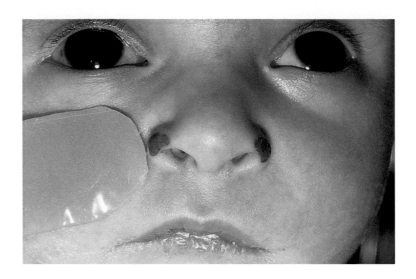

▶ **9.12 Female aged 5 months**

This infant with a carpet burn on her nose was admitted to hospital seriously ill. Investigation showed an acute subdural haematoma and the infant was ventilated. At follow-up she has severe developmental delay.

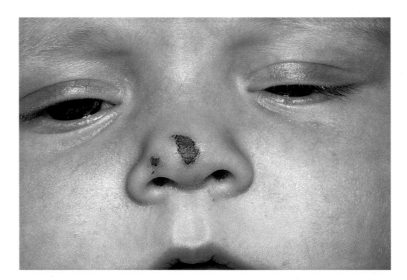

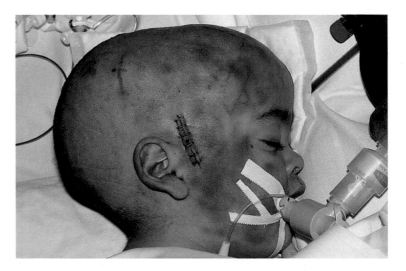

▲ **9.13–9.17 Male aged 2 years**

He was admitted to hospital after his mother had returned home and found him unconscious with a badly bruised face. He had been looked after by 11 and 13 year olds during the evening and they said he had fallen from the landing through the banister.

▲ **9.14, 9.15**

He was extensively bruised and a Star of David was inscribed on the right side of his forehead with a broken biro.

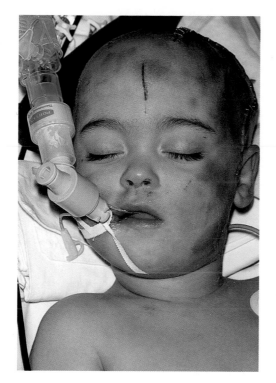

▲ **9.15**

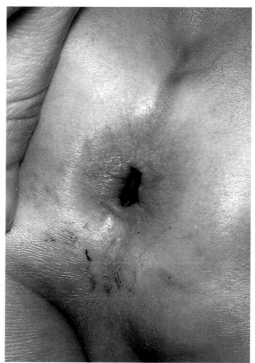

▲ **9.16**

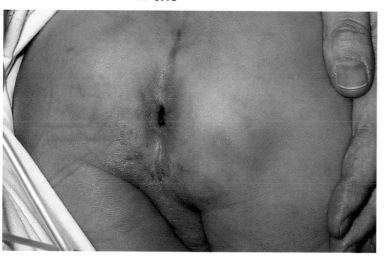

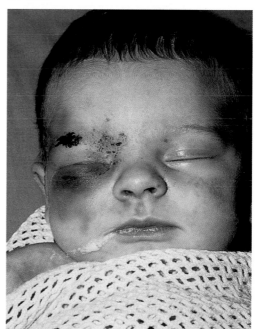

▲ **9.16, 9.17**

He had a markedly dilated anus, which reverted almost to normal over the first five days on the Intensive Care Unit. The aggressors admitted to causing injuries which included kicking and inserting a torch in the child's bottom. The child's younger sibling was also seen and he had a burn on the back of his hand. The mother of the babysitters had looked after him and she had put the child's hand on the fire to show him not to do it in future. In the past history her own daughter, when 4 years old, had been badly burned when she was put in front of the fire to punish her for allowing her young sister to be burned. The boy involved in the assault had earlier tried to hang himself. To summarize therefore, this boy had been physically and sexually assaulted by two older children. He has made a very poor recovery and has only limited movement in his left side, being able to hold a beaker and sit propped. He continues to have convulsions. His language is very limited. After a period in foster care he was rehabilitated home with his two younger brothers. It is worth noting that this child had an abnormal anus whilst on the Intensive Care Unit but there is also a good history of anal penetration.

▲ **9.18 Female aged 2 months**

This child was allegedly dropped by her father when coming downstairs. Examination showed that there was facial, ear and mouth bruising as well as a burn on the right cornea. She had a fractured skull. The injuries were not compatible with the history given.

▶ 9.19 Male aged 9 years

The child was bouncing up and down on his bed; his father told him to stop and when he didn't he lifted the boy bodily and threw him onto the bed. His scalp was then lacerated on the bed springs. The photograph shows a long, irregular, deep laceration of the scalp. This is an unusual, worrying history and injury.

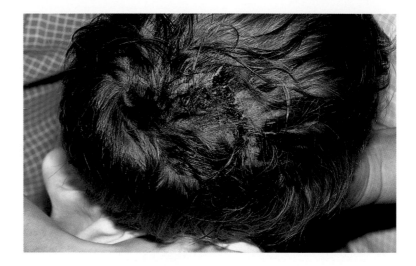

▶ 9.20 Male

This boy was shaken by his father when aged 4 months old. He unfortunately as a result has cerebral diplegia, impaired vision with an amblyopic right eye, and severe learning problems.

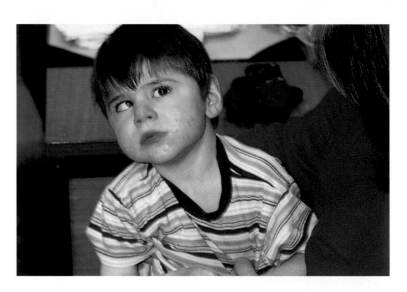

▶ 9.21 Female aged 3 years

The history given was that she fell off a settee. Her parents admitted giving her alcohol. She was drowsy with bleeding from the ear and bruising around the right eye. Fracture of the base of the skull was considered, but bleeding was in fact due to a ruptured eardrum. The diagnosis was physical abuse.

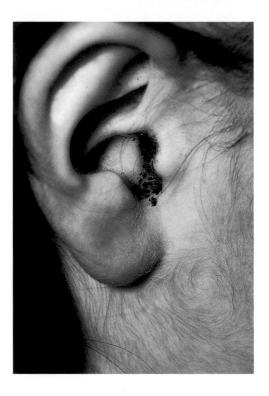

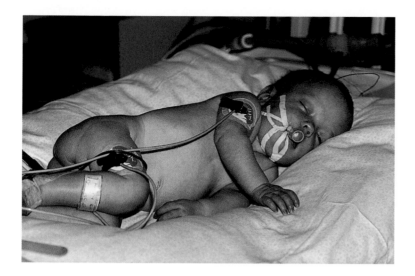

◀ **9.22,**◀ **9.23,**◀ **9.24**
Female aged 4 months
The child was brought into hospital collapsed and was resuscitated. She was ventilated but died several days later of massive head injury. The only bruises were one small bruise to the side of the spine (Fig. 9.24) and a similar one behind the ear. Further examination showed retinal haemorrhages and the CT brain scan showed gross cerebral swelling and subdural haematoma. Skull X-ray showed a complex skull fracture. The clinical findings are consistent with a shaking and impact injury. Neuro-imaging and the 'shaken/impact baby syndrome' (BBS). (Courtesy of Dr John Livingston, Consultant Paediatric Neurologist at The General Infirmary, Leeds.)

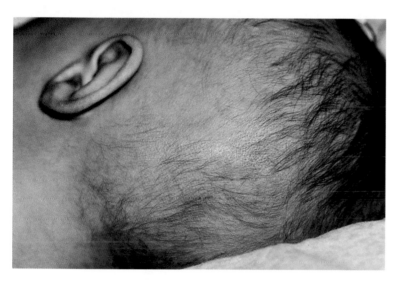

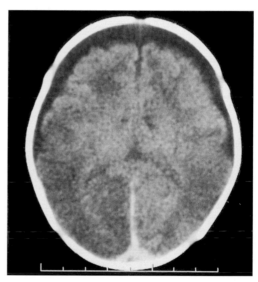

▲ **9.25**
Acute and chronic subdural haematomas in a CT brain scan showing the typical changes of the BBS. There is acute (recent) subdural haemorrhage in the interhemispheric fissure most marked posteriorly and around the occipital lobes. Over the frontal lobes there is a peri-cerebral collection of a different attenuation to cerebrospinal fluid (CSF) indicating a subdural effusion, suggestive of a previous or old injury. There are parenchymal changes in the brain in the right posterior region.(With permission of Dr J. Livingston.)

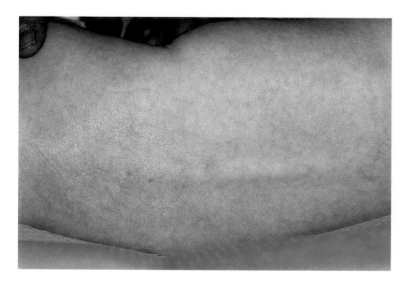

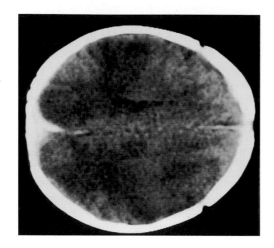

▲ **9.26**

This scan shows the consequences of a severe shaking/impact injury. The CT brain scan demonstrates an acute, but subtle collection of subdural blood in the posterior interhemispheric region. There is also severe parenchymal damage with the loss of white/grey distinction bilaterally. This indicates severe brain injury and a poor prognosis. (With permission of Dr J. Livingston.)

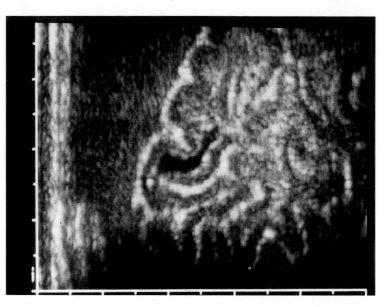

▲ **9.27**

This coronal ultrasound scan of the brain shows the typical appearance of a subcortical tear, which may not be visible on a CT brain scan. This sign is pathognomanic of a non-accidental brain injury. (With permission of Dr J. Livingston.)

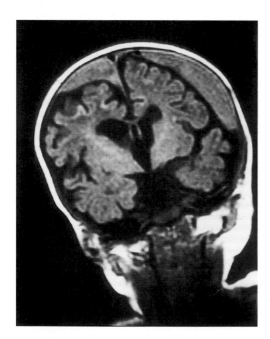

▲ **9.28**

This is a coronal MRI T₁ scan showing a chronic (old) subdural effusion. Note the clear distinction of subarachnoid space from the subdural space. There is cerebral atrophy due to the effect of a previous shaking injury.(With permission of Dr J. Livingston.)

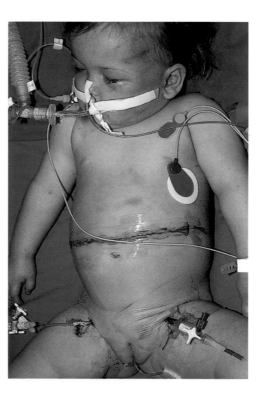

◄ **9.29 Female aged 2 years**

She was admitted with a history of 'collapse' by the A&E Department. She had bruising to the face, upper abdomen and chest. She was extremely ill and at laparotomy an extensive laceration of the liver was seen. She made an apparently good recovery following this severe blunt trauma to the abdomen.

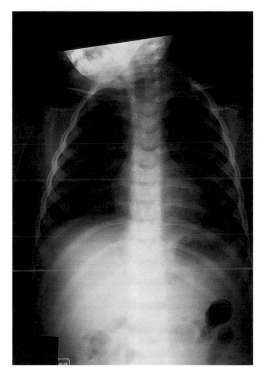

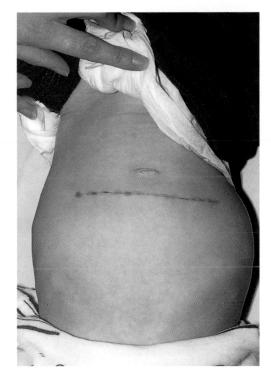

▲ 9.30, ▲ 9.31 Male aged 20 months
He was admitted via the A&E Department at the hospital following a 48-hour history of vomiting and diarrhoea. He was moribund on admission to hospital and investigation showed free air under the left diaphragm. The duodenum was torn. The child made a good recovery but was clearly very scared when visited by his family.

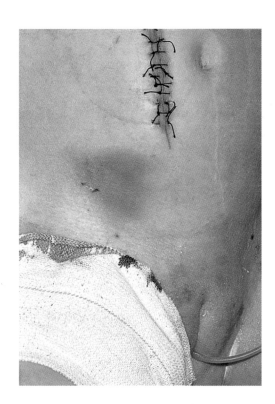

▶ 9.32 Female aged 2 years
This child was admitted via the A&E Department with a history of vomiting. There was bruising on the abdomen and the history was that she had fallen across a table. She had a duodenal rupture and was very ill although subsequently made a good recovery.

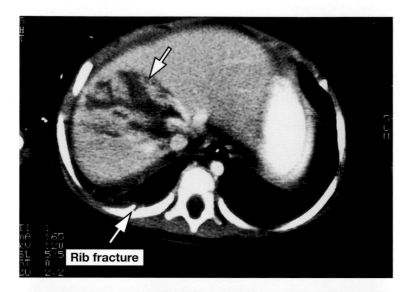

Rib fracture

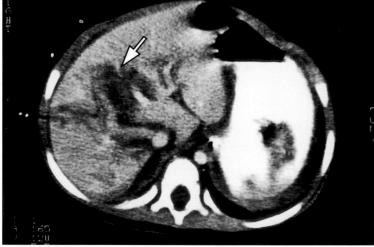

◀ **9.33–9.36 Female aged 15 months**
She was admitted to hospital moribund with a ventricular tachycardia. Investigation showed that she had extensive lacerations of the liver with fractured ribs overlying the liver injury. The fractures were new. There was also a cigarette burn on the foot. Facial bruising was present. The liver scans showed the injuries clearly (arrows). Examination of the anal area showed that she had a marked vulvitis with labial fusion. The labial fusion was divided in order to catheterize the child. The hymen looks swollen and relatively narrow given her age. The anal sphincter was lax with a halo of veins, prolapsing mucosa with deficits in the anal margin at 10, 1, 2, and 7 o'clock; there was also uniform reddening perianally. In the ano-genital area the physical signs would suggest penetrative abuse.

◀ 9.34

◀ 9.35

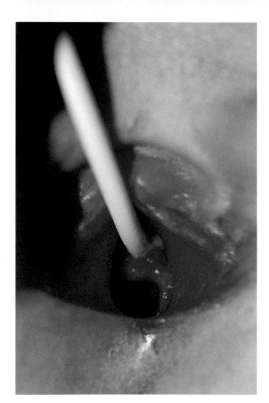

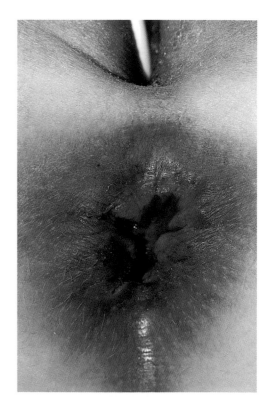

Chapter 10

Fatal Abuse

	Number	Offences per million children
Infants (under 1 year)	38	48
Toddlers (1 to 4)	25	8
Children (5 to 15)	40	5
Total Children (<16)	103	9

**The risk of death increases with diminishing age
UK Child Homicides in 1992**

Clinical presentation of fatal child abuse
1. Severely battered infant or child (head or abdominal injury).
2. Unexpected death where occult injury found.
3. Cot death presentation (death due to suffocation).
4. Neglect – child deliberately or passively left in dangerous situation, e.g. drowning, house fire.
5. Deliberate poisoning.
6. Recurrent unexplained deaths (factitious illness, Munchausen syndrome by proxy abuse).
7. Child death associated with sexual assault (always inspect genitalia and anus).
8. Suicide in older child.

Investigation of suspicious death
- Post-mortem examination should be performed by a pathologist who has training in both forensic and paediatric pathology.
- Post-mortem may show little in cases of suspected abuse in young children. In particular, smothering and drowning cannot always be excluded.
- Medical and social history plays a major role in the interpretation of the necropsy findings.
- Severe head trauma can occur without fractures or obvious impact injuries to head.
- The parents may cover up previous deaths (of siblings), injuries, abuse or admissions to care. There are links with factitious illness by proxy (Munchausen syndrome by proxy abuse).
- Current crises should be sought in the parents' personal lives.
- The need for toxicology or electrolyte samples to check for inappropriate drug or salt ingestion should be considered. Samples of vitreous humour, blood, urine, stomach contents and various tissues can be sent for analysis.
- Site of death examination may involve police, pathologist and forensic scientist.

- Post-mortem skeletal surveys may reveal occult bony injury but detailed histology/specimen X-rays is more sensitive in detecting trauma.
- A confidential professional inquiry to share information concerning a child's death may conclude that factors were present in the care of the child which contributed to the death of the child.

Such information may assist professional agencies in providing care to the family if a further child is born.

Clinical features suggesting suffocation
- Sudden and unexpected deaths in previous siblings.
- 'Near miss cot death' presentation.
- Petechiae on face or mouth, bruises to neck (minority). History of bleeding from nose or mouth.
- Survival with handicap a possibility.
- Recurring apnoeic attacks which failed to reveal a cause on extensive investigation.
- Mother (carer) present when child collapses.

Unexpected death where occult injury is found
'Unexpected deaths' can be defined as deaths occurring before arrival at the hospital or unrelated to any previously known congenital anomaly or medical condition.

Suspicious features include the following:
- Injury only discovered at autopsy.
- If the child demonstrated inflicted or unexplained trauma.
- If there had been inadequate supervision.
- If there was probable delay in seeking care.

Deaths following falls
- Children who fell 3 house storeys: all survived.
- Children who fell 5 house stories: 50% died.
- Children who fall downstairs, are dropped from parents arms, who roll off settees and coffee tables do not die.

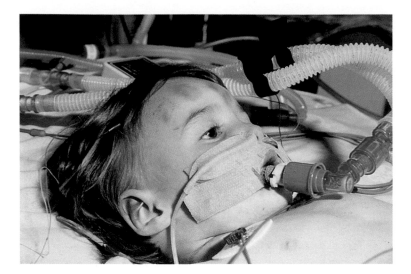

◀ **10.1–10.6 Male aged 2 years**

He was in pre-adoptive placement. Foster mother had problems coping with his feeding and he started to wet again. Photographs show extensive bruising of the forehead, right ear and extensive bruising on the buttocks (Figs 10.1, 10.2). This is where he had been 'smacked' for wetting himself earlier. Examination of the mouth showed bruising on the inner aspect of the upper lip and a torn frenulum (Fig. 10.3). He had extensive bruises around the knee and a bruise at the base of the penis and also distally (Fig. 10.4).Post-mortem examination showed the bleeding into the deep tissues of the buttocks (Fig. 10.5). He died of his head injury (Fig. 10.6).

▲ **10.2**

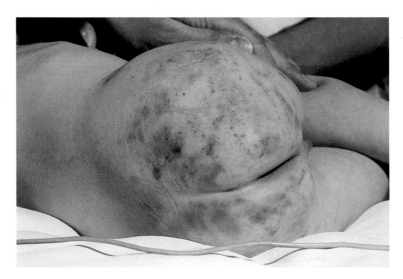

▲ **10.3**

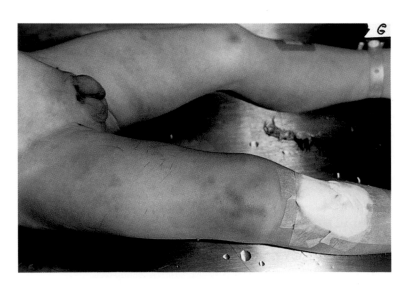

▲ **10.4**

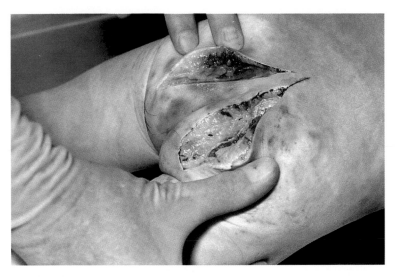

▲ 10.5

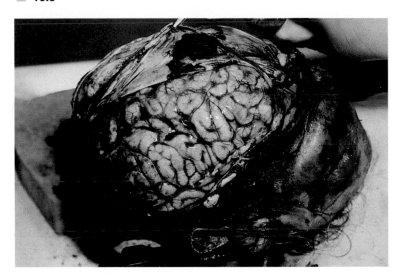

▲ 10.6

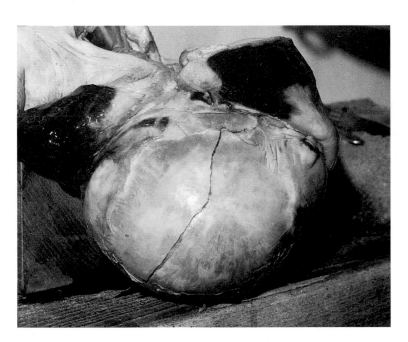

◀ **10.7 Female aged 3 months**
The child was brought to hospital having stopped breathing. The given history was that she had rolled off the settee. She was dead on arrival at hospital. The skeletal survey showed fractured ribs and a skull fracture. At post-mortem it was seen that the child had a long, wide, parietal fracture. Initially it was accepted that this was an accident but the mother later injured a child whilst babysitting and admitted to the murder of her baby.

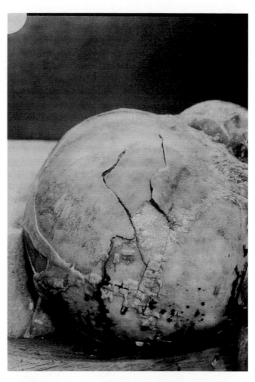

▶ **10.8 Male aged 6 months**

The child was brought to hospital after an emergency call. There was extensive bruising on the face (cheek and behind the ear), the front of the chest and around the knees, and subhyaloid haemorrhages. He had cerebral swelling and coning and died after 48 hours. There was a single old rib fracture, and multiple and complex skull fractures including a depressed fracture leading from the parietal into the occipital bone. The adoptive mother admitted to the murder of the baby.

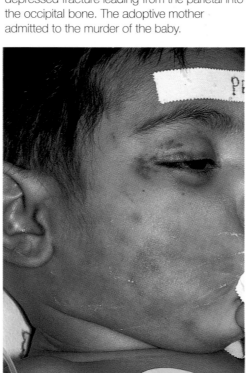

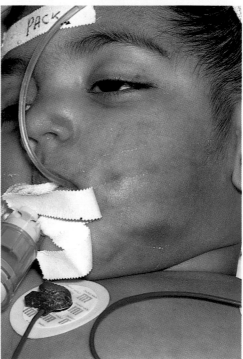

▲ **10.9–10.13 Female aged 6 months**

She was taken to the A&E Department after having a respiratory arrest at home. She had theoretically rolled off the bed (or settee). She was resuscitated and transferred to the intensive care unit where she was ventilated for several days but died. On examination she had bruising of both upper eyelids and bruises of the cheek. There was bruising of the lower left mandible. She had Mongolian blue spots on her back. Her genitalia and anus were examined because she had a green vaginal discharge; no pathogens were grown. She also had a congested anus and the post-mortem examination findings showed a dilated anus. She had an extensive occipital skull fracture which was clearly evident at autopsy (Fig. 10.12). CT scan shows marked cerebral oedema and the 'acute reversal sign'. No charges have been brought for these injuries.

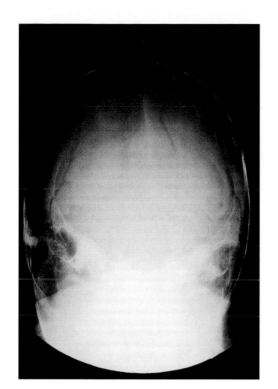

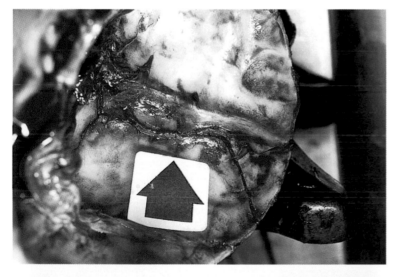

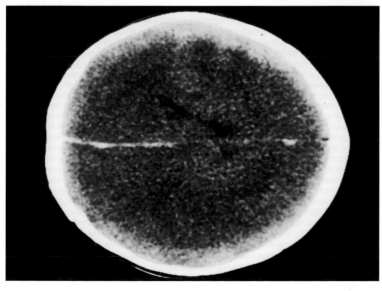

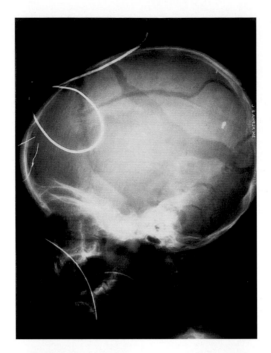

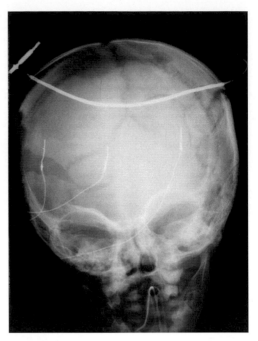

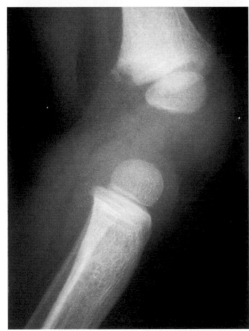

▲ **10.14,** ▲ **10.15,** ◀ **10.16**
Male aged 15 months

The child was admitted as an emergency to hospital. He was a thin, underweight child, failing to thrive. There were bilateral retinal haemorrhages, and 34 bruises over the face and body and a torn frenulum. A subdural haematoma was treated surgically. He had five skull fractures in the parietal bones and occiput. There was also a metaphyseal fracture at the lower end of the femur. The child died and the mother later admitted to his murder.

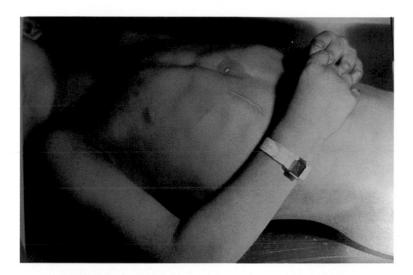

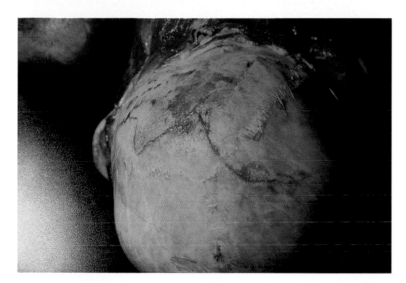

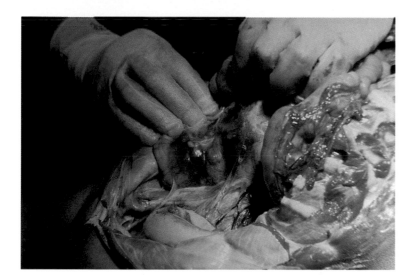

◁ **10.17,** ◁ **10.18,** ◁ **10.19**
Male aged 4 years
The child was brought to hospital dead. The history given was that he had slipped in the bath and banged his head. On examination he was thin and wasted and had unexplained marks on his body. At post-mortem he had a complex parieto-occipital fracture. He also had bleeding into the base of the mesentery. Ordinary falls such as falling in the bath do not cause complex skull fractures including the occiput. This child died of a massive head injury, and there were also signs of previous injury, including bilateral healing fractures of the distal part of the radius and ulna. He was also thin and wasted. A police prosecution for manslaughter was successful.

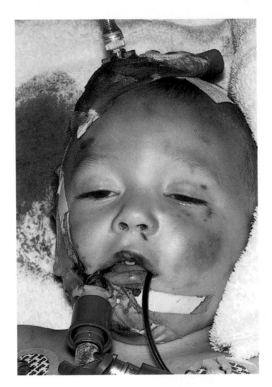
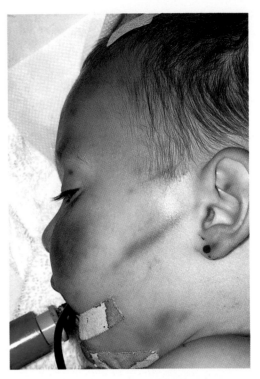
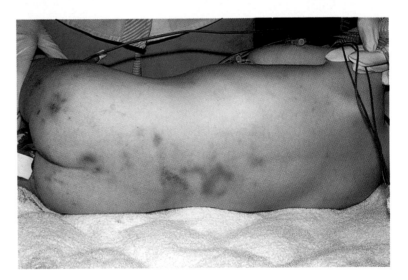

▲ **10.20,** ▲ **10.21,** ▲ **10.22 Male aged 2 years**
This child was brought to the hospital having been beaten up by his mother's partner. Examination showed extensive bruising to face, mouth, linear marks on side of face with bruised ear and bruising across the angle of the jaw. Extensive bruising on back including linear marks suggested he had been hit with an implement. There was also bruising of the penis.

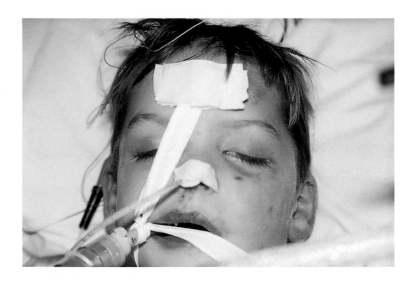

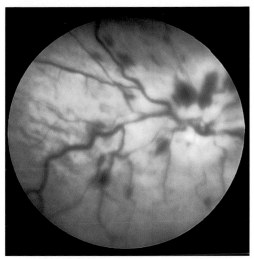

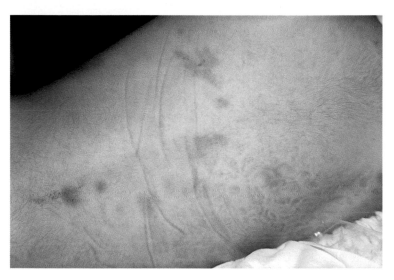

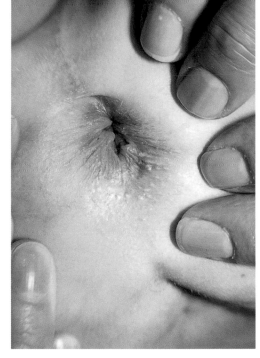

▲ **10.23,** ▲ **10.24,** ▲ **10.25,** ▶ **10.26 Male aged 4 years**
The child arrived at hospital after an emergency call but was dead on arrival. He was resuscitated but died several hours later. His injuries included facial bruising, bruising to the back, bilateral retinal haemorrhages and an abnormal anus. The CT scan showed gross cerebral oedema. The bruising on the back has the appearance of fingertip bruising. The anus showed some perianal reddening, a very irregular margin and dilated veins. This boy died of a shaking injury. The bruises on his back, retinal haemorrhages and cerebral oedema are consistent with this diagnosis. The anal changes and an acute anal fissure seen at post-mortem are consistent with recent anal penetration.

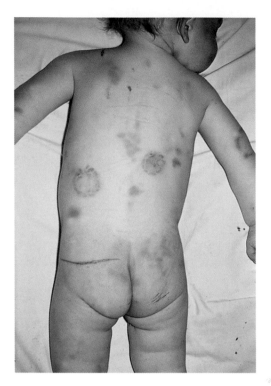

◀ **10.27 Female aged 18 months**
The child was brought into the hospital emergency department dead. Resuscitation was unsuccessful. Her body and limbs were covered in bites, bruises and lacerations. (This is an old photograph and signs of sexual abuse were not sought.) Post-mortem showed signs consistent with suffocation. (With permission of Dr MFG Buchanan).

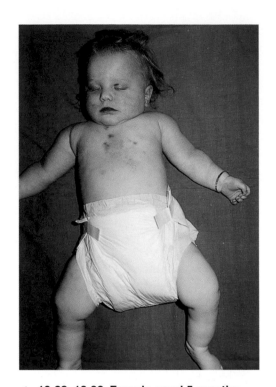

▲ **10.28–10.32 Female aged 5 months**
The child was brought in to the hospital emergency department dead. The photographs show new and old bruises around the face and trunk, including pinch marks on the front of the chest and a torn frenulum. A skeletal survey showed a fractured skull and fractured ribs. Post-mortem revealed she had died of a massive head injury. (Note: this infant had labial fusion (Fig. 10.31) which is not uncommon in infancy but is long and thick in this child.) The apparently abnormal anal findings (Fig. 10.32) are due to post-mortem changes. An older sibling had been sexually abused.

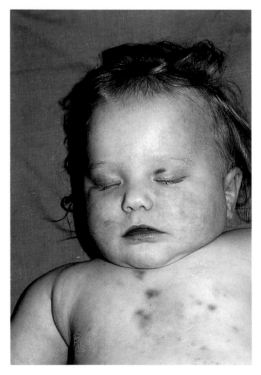

▲ **10.29**

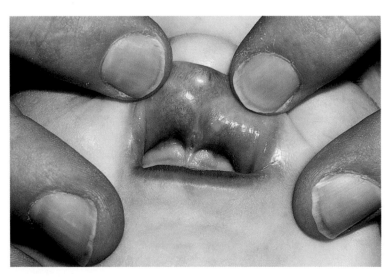

▲ **10.30**

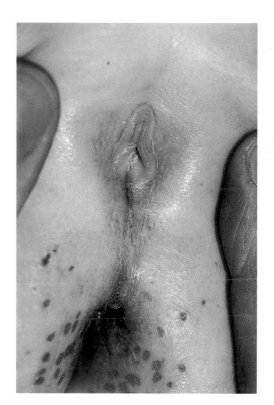

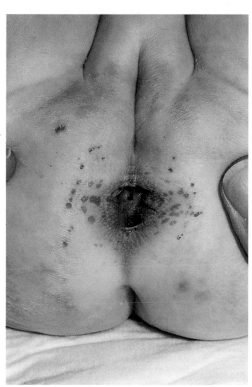

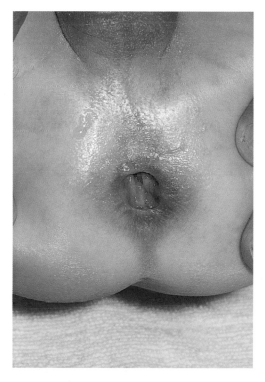

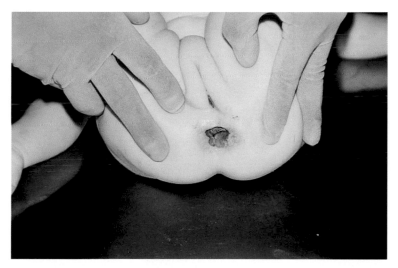

▲ **10.34 Female aged 3 months**
The child was brought into the hospital emergency department dead. The post-mortem suggested a diagnosis of sudden infant death syndrome but the pathologist was concerned about the anus. A further history was obtained from the parents who said that the baby had been constipated and they had used a spoon to remove faeces from the rectum. (With permission of Dr S. Siva.)

▲ **10.33 Male aged 8 months**
The child was brought into the hospital emergency department collapsed and was resuscitated, but died several days later of a massive head injury. The photograph shows a markedly dilated anus with some venous congestion. This slide was taken before death. The question of possible sexual abuse was raised but not investigated, and remains unanswered.

▶ **10.35 Female aged 2 years**

The child was admitted to hospital collapsed with a history that she had fallen across a loudspeaker. On examination there was bruising on the lower abdomen and at laparotomy a ruptured duodenum. This injury is caused by blunt force to the abdomen. The duodenum is vulnerable because it is located near the bony spinal column.

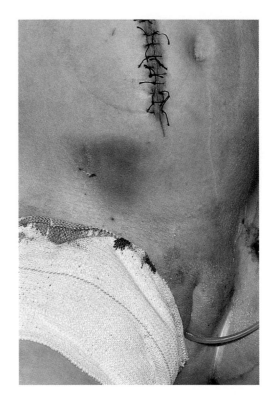

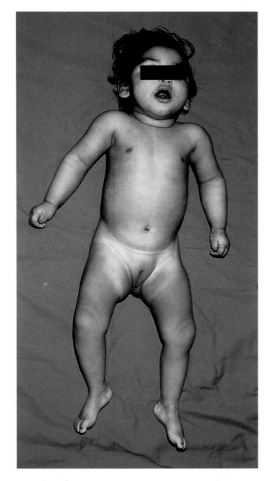

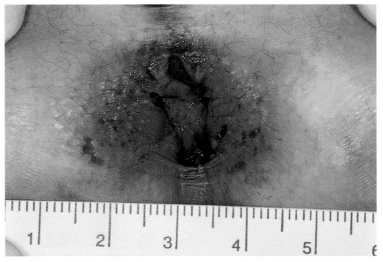

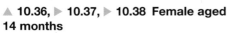

▲ **10.36,** ▶ **10.37,** ▶ **10.38 Female aged 14 months**

This child, with microcephaly and severe learning problems and failure to thrive, was brought to the hospital moribund. Dilated torn anus with bleeding and small skin excoriations. Mucosa prolapsing. Unexplained traumatic lesions on right foot. The cause of the death was recorded as pneumonia. The anal signs would be consistent with recent traumatic penetration. There was no history of bowel disease or treatment for constipation, etc. The lesions on the feet also remain unexplained.

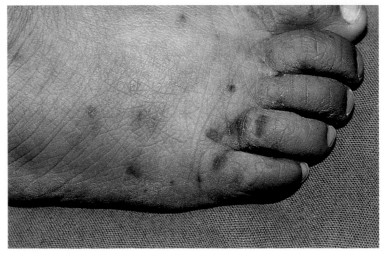

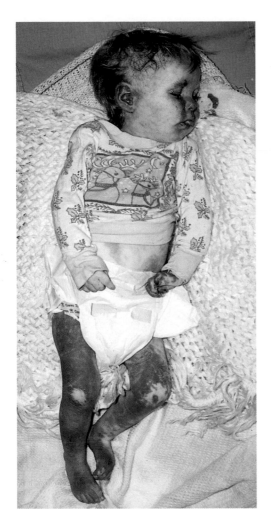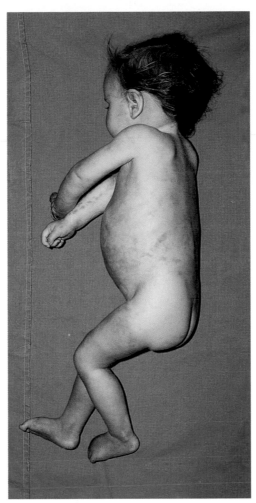

▲ 10.39, ▲ 10.40 Female aged 8 months

This emaciated child was brought to hospital by ambulance after the parents found her dead in her cot. Resuscitation was not possible. Her general skin care was poor. A growth chart showed that she had a birth weight just below the 50th centile and she continued to grow along the 50th centile until she was 3½ months when she fell to the 10th centile. However, by the time of death she weighed just over 5 kg, i.e. the weight she had been at 3 months. Her head circumference had fallen from the 90th centile to the 10th centile. She was the third child in a family that had moved to Leeds from elsewhere. There were multiple social problems. The family were not under the care of a health visitor or general practitioner for the last two months of the child's life. The pathologist commented that the signs of the chest infection were not enough to account for her death.

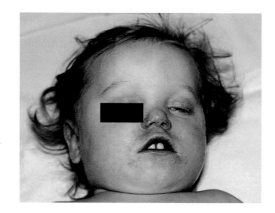

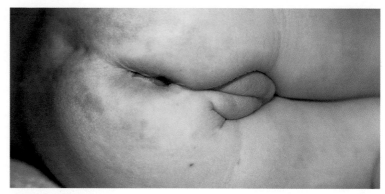

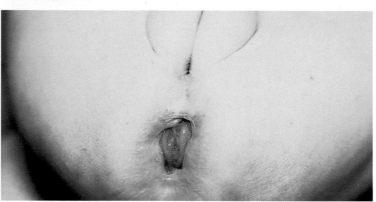

▲ 10.41, ▶ 10.42, ▶ 10.43, ▼ 10.44
Female aged 14 months

The child began to fail to thrive from around 1 year. She was brought into hospital dead. The history given was that she slipped in the bath and drowned. Her hair was dry on admission to hospital and she was very cold. She had bruising round the mouth, several fingertip bruises round the knees and a grossly gaping dilated anus (Figs 10.41, 10.42 and 10.43). A skeletal survey showed an old healing mid-shaft fracture of femur (which had never been presented clinically).

The growth chart (Fig. 10.44) showed failure to thrive. Her 2-year-old sister had had a recent burn on the back of her hand and following the death of their sister this child and the 5-year-old brother both disclosed sexual abuse. The post-mortem findings were consistent with suffocation but not drowning. The interpretation of the anal signs is difficult but in view of the history of penetrative sexual abuse involving the older siblings abuse has to be considered.

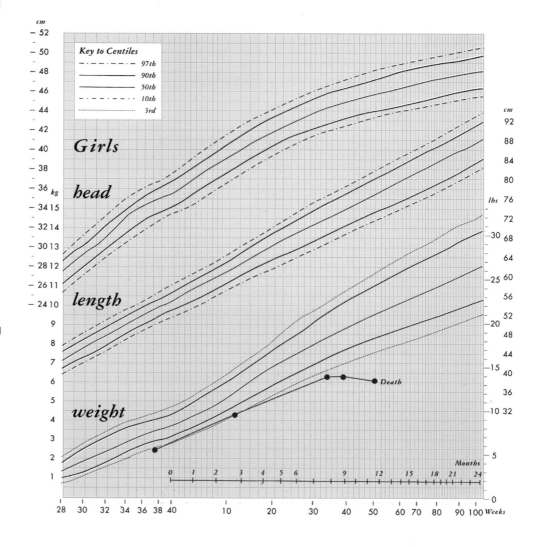

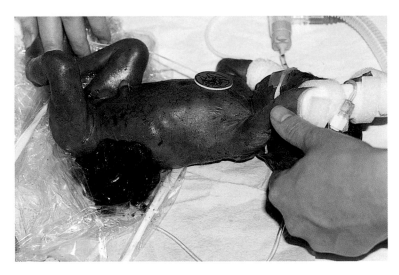

▲ **10.45 Extremely pre-term infant**
The baby was born by Caesarean section after the mother was admitted to hospital having been stabbed in the abdomen. The baby's abdomen was perforated and the guts eviscerated. The baby died some days later. This is a form of pre-natal child abuse. (With permission of Dr K. Brownlee.)

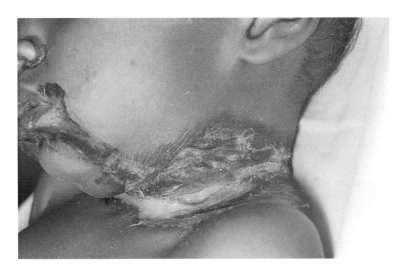

▲ **10.46 Male aged 2 years**
The child was brought to hospital collapsed. On examination there were deep full skin thickness burns from the side of the mouth round the neck. This child had been given a corrosive substance to drink and died of the injuries.

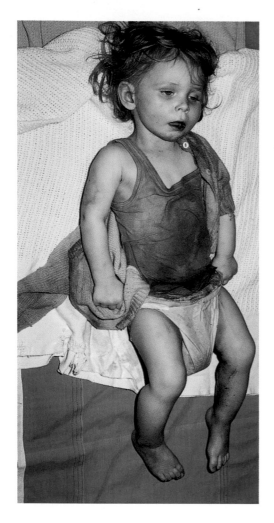

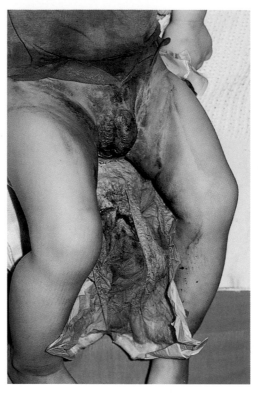

◀ 10.47, ▲ 10.48 Male aged 18 months
The child was brought into hospital dead following an emergency call. The child was of normal nutrition but was very cold, wet and the nappy contained the equivalent of 4 days of normal stool. The nappy area showed evidence of post-mortem gangrene. The mother was a drug addict and the baby had been last seen alive 4–5 days earlier.

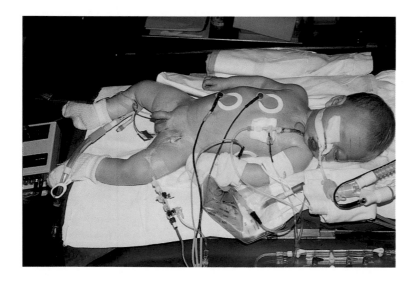

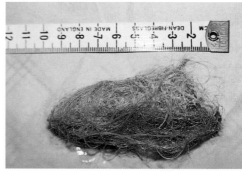

◀ 10.49, ▲ 10.50 Male aged 6 months
The child was brought into the hospital emergency department dead. He was resuscitated but died several hours later of anoxic brain damage. A ball of nylon fibres was retrieved from the posterior nasal space (Fig. 10.50). The fibres were thought to have come from a toy. This was treated as an accidental death.

Chapter 11

Fractures

◆ These serious injuries result from the more extreme forms of violence.

◆ They may coexist with other injuries, e.g. bruises, scratches, or internal, e.g. subdural haematoma, retinal haemorrhage or ruptured gut, or be an isolated injury.

◆ They may occur with or without associated bruising at the fracture site.

◆ They may occur in any bone, single or multiple, clinically obvious or occult (detected only on radiography).

The younger the child the greater the likelihood that a fracture has occurred abusively e.g. 39% of all fractures in infants less than 12 months of age were abuse (Leventhal JM et al, 1993).

History

◆ In infants and toddlers in falls from up to 3–4 feet the chance of fracture is low at 1–2% or less.

◆ About half are uncomplicated single linear fractures of the skull.

◆ Falls downstairs: less than 10% with a fracture, limb distal, femoral fractures very unusual.

Does the type of injury observed and the proposed mechanism fit with the known mechanisms required for its production?
Presentation
Accident

◆ History of injury given.

◆ Prompt presentation for treatment.

◆ Immediate pain, loss of function and swelling.

Abuse

◆ History vague, inconsistent or absent.

◆ Medical attention sought for swelling, loss of function often after a period of time.

◆ Pain may be minimized or ignored.

◆ Fracture may be unexpected or discovered incidentally or on skeletal survey.

Specificity of fracture types of abuse (Klehman PK, 1998)
High
1. metaphyseal lesions;
2. posterior rib fractures;
3. scapular and sternal fractures;
4. spinous process fractures.
Moderate
1. multiple fractures, especially bilateral;
2. fractures of different ages;

3. epiphyseal separations;
4. vertebral body fractures and subluxations;
5. digital fractures;
6. complex skull fracture.
Low
1. linear parietal skull;
2. shafts of long bones;
3. clavicle.

NB most abusive fractures are of low specificity. Diagnosis is made by comparing the history to the injury.

Simple mechanics of fractures
◆ Transverse – angulation, e.g. following a direct blow.

◆ Oblique transverse – angulation (or bending) with axial loading (or compression).

◆ Spiral – axial twists with or without axial loading.

◆ Oblique – angulation and axial twisting in the presence of axial loading.

When to do a skeletal survey
◆ Presentation with a fracture which suggests abuse.

◆ Physically abused child under 2 years of age (abusive fractures are uncommon after this age).

◆ Older child with severe soft tissue injury.

◆ Localized pain, limp or reluctance to use a limb.

◆ Previous history of recent skeletal injury.

◆ Unexplained neurological symptoms or signs.

◆ Child dying in suspicious or unusual circumstances.

Ageing fractures
◆ A fracture without periosteal new bone formation is usually less than 7–10 days old and seldom as much as 20 days old.

◆ A fracture with definite but slight periosteal new bone formation could be as recent as 4–7 days old.

◆ A 20-day-old fracture will always have well-developed periosteal reaction and typically soft callus.

◆ A fracture with well-developed periosteal new bone formation or callus is more than 14 days old.

References
Klehman PK Diagnostic Imaging of Child Abuse 1998 London: Mosby

Differential diagnosis of skeletal disorder

Condition	Features	Radiology	Investigations
Normal variant pseudofracture	e.g. aberrant skull suture symmetrical periosteal reaction minor abnormality	Often symmetrical identical to changes of trauma	Consult specialist, large textbook
Birth trauma	Clavicle, humerus, femur, rib, depressed skull, etc.	Absence of callus after 2 weeks = not birth trauma	Check history at birth
Osteogenesis imperfecta Heterogeneous rare condition Types I–IV	Fractures with minimal trauma, blue sclerae, deafness, family history, wormian bones, dental changes, easy bruising, growth retardation, scoliosis	Osteopenia, thin cortices, angulation and bowing of fractures	Diagnosis on clinical and radiological features. No laboratory test available
Osteoporosis	Heparin, disuse, e.g. cerebral palsy, osteogenesis, copper deficiency	Poor mineralization	History, clinical and radiological diagnosis identified cause
Copper deficiency	Rare, temporary. Features: sideroblastic anaemia, neutropenia, hypotonia. Occurs in preterm, low birth weight, fed by TPN	Osteoporosis, cup-shaped and frayed metaphysis, sickle-shaped spurs, symmetrical, fractures	80–90% Hb < 10.0 g/dl. neutropenia <1.0 × 10^9/l plasma copper <40 µg/dl caeruloplasmin <13 mg/dl
Osteomyelitis congenital syphilis	Systemic signs and symptoms variable in early infancy. Local signs may predominate	Multifocal metaphyseal lesions, periosteal reaction, no corner fractures, bone destruction	Blood cultures, aspirates positive for *Staph. aureus*, coliforms, group B strep. Meningococcus syphilis serology positive mother and baby
Caffey's disease	Rare disease of infants painful periosteal thickening in multiple bones	Any bones, especially mandible, clavicle and ulna. No fractures or metaphyseal irregularity	Clinical diagnosis course of disease
Rickets	Premature infant, TPN confusion after discharge from neonatal unit. Older child–fractures unusual	Cupping, fraying costochondral junctions and metaphyses. Decreased bone density, Looser's zones	Low serum calcium, low or normal phosphate, raised alkaline phosphatase. Low 25-hydroxyvitamin D
Scurvy, vitamin A intoxication	Rare, related to bizarre feeding practice	Periosteal and metaphyseal changes	Vitamin A or C levels in blood

(With permission from Hobbs CT. Child Abuse. In: Addy D.P. Investigation in Paediatrics. London: WB Saunders.)

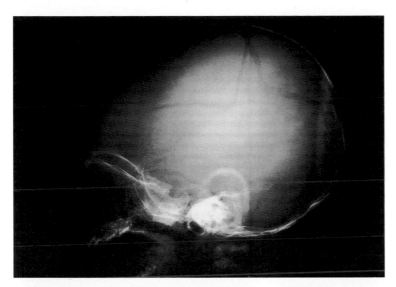

◁ **11.1 Male aged 4 months**
The child was brought to the hospital following a 'fall from father's arms'. A skeletal survey showed bilateral parietal skull fractures. The fractures were wide. The history given was not compatible with the injury found, i.e. there are two fractures implying there must have been two impact injuries. The only exception would be a fall from around 2 metres on to the vertex. Bilateral parietal fractures may result from a fall of more than 2 metres but the fractures are narrow and symmetrical, not as shown here. This case suggests two impact injuries.

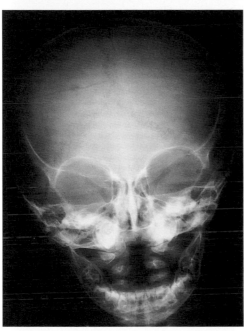

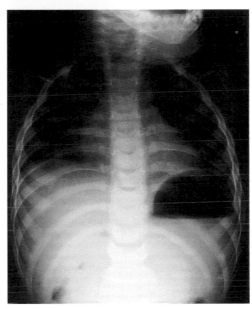

◁ **11.2,** ◁ **11.3 Female aged 9 months**
This infant presented following a fall from a settee. Investigations showed a narrow parietal fracture but also fractured ribs. The rib fractures show early signs of healing, i.e. callus formation. A parietal fracture is the commonest skull fracture seen in child abuse. It is very unlikely that this fracture was caused by the child rolling off a settee, i.e. 1–2 feet, onto a carpeted floor.

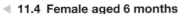

◁ **11.4 Female aged 6 months**
An infant was said to have been dropped onto a concrete floor in a DIY warehouse. An extensive haematoma formed across the child's head. X-ray showed a long fracture which was continuous and which extended into both parietal bones. There was a depression of one limb of the fracture. There were no other injuries, including brain injury. The injury was thought to be accidental.

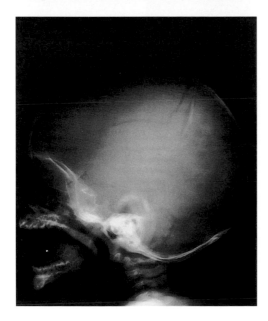

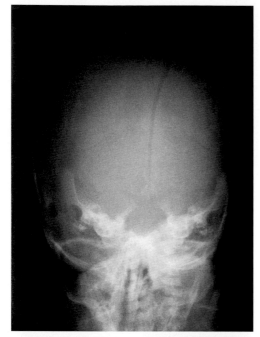

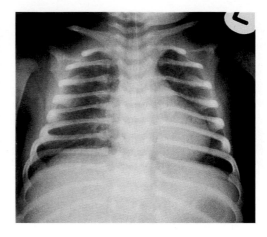

◀ 11.5, ▲ 11.6 Infant aged 6 weeks

An infant presented with a respiratory arrest at the local hospital. Investigation showed an extensive linear fracture across the occipital bone. Skeletal survey showed fractured ribs. This was severe physical abuse.

◀ 11.7 Female aged 3 months

She was brought by her parents to the hospital emergency department with a serious head injury. The radiograph shows a healing fracture of the left clavicle with well-developed callus. There is a possible fracture of the posterior end of the 5th and 6th ribs on the left side. The opinion of a paediatric radiologist is essential in assessing cases such as this. The question of possible birth injury will be raised concerning the clavicle, but the additional skull fractures and head injury made the diagnosis of non-accidental injury a clear one (see Fig. 11.8). The child survived the injuries and at the age of 10 years has a moderate learning difficulty, a mild right hemiparesis but good vision in spite of occipital contusion.

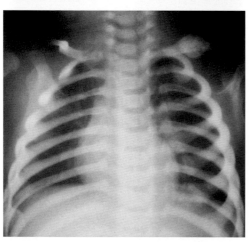

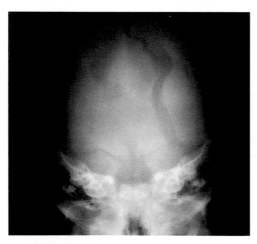

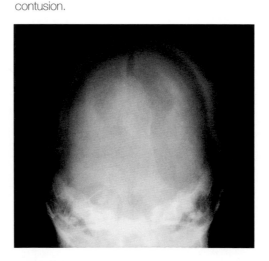

▲ 11.8 Female aged 3 months

The same child as in Fig. 11.7. This radiograph shows an extensive occipital fracture, measuring up to 0.5 cm in width.

▲ 11.9 Female aged 3 months

The same child as in Figs 11.7 and 11.8. This is a follow-up skull X-ray 2 weeks later showing that the occipital fracture has now grown in width, i.e. this is an example of a growing skull fracture in infancy.

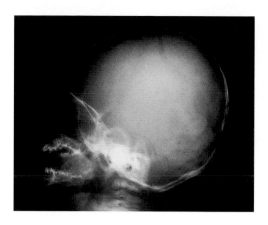

▲ **11.10 Male aged 2 months**
His mother, while suffering from severe post-natal depression, threw him on the floor, hitting his head on a stone fireplace. A long wide linear parietal fracture can be seen extending into the occiput. This was a severe intra-cranial injury from which the child died.

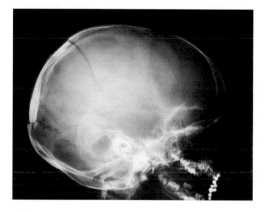

▲ **11.12 Female aged 18 months**
The same child as in Fig. 11.11, showing the occipital fracture clearly. Depressed occipital fracture in infancy is virtually pathognomonic of abuse.

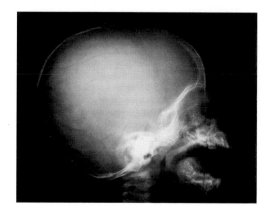

◄ **11.14 Female aged 8 months**
She had tipped herself up attempting to go downstairs in a baby walker. Long linear parietal fracture is seen, with maximum width of 2 mm. There is no intra-cranial injury. This was accepted as an accidental fall.

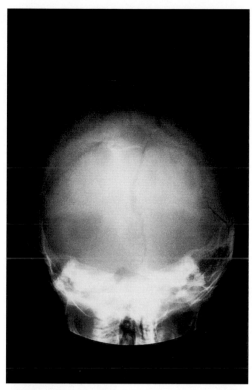

◄ **11.11 Female aged 18 months**
She was taken to the hospital emergency department by her parents who said the child had fallen off a chair. Multiple bruises on the buttocks and back were seen, as well as a right parietal/occipital fracture with a large depressed segment of the skull. The child had a persistent right hemiparesis.

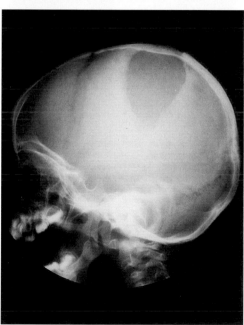

◄ **11.13 Male aged 18 months**
He was referred to neurosurgeons with a large fluctuant swelling over the left parietal region and minimal weakness in the right arm. At the age of 7 months he had been dropped down the stairs by his sister, and was seen in the hospital emergency department with a 4 mm wide linear parietal fracture. Surgical repair was required at 18 months. (Note: this is an unsatisfactory history, i.e. at presentation the infant had a wide fracture implying that considerable force had been applied to the skull. Fuller investigation at the time of initial presentation was needed.)

▶ 11.15 Male aged 10 months

He had a history of being dropped onto the corner of a central heating radiator. There is a localized depressed fracture of the parietal bone, with no intra-cerebral injury. This was accepted as an accidental injury.

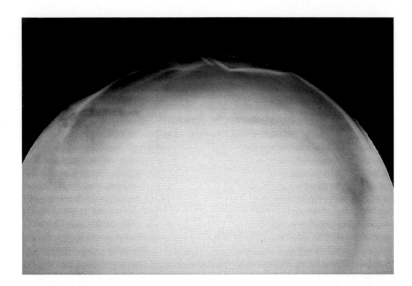

▶ 11.16 Female aged 19 months

She received a significant head injury aged 4 months when the wind blew her pram over a ledge and she fell 5 feet (1.5 m) onto concrete. She initially showed localized neurological signs with focal fits. The child was followed up and the computed tomography (CT) brain scan at 19 months shows a 1.5 cm × 8 cm deficit in the skull. At operation the dura was adherent to the pericranium at the skull edge. The brain was gliotic, the arachnoid herniating and pulsating and probably connected to the lateral ventricle. A repair was undertaken but the child has continued to have convulsions.

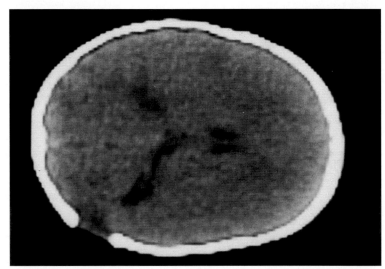

▶ 11.17 Female aged 6 weeks

Her grandfather was said to have dropped her onto a linoleum-covered floor while he was feeding her. Bilateral linear parietal fractures are evident up to 2.5 mm in width.
(Note: non-accidental injury was not suspected at the time of presentation, but at 16 months the child sustained 6% scalds to the neck, chest and upper arm from spilt tea, and at 2½ years was hit across the buttocks and back resulting in severe non-accidental bruising.)

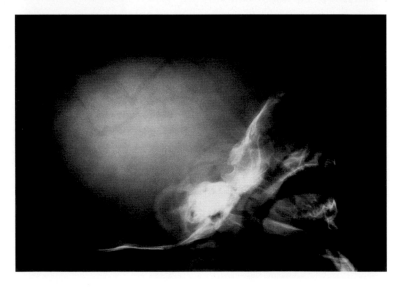

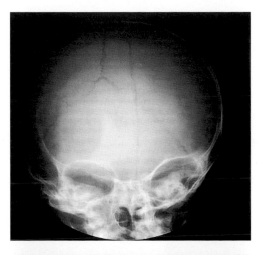

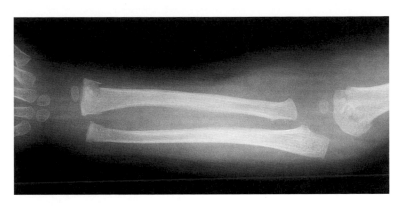

◄ 11.18, ▲ 11.19, ◄ 11.20 Female aged 14 months

She was left unsupervised and fell through a gap in a broken banister from the first floor landing to the floor below. The distance of the fall was estimated to be 10–12 feet (3–3.5 m). There was bruising to the forehead and a linear frontal fracture. The skull X-ray shows a long, narrow, mid-line frontal fracture (Fig. 11.18). The X-ray of the right forearm (Fig. 11.19) shows a fracture of the distal end of the radius and also an epiphyseal fracture of the humerus. Bruising of the upper eyelid (Battle's sign) is seen in Fig. 11.20. This was a preventable accident, due to neglect.

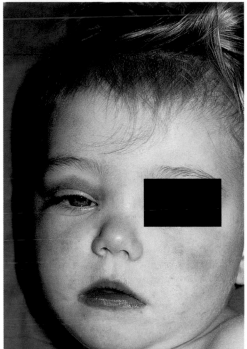

◄ 11.21 Male aged 19 months

He fell 13–14 feet (approx. 4 m) from a first floor window onto the garden below. He was taken straight to hospital where he was found to be drowsy and bleeding from the ear. The radiograph shows a linear parietal/temporal fracture involving the base of the skull, 2 mm maximum width × 9 cm in length. The child spent 3 days in hospital and made a full recovery. (Note: children falling from one or two stories frequently escape major injury: at four to five stories there is a real threat to life.)

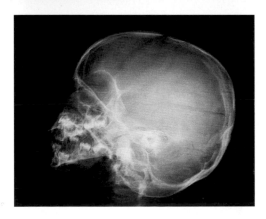

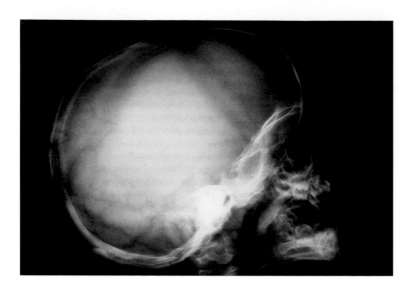

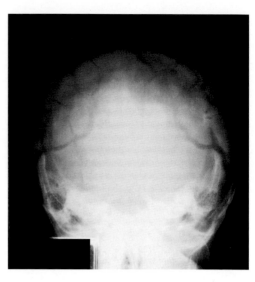

▲ 11.22, ▲ 11.23 Male aged 11 months

He was taken to the hospital emergency department where it was claimed he had fallen from a settee. The skull X-rays show multiple, convoluted crazy-paving fractures of the parietal and occipital bones with a parietal fracture measuring 11.5 cm long and 0.8 cm wide. The injury was complicated by intra-cerebral haemorrhage resulting in hydrocephalus and 6th nerve palsy. The child's father admitted to causing the injury.

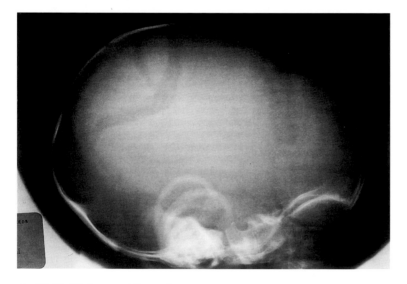

▲ 11.24 Male aged 6 weeks

It was claimed that he had fallen from a bed onto the floor. The radiograph shows two parietal fractures towards the vertex, 4 cm and 3.5 cm long with a maximum separation of 0.4 cm. The CT brain scan showed cerebral contusion to the left parieto-occipital areas. A skeletal survey showed fractured ribs and ulnar fracture – the father admitted to injuring the baby.

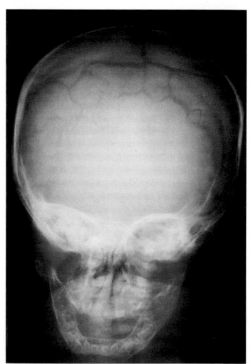

▲ 11.25, ▶ 11.26 Female aged 5 months

She was brought by her parents to the hospital emergency department having died. The skull X-rays show multiple, bilateral skull fractures with crazy-paving appearance (parietal bones). In addition to the fatal head injury she had a torn frenulum and multiple bruises over her body. In addition there was gross abnormality of the anus consistent with anal abuse.

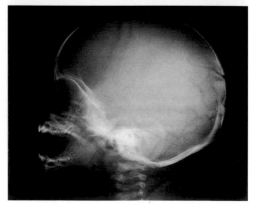

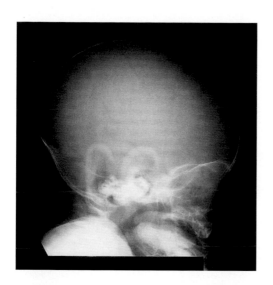

11.27 Male aged 4 weeks

His mother was feeding him when an angry male neighbour ran into the house to assault her but hit the baby instead. A long parietal fracture is seen extending the width of the parietal bone. There is a smaller parallel parietal fracture at the vertex. The infant was unwell with focal fits but subsequently made a good recovery.

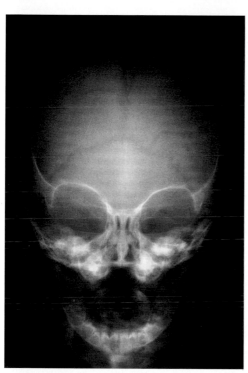

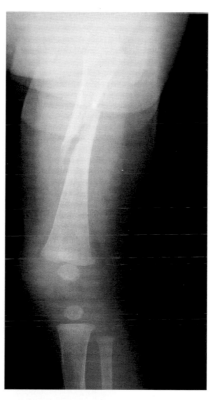

11.28, 11.29 Female aged 6 months

She was brought to the hospital emergency department with multiple unexplained injuries. The skull X-ray (Fig. 11.28) shows bilateral linear parietal fractures, and the sutures may be slightly widened. Other injuries included a rib fracture and a long bone fracture (Fig. 11.29). The pattern of injuries is typical of severe physical abuse in infancy.

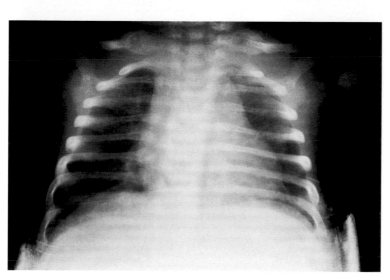

11.30 Female aged 8 months

This infant was admitted to hospital and found incidentally to have healing fractures of both clavicles.

▶ **11.31 Male aged 3 months**

It is not acceptable practice to ask the radiographer to do a 'babygram'. This inevitably leads to the need for re-X-raying as the radiographs are not adequate. This X-ray shows healing bilateral fractures of the ribs and a recent spiral fracture of the right humerus.

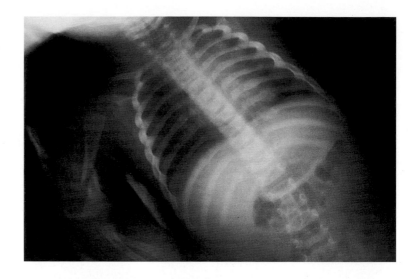

▶ **11.32,** ▶ **11.33**
Male aged 5 months

This infant was admitted with a chest infection. Follow-up chest X-ray to check progress of the pneumonia showed bilateral healing rib fractures. Rib fractures are not caused by physiotherapists!

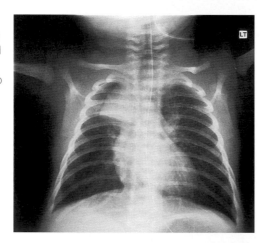
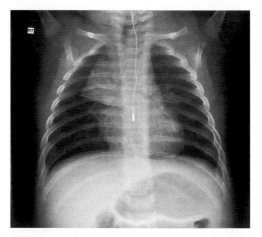

▶ **11.34 Male aged 3 days**

Newborn infant with fractures of the right 6th and 7th rib. This appears to have been a birth injury. This is very rare for a term infant. (Figure provided by Dr Margaret Crawford.) Note: birth injuries (fractures) are uncommon. Clavicle fracture is the most common site. Of the long bone fractures, the humerus is the most likely injury; femoral fractures are seen occasionally. Fractures seen in abuse are usually posterior.

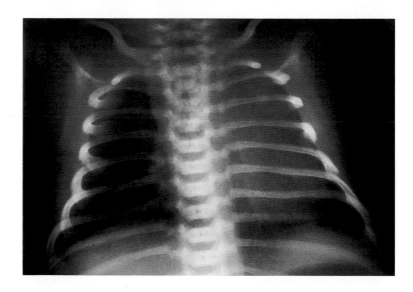

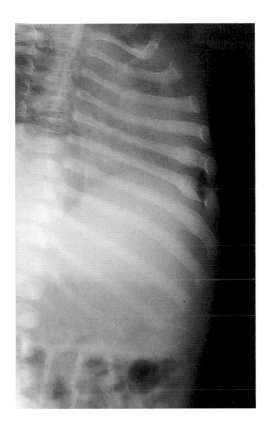

11.35 Female aged 3 months

She was brought by her parents to the hospital emergency department with a serious head injury. The radiograph shows healing fractures of the 5th, 6th and 7th ribs, with wel-developed callus so that the fracture line is not visible. This is a typical shaking/crush injury – injuries of this order are only seen in serious non-accidental injury and crush injuries such as in road traffic accidents.

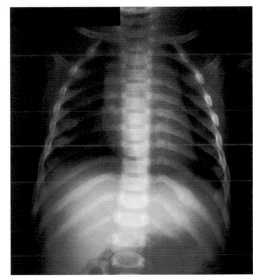

11.36 Male aged 4 months

He presented as a battered baby, with multiple rib fractures. Note the recent fracture of the right 5th rib with the fracture line visible and healing fractures of the left 10th and 11th ribs with marked callus formation and the fracture line just visible.

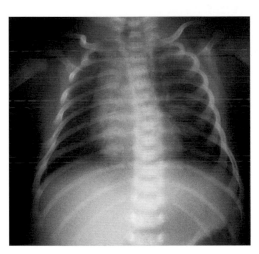

▲ 11.37 Male aged 4 months

He presented with bilateral rib fractures of the left 6th and 7th and the right 7th, 8th and 9th ribs.

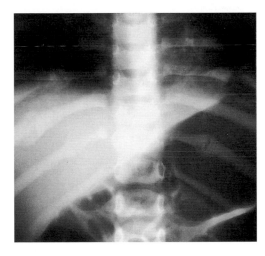

▲ 11.38 Male aged 18 months

The health visitor referred the child to hospital after she had seen him with an untreated scald on the forehead when visiting at home. When examined the child also had multiple bruises of different ages and therefore a skeletal survey was performed. The chest X-ray shows bilateral rib fractures. The clinical picture is one of clear non-accidental injury.

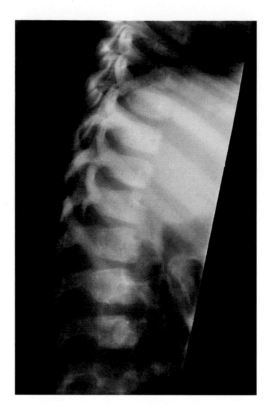
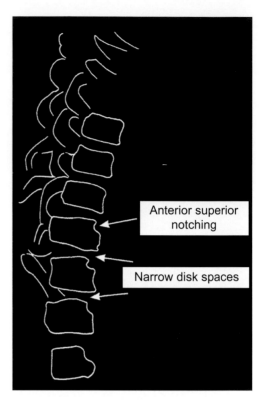

Anterior superior notching

Narrow disk spaces

▲ **11.39,** ▲ **11.40 Female aged 6 years**
She was taken to see her doctor because of abdominal pain and was referred to hospital for investigation. The clinical picture was one of chronic pancreatitis. Further examination showed evidence of bony injury with an old fracture of the humerus and characteristic notching of the anterior/superior surface of the vertebral bodies and narrowed disc spaces, the result of a spinal injury. (Reproduced with permission from Meadow S.R. (ed.) (1989) *ABC of Child Abuse*, British Medical Journal, London.)

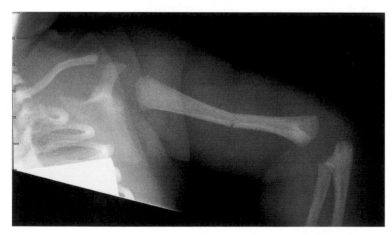

▲ **11.41 Male aged 4 months**
Infant with transverse fracture to left humerus. It is likely to have been caused by a horizontal blow.

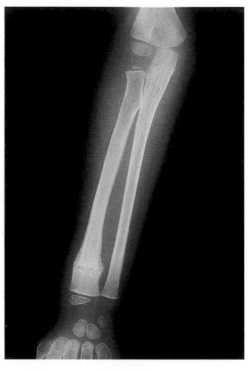

▲ **11.42 Male aged 4 years**
This child has a healing right radial fracture. The history given was that he had been hit with a bone cane across the lower arm.

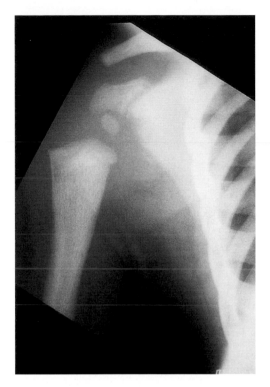

▲ **11.43 Male aged 6 months**
Young child with fracture of scapula. This particular fracture is highly specific for child abuse.

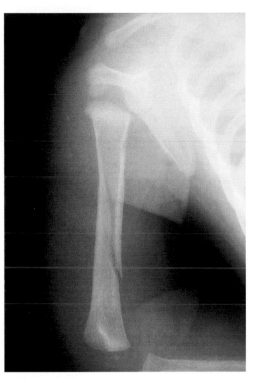

▲ **11.44 Female aged 3 months**
Extensive spiral fracture of right humerus. Fractures of the humerus and femur in infancy are highly correlated with abuse.

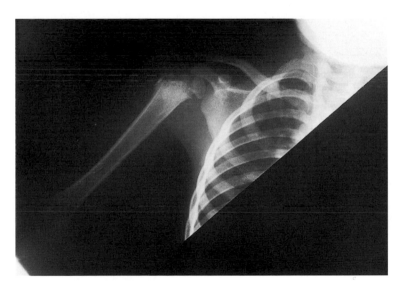

▲ **11.45 Male aged 4 years**
This foster child had multiple injuries, including this old bony injury to the right shoulder.

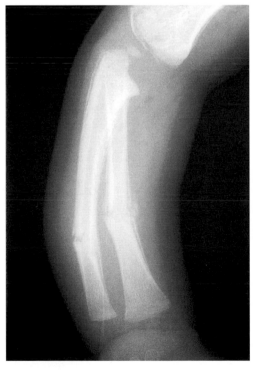

▲ **11.46 Female aged 2 years**
Horizontal fracture to radius and ulna and marked periosteal reaction extending round to the humerus. These injuries were unexplained.

▶ **11.47 Male aged 11 months**
Metaphyseal fracture of the lower end of the right humerus. The fracture is seen in the A-P and lateral views. These fractures are highly indicative of abuse in the absence of severe bony disease.

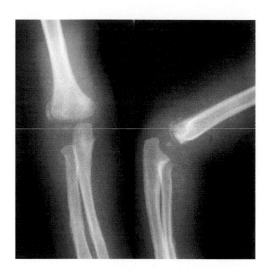

▶ **11.48 Male aged 2 months**
Stages of healing in the humeral fracture in an infant. Spiral fractures are highly correlated with physical abuse in infancy

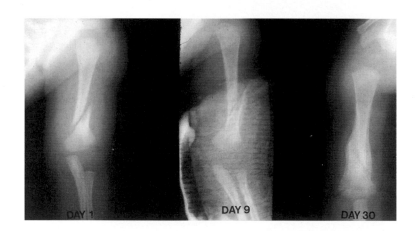

▶ **11.49 Female aged 5 months**
Her parents took her to the hospital emergency department as she was not moving her left arm. A recent fracture of the left humerus and healing fractures of the radius and ulna can be seen. (Note: although spiral fractures of the humerus are the more usual fractures in non-accidental injury transverse fractures may also be seen.)

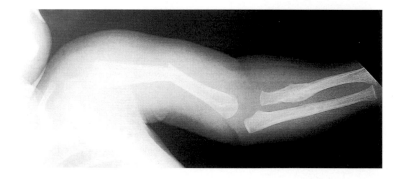

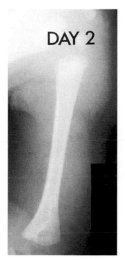

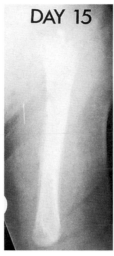

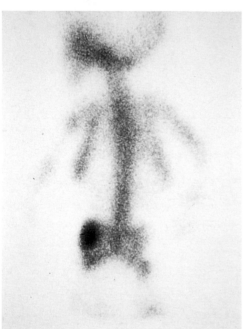

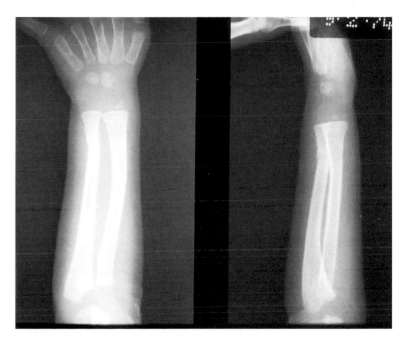

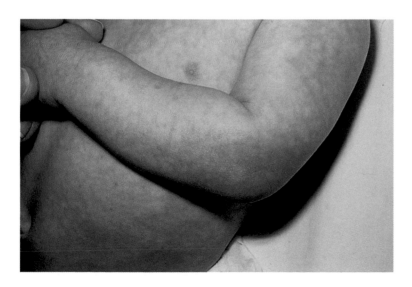

◀ **11.50,** ◀ **11.51 Male aged 3 months**

He presented in the hospital emergency department with his parents who said he would not move his left arm and seemed to have pain on movement. The initial X-ray showed no abnormality but by Day 15 a clear periosteal reaction can be seen. A radioisotope bone scan (Fig. 11.51) was done on Day 3 which showed increased uptake of ^{99m}Tc. The injury was due to the arm being twisted, causing damage to the periosteum.

▲ **11.52 Male aged 3 years**

His history was of tripping and falling onto his outstretched arm. The X-ray shows a greenstick fracture of the ulna. This was an accidental injury.

◀ **11.53 Male aged 3 months**

He was taken to the hospital emergency department because of a red, painful arm. The photograph shows a reddened painful swollen elbow; the child resisted movement. The diagnosis was of a pulled elbow. The child was subsequently seriously physically abused (skull fractures and bruised face).

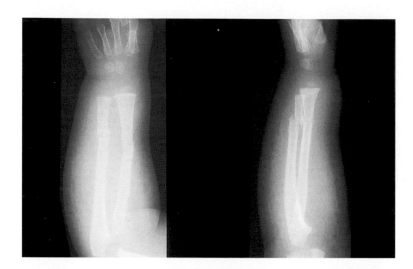

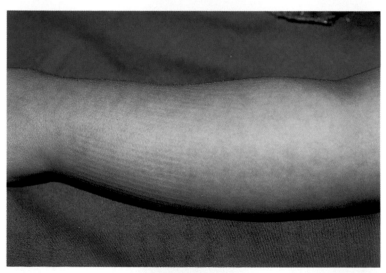

◀ **11.54,** ◀ **11.55 Male aged 14 months**
His mother took him to the hospital emergency department 3 days after he had received contact burns to the abdomen. On examination he also had multiple bruising to the face, body and legs and bilaterally swollen forearms which were non-tender. He also had penile abrasions. He was failing to thrive. The X-ray shows fractures of both forearms with some healing reaction; possibly fractures have occurred at different times and healing has started. Swelling of the forearm is evident in Fig. 11.55. The diagnosis is a multiply injured emotionally abused child who is failing to thrive.

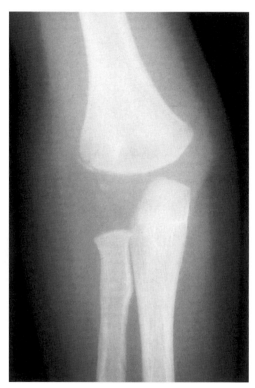

▲ **11.56 Male aged 2 years**
He was taken to the hospital emergency department by his parents when he 'wouldn't stand up'. A metaphyseal fracture of the lower end of the humerus is seen on the radiograph. There was also a spiral fracture of the tibia. The usual mechanism for these fractures is rotation or wrenching. These two unexplained fractures were due to non-accidental injury.

▶ **11.57 Male aged 2 years**
He was taken to the hospital emergency department by his mother because he was not using his arm. Bruises were seen on his ear, face and trunk. The X-ray shows a metaphyseal fracture (bucket-handle type). This was diagnosed as a non-accidental injury. This type of fracture is thought to be almost pathognomonic of abuse. The child had also been sexually abused.

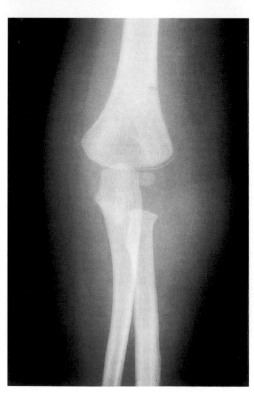

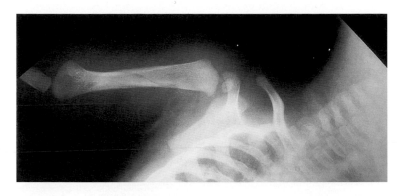

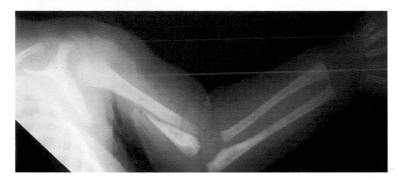

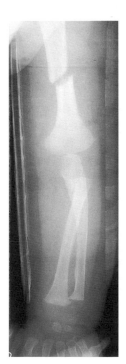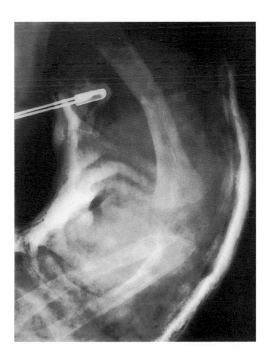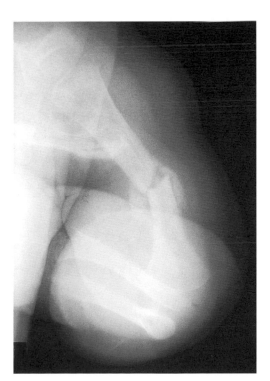

◀ 11.58 Female aged 4 months

She was taken to the hospital emergency department by her father because she seemed to be in distress when her arm was moved. He gave a history that the previous day he had been bathing her when she slipped and he grabbed her by the arm. The radiograph shows a spiral fracture of the right humerus. There were also healing fractures of the right 5th rib. Spiral fractures of the humerus are highly correlated with physical abuse. The combination of a spiral fracture of the humerus and rib fractures is physical abuse. (Note: originally the child was sent away from hospital until the radiologist noted the rib fractures, which were beginning to heal.)

▲ 11.59 Female aged 6 weeks

Her mother claimed she felt her arm 'give way' when she put it through the sleeve of a babygrow. A spiral displaced fracture of left humerus is evident. Skeletal survey showed that the baby also had a linear parietal fracture which was unexplained. The diagnosis is non-accidental injury.

▲ 11.60, ▲ 11.61, ▲ 11.62 Male aged 5 months

He was taken to the hospital emergency department, 2 days after having been picked up from his cot by his father in the middle of the night. The father complained that the child disliked his arm being moved. The X-ray (Fig. 11.60) shows a transverse fracture of the left humerus with displacement (Day 2). The X-ray taken on Day 11 shows early healing (Fig. 11.61). Figure 11.62 taken on Day 23 shows marked callus formation. The child also had a fractured left clavicle. The father later admitted to having performed a karate chop on the child's arm.

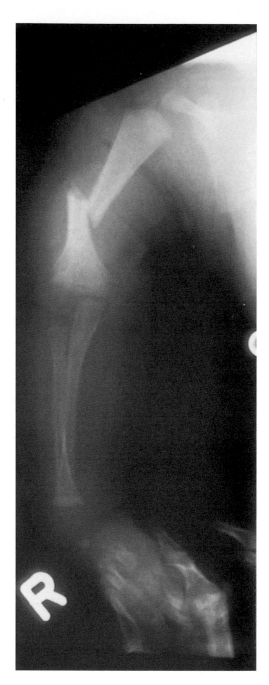

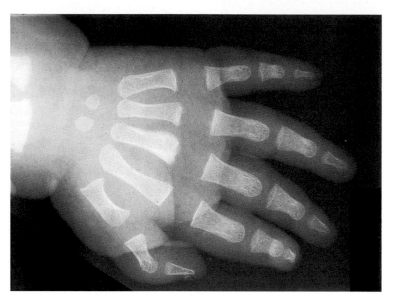

◀ 11.63 Male aged 3 months

He was taken to the hospital emergency department because he seemed in pain when he was picked up. The baby had been well in the mother's care earlier that morning but he was irritable and crying when she came home. The X-ray shows a spiral fracture of the right humerus. The parents vehemently denied causing any trauma to their baby, but spiral fracture of the humerus is almost always due to non-accidental injury and in a 3-month old there is little space for an alternative diagnosis.

▲ 11.64 Male aged 9 months

He had been admitted to hospital two weeks earlier with a skull fracture after a fall. Subsequently he was seen with facial bruising by a health visitor. Investigation following the second admission showed rib fractures and an old healing fracture of the second left metacarpal. The skull fracture, the rib fractures, the finger fracture and the facial bruising all indicate non-accidental injury. Fractures involving the hands and feet are uncommon and probably represent a very sadistic injury.

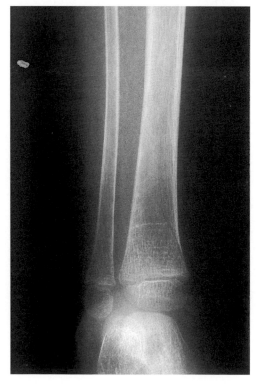

◀ 11.65 Male aged 21 months

Toddler fracture, i.e. an oblique undisplaced hairline fracture of the lower third of the tibia. This fracture usually occurs between 9 months and 3 years and is associated with a history of minor trauma such as running and falling awkwardly.
This child was subsequently shown to have a mild form of osteogenesis imperfecta.

▶ **11.66 Female aged 6 months**
Oblique fracture of the femur in an infant. The child was failing to thrive. The fracture was unexplained.

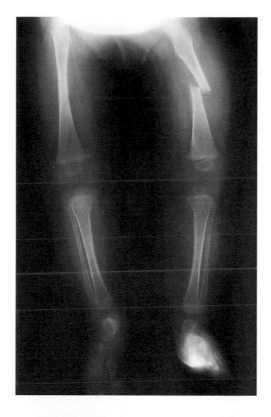

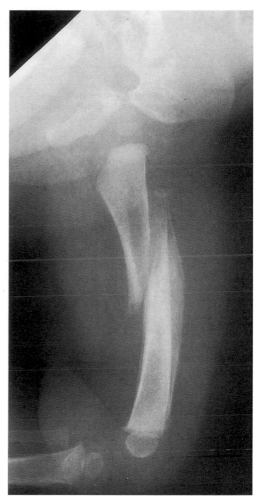

▲ **11.67–70 Female aged 5 months**
Infant presented at A&E Department because of a swollen thigh. She also had linear red marks on the limbs. A home video filmed two days earlier showed the child weight bearing without discomfort. The X-ray therefore shows a recent and healing fracture through the femur. Three weeks later the X-ray shows fresh callus as well as signs of early healing.

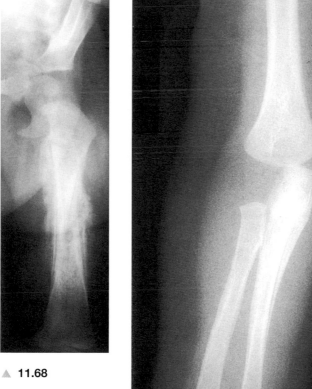

▲ **11.68**

◀ **11.69**
A healed fracture of the proximal end of the ulna. This healed fracture was found at the same time as the refracturing of the femur.

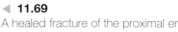

▶ **11.70** lateral view of Fig. 11.69.

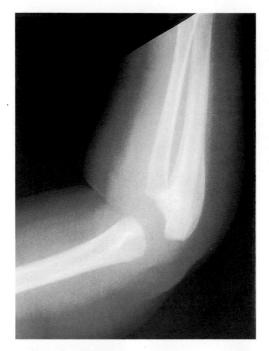

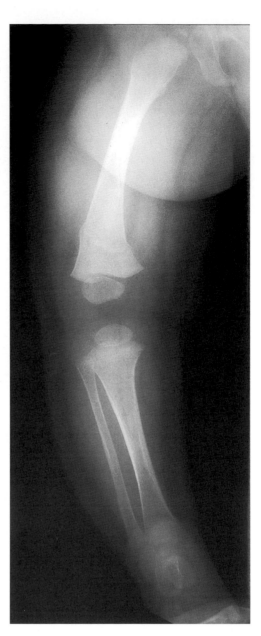

▶ **11.72 Female aged 5 years**
Oblique fracture of the tibia. Long bone fractures are highly correlated with abuse in infancy. Non-accidental fractures may be caused by a pull and twist, direct blow and even shaking (metaphyseal fractures).

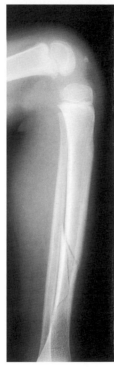

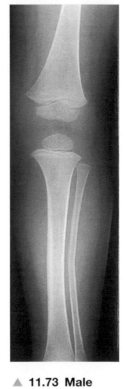

▲ **11.71 Male aged 10 months**
Fracture of the lower end of the femur, which is a worrying injury in infancy.

▲ **11.73 Male aged 4 years**
A foster child said to have fallen over a cement step. X-ray shows horizontal greenstick fracture of radius and ulna. Subsequently this child was killed by his foster father. The history of a fall had been accepted previously.

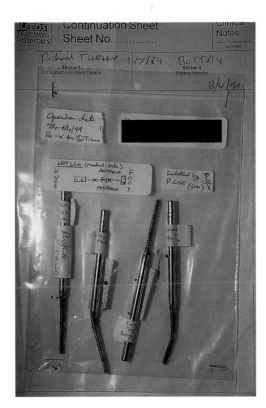

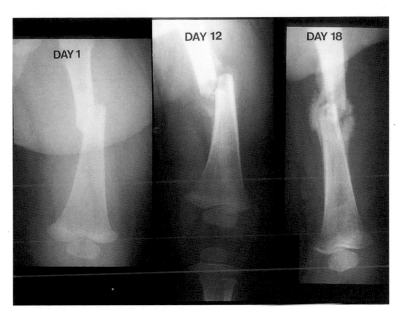

▲ **11.75 Male aged 12 months**
Healing femoral fracture. Radiographs of a displaced fracture of the femur showing stages of healing over the first 18 days.

▲ **11.74 Male aged 15 years**
He had a compound fracture of the tibia. He and his siblings were on the Child Protection Register because of neglect. He was allowed home with steel pins holding the fracture but was readmitted from the pub with the pins removed.

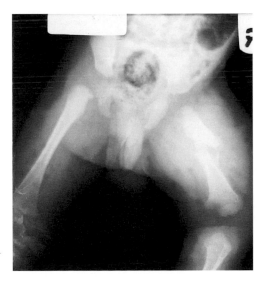

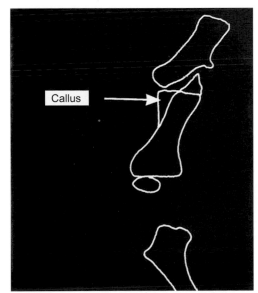

▲ **11.76,** ▶ **11.77 Male aged 2 months**
He was taken to the hospital emergency department by his parents who noticed that his right leg was swollen. A fracture of the right femur can be seen through a previous fracture which had started to heal. This was a non-accidental injury. The child had initially been seen by an orthopaedic surgeon who had discharged him home without taking any child protection initiatives.

▶ **11.78 Male aged 4 months**
Social services referred the child to a
paediatrician after he had been seen with
multiple facial bruising. A skeletal survey
revealed a fracture of the right pubic ramus.

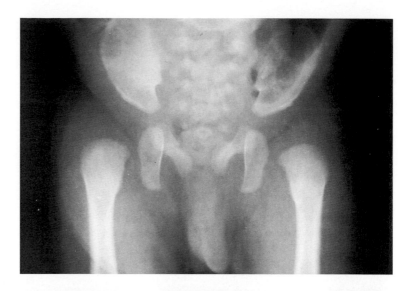

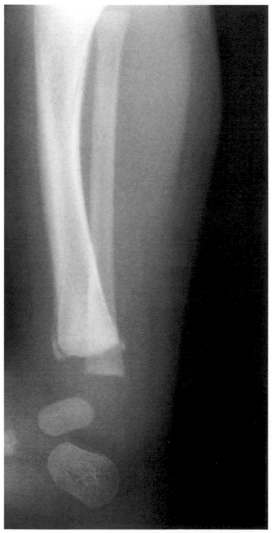

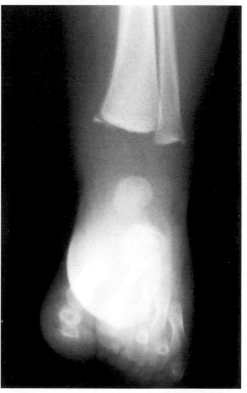

◀ **11.79,** ▲ **11.80 Female aged 3 weeks**
She was taken to the hospital emergency
department because she was crying
inconsolably. A skeletal survey was performed
because bruises were seen on the child's face.
The X-rays revealed a long undisplaced spiral
fracture of the left tibia extending to include the
metaphysis, and a second fracture. Also shown
are distal metaphyseal fractures at the lower
end of the tibia and fibula. These indicate
physical abuse of a young baby.

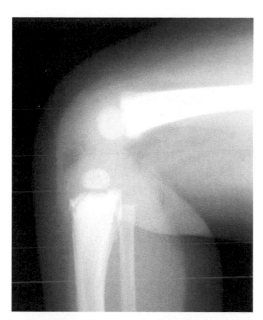

◄ 11.81 Male aged 5 months

The parents brought the child to the hospital's emergency department because of a lack of movement of the arm. A skeletal survey revealed a metaphyseal fracture of the upper end of tibia. There was a total of 25 separate injuries in this child, which indicates serious physical abuse of a young baby.

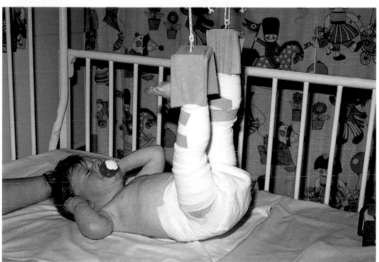

◄ 11.82, ◄ 11.83 Male aged 12 months

The history given by his mother was that he had been jumping up and down in his cot, but later she had found him sitting in the cot on his legs and with a bleeding mouth. Investigation revealed a fracture of the lower end of the shaft of the femur. Further investigation showed a recently torn frenulum, an old bite mark and bruising to the right arm; he was also failing to thrive.

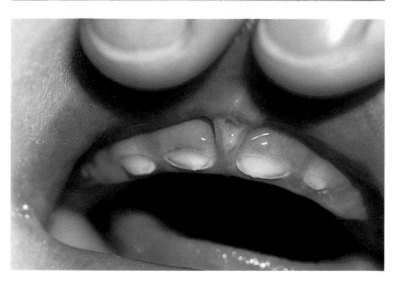

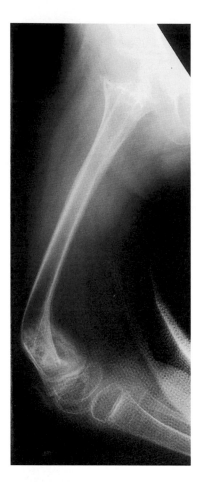
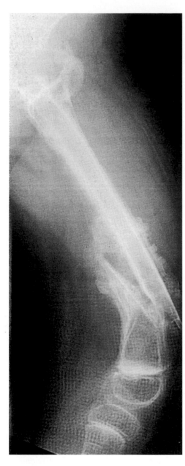

◄ **11.84,** ◄ **11.85**
**Female aged
8 years**

The mother found her daughter, who was handicapped with cerebral palsy, sitting in an unusual position on a beanbag. The child's hips were adducted normally but she was described as sitting 'ordinary fashion'. The child appeared to be both miserable and in pain. The X-rays were taken several days later and show bilateral fractures of the femur with different rates of healing. She was diagnosed as having markedly osteopenic bones.

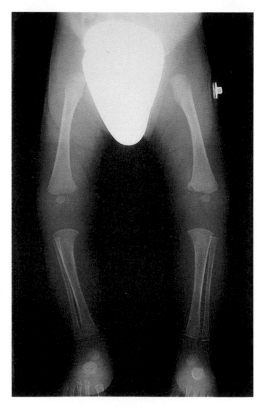

◄ **11.86 Male
aged 8 months**

He was brought to hospital unconscious by his parents after he had had 'a fit' at home. Investigation showed that he had retinal haemorrhages and a subdural haematoma.
A skeletal survey showed metaphyseal corner fracture at the distal end of the left femur. The combination of severe head injury and fractures is diagnostic of abuse.

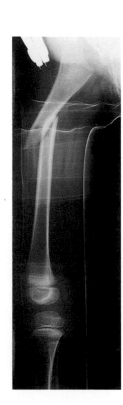

◄ **11.87 Male
aged 4 years**

The history initially given in the hospital emergency department was that the child had fallen downstairs. Later the father admitted grabbing at the child as he ran away from him down the stairs. The child had been seen previously because of failure to thrive, unexplained burns and apnoeic attacks in early infancy. The X-ray shows a spiral/oblique fracture of the right femur. This was probably a non-accidental injury.

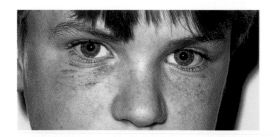

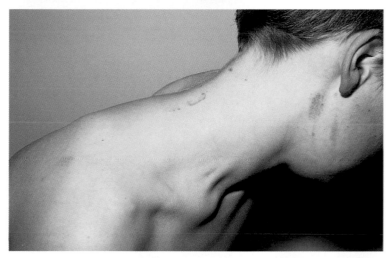

11.88, 11.89, 11.90 Male aged 13 years

He had gone to his uncle's house to say that he was fed-up of being beaten up by his father. His injuries included a bruised right eye, injury to the side of his face and neck and recent bruising to his legs caused by kicks. Investigation confirmed an old fracture to his clavicle. The boy had suffered repeated physical assaults by his father. Assaults on teenagers should be taken very seriously.

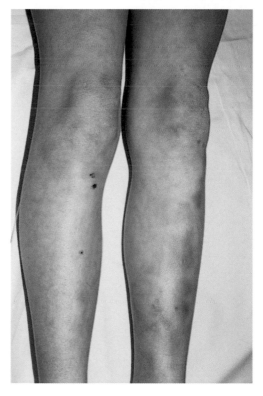

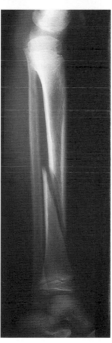

11.91 Female aged 5 years

Spiral tibial fracture. Child said to have fallen from top bunk. Found the following morning asleep, reluctant to move leg.

Chapter 12

Contact burns

There are features which assist in the recognition that a burn is a 'contact burn':

- shape conforms to the object;
- sharply delineated margins;
- square and straight edges;
- depth variable but generally uniform;
- dry, scabbing.

Common causes of contact burns include contact with various hot metal objects: metal is a good conductor of heat and so a burn may result if the object is sufficiently hot.

Common objects include:

1. domestic iron;
2. fire or fire surround/fire guard;
3. various tools – soldering iron, curling tongs, pokers;
4. cooker and cooker hot plate;
5. object that is not normally hot – it may be either intentionally or unintentionally heated, e.g. cutlery, belt buckle in car seat (car in sun);
6. exhaust pipes, e.g. on motor cycles;
7. hot water radiators.

- Heat is transferred by conduction. Because of the high thermal conductivity of most metals, the object is uniformly hot and so contact produces a burn of uniform depth.
- In most situations contact between the object and skin is brief.
- Reflex withdrawal to pain occurs, removing the limb or body from the source of the heat.
- In abusive burns the skin is maintained in contact with the object for longer, resulting in deeper or more severe extensive injury.
- The extent of the injury also tends to be greater as held on contact favours a larger surface area.
- The temperature of the object enables an estimate of the time in which the object was in contact with the skin to be made.

Common sites for abusive contact burns include the hands (especially the dorsum) and feet but also the limbs and face.

DIAGNOSIS OF NON-ACCIDENTAL BURNS

General features

- Delay in presenting the child for treatment/present after a delay if a complication develops.
- Presence of other injuries, old and new.
- Pattern of repeated burns/scalds to children in the family.
- Evidence of neglect, including non-organic failure to thrive.
- Responsible adults allege that there were no witnesses to the 'accident' and that the child was merely discovered to be burned, thus hoping to discourage any further inquiry.
- Scald attributed to action of sibling or other child.
- Child reported to cry little/experience little pain at the time of injury or to show unusual response to the injury/treatment.

The investigation

- Full detailed history of the injury, including time and place, witnesses, precise detail of the events surrounding the injury, action taken following the injury and child and parent's responses.
- Full paediatric history, including family and social history, history of siblings, previous injury, including other burns, child's behaviour.
- Full examination of the child for any injury. Detailed drawing of the burn, including measurements, site, pattern (consider position child was in at the time of injury), depth of injury (in conjunction with surgical team). Is there sparing, e.g. soles/palms in immersion injury? Consider effects of clothes.
- Obtain consent for genital and anal inspection (links with sexual abuse).
- Assess child's development and ability to act in the way stated, e.g. can this child turn on a tap or climb into a bath?
- Ask to see appliance/heater alleged to have injured. Does it fit? What was the likely temperature at time of alleged injury? May ask to see clothing.
- Assess likely time of contact from temperature (if known) time graph.

- Arrange photographs of injury, appliance, environment, etc.
- Attend strategy meetings, work closely with police, social services, surgical team and family. Information must be freely shared and discussed. A series of meetings at different stages of the investigation may be helpful in some cases.
- Visit the home to view the scene of injury. Re-enact the scene according to the description of the carer present at the time of injury. This can be a very revealing exercise as well as a distressing time for the carer and needs to be handled with care and sensitivity. Exact details of temperature and time should be obtained as well as heights, depths of water, nature of materials. Scientific advice, manufacturers data, etc., may be required.

Summary

1. Accidents follow brief lapses in protection, neglect as part of a pattern of inadequate parenting and abuse when injury is deliberately inflicted.
2. Burns and scalds following abuse are under-reported.
3. Evaluation is difficult, requiring a careful and detailed history. A visit to the home may be necessary.
4. Non-accidental thermal injuries include forced immersion and pour scald, contact, friction and chemical burns.
5. Sites in abuse particularly include backs of hands, buttocks, genitalia and feet. No site is exempt.
6. Significant points in the history are un-witnessed incidents, delayed presentation, minimization of severity of injury, surprising lack of pain, repeated burns.
7. Differential diagnosis includes other skin pathology, especially infections.
8. There is a particular association between sexual abuse and burns.
9. Repeated burns are a dangerous form of neglect.
10. Burns may be associated with any form of abuse.

'it is often alleged in abusive burns that the child felt no pain'

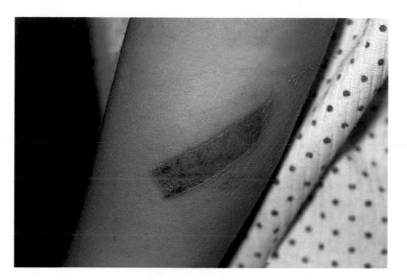

▲ 12.1 Female aged 4 years
Unexplained contact burn. This child was taken to the A&E Department with this unexplained injury and the history that there had been no pain. This clearly warrants further investigation. Burns are exquisitely painful.

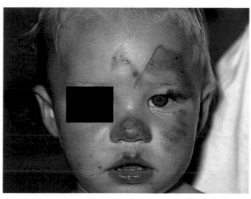

▲ 12.2 Female aged 18 months
She was taken to the A&E Department with a history of having leaned against an old refrigerator which had been left outside the house. It was a hot summer's day which was the explanation as to why the fridge was hot and thus burned the child. Marks of an iron are clearly seen.

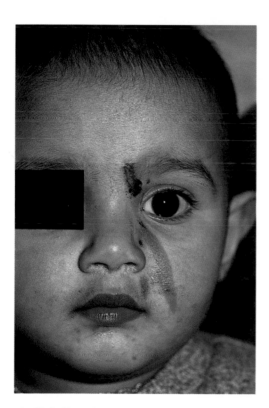

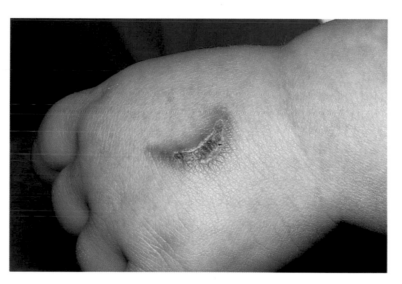

▲ 12.4 Male aged 14 months
He had been left in the care of a 35-year-old female babysitter, who claimed that he had touched the fire with his hand. (The babysitter's own daughter had been deliberately burned by being made to stand too near to the fire at 5 years of age.) A curved healing contact burn is seen on the dorsum of the left hand, probably an inflicted injury.

▲ 12.3 Female aged 2 years
She presented with an iron burn to the face. Her mother was ironing on the floor and the iron was said to have fallen over on top of the child.

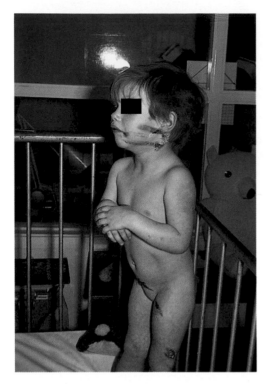

▲ **12.5 Female aged 2½ years**
She was burned with a poker. Linear burns are seen to the side of the face, lower abdomen and thigh. The distribution would suggest sexual abuse but this was not investigated. The diagnosis is an inflicted, extremely sadistic injury.

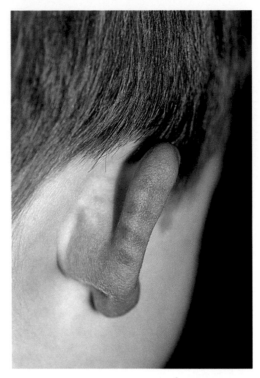

▲ **12.6 Male aged 5 years**
He told his teacher that his father had heated a fork and applied it to his ear, while laughing. The photograph shows four parallel superficial contact burns on the outer aspect of the pinna. This indicates sadistic abuse.

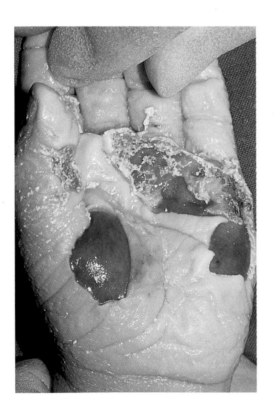

◄ **12.7 Male aged 2½ years**
He was taken by his parents to the hospital emergency department, because he 'put his hand on the convector heater'. There was a past history of neglect and physical abuse. He was in the sole care of his father at the time of the incident. The photograph shows a superficial contact burn to the palm of the hand. It was taken on the ward after 24 hours of treatment and consequently resembles a scald rather than a contact burn. The cause of the burn remained unexplained but abuse was suspected.

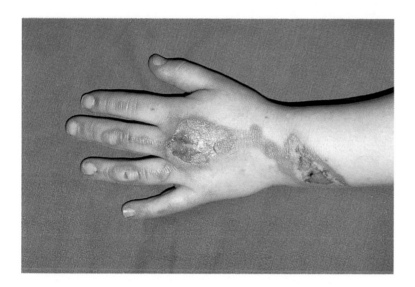

12.8 Female aged 7 years

She went to school with her hand wrapped in a dirty bandage; her parents subsequently speculated that while she was doing the ironing she must have burned herself on the back of the hand. The girl had moderate learning difficulties. There was no history of the child complaining of pain, but on examination there were also signs consistent with sexual abuse. There was also previous serious physical abuse to a sibling. The photograph shows an extensive burn over the dorsum of the fingers, hand and wrist with a full thickness burn over the wrist. The injury is too severe and extensive for the history given and the response of the child and the parents is inappropriate. This is likely to be an inflicted injury by a hot iron, rather than an accidental injury.

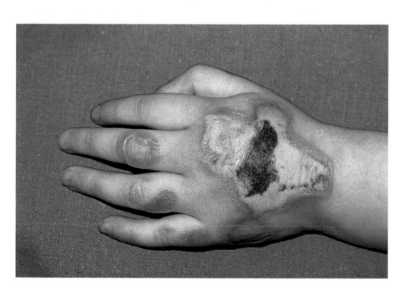

12.9 Female aged 2 years

Her mother speculated that the 7-year-old brother had put the iron on his younger sister's hand while she was out of the room. The brother denied doing this. He also had a history of soiling and emotional difficulties. The girl also had physical signs consistent with vaginal and anal abuse. The photograph shows an extensive full thickness burn on the dorsum of the hand and more superficial burning on the dorsum of the fingers. Grafting was needed. The diagnosis is an iron burn: probable abuse.

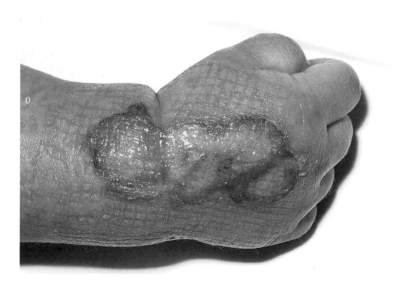

12.10 Female aged 8 months

The history given was that whilst in the care of teenage siblings she was sitting by the side of the hot stove and reached out and touched it. A contact burn of variable thickness can be seen over over the dorsum of the hand and wrist. (Note: when children explore and grasp it is usually the palmar surface of the hand which comes into contact with the hot surface. Burns on the dorsum of the hand are thus always suspicious.)

▶ **12.11 Male aged 4 years**
Contact burn caused by poker. The child was said to have been playing with the poker and this was an 'unfortunate accident'. These are inflicted burns.

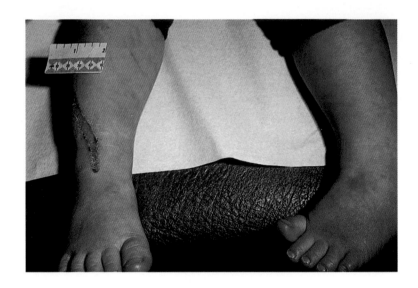

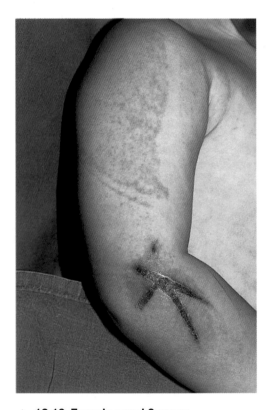

▲ **12.12 Female aged 3 years**
This child presented in the A&E Department with a totally unexplained old contact burn.

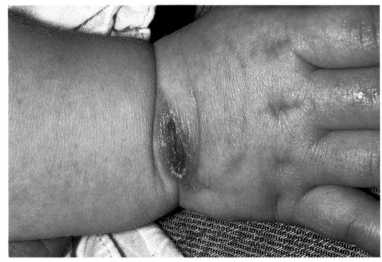

▲ **12.13,** ▶ **12.14**
Female aged 15 months
She presented with an old infected burn to the back of the wrist and flexor aspect of four digits. In spite of the late presentation and neglect, further investigation wasn't thought necessary by statutory agencies.

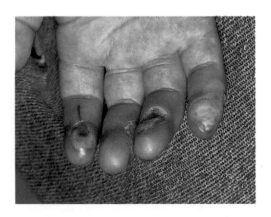

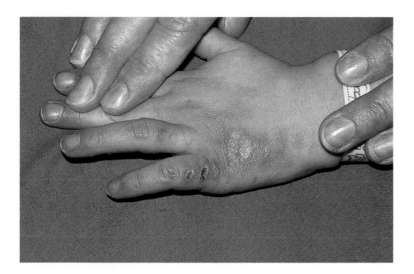

◀ 12.15, ◀ 12.16 Male aged 5 years

He was profoundly deaf, hyperactive and with difficult behaviour. He presented with burns of different ages on his hand and buttock. Figure. 12.15 shows three parallel healing burns on the dorsum of the left little finger and a healing burn extending onto the dorsum of the hand. Figure. 12.16 shows an extensive burn on the right buttock demonstrating a grill pattern. This child has had at least two burns due to contact with the grill of a portable room heater. (Note: as with burns on the back of the hand, burns on the buttocks are always suspicious; in this case there was no history of a witnessed injury but repeated burns imply neglect or inflicted injuries.)

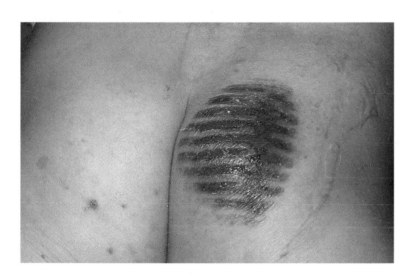

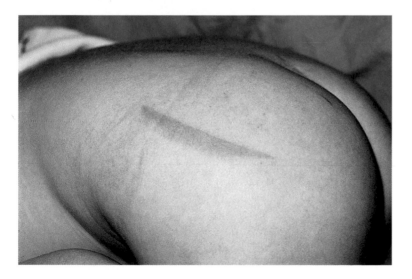

◀ 12.17 Male aged 5 years

His parents said that he had inflicted this burn deliberately by holding himself against a radiator. Superficial contact burns of the outer aspect of the left buttock can be seen. This boy had also been seen on several previous occasions with unexplained bruising and his younger sister was found to have been sexually abused. If this burn was self-inflicted, i.e. self-mutilation, it is of extreme concern, and further investigation is clearly warranted.

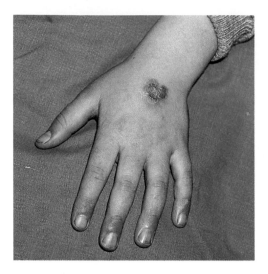

▲ 12.18 Male aged 8 years

He had an unexplained mark on the back of his hand seen while the family were visiting a child welfare charity family unit. The photograph shows an irregular-shaped healing burn on the dorsum of the left hand, possibly caused by multiple cigarette burns. (Note: it is not always possible to establish the cause of a burn, but unexplained burns on the back of the hand are always of concern.)

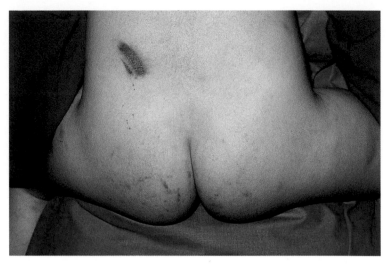

▲ 12.19 Female aged 3 years

Her nursery nurse noted a burn and an excessive number of bruises during routine care in a day nursery. A clearly demarcated arc with an inner parallel burn, of uniform thickness, of several days duration is seen on the left lower back. Scattered petechial bruising over both buttocks and bruises were also noted on the left thigh and right loin. All the marks are unexplained, but the burn suggests contact with, for example, a kettle, and the petechial bruising over the buttocks suggests a hand slap.

▶ 12.20 Female aged 5 years

Her mother said the child had fallen backwards against a heated towel rail while getting ready for her bath. The mother is schizophrenic, and became very agitated when the 'accident' was discussed. The photograph shows a superficial burn of the left buttock, with surrounding erythema and signs of recent blistering. This is consistent with the history, but the reason for the fall is unclear.

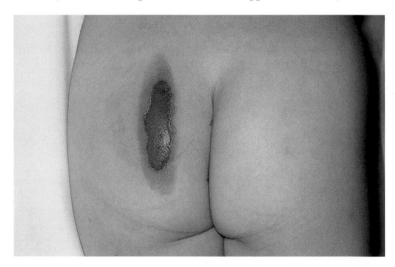

▶ 12.21 Female aged 3 years

The grandmother was caring for this child and her brother when she found the children had bruises on their faces and burns on their hands and contacted a child welfare charity. The photograph shows multiple contact burns over the lower legs and feet in various stages of healing. (Note: the similar shape of all the burns – the inflicting implement was not discovered. The older brother had signs consistent with anal abuse.) These were sadistic inflicted burns; there is a high correlation between injuries like this and sexual abuse.

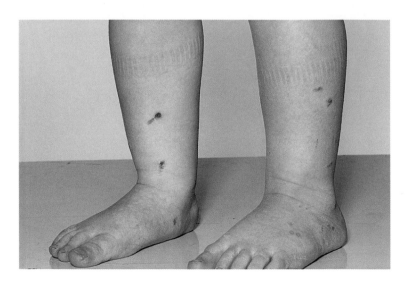

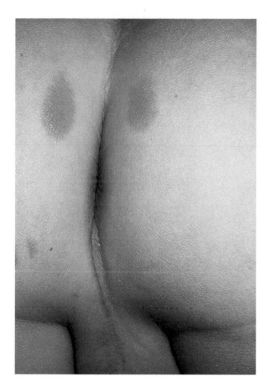

▲ 12.22 Male aged 4 years
He returned home after an access visit with his
father with two black eyes and multiple burns.
Paired superficial contact burns on the buttocks
are seen. There were similar burns on the
scrotum and legs. The child subsequently gave
a very clear history of sexual abuse and
deliberate burning by his father.

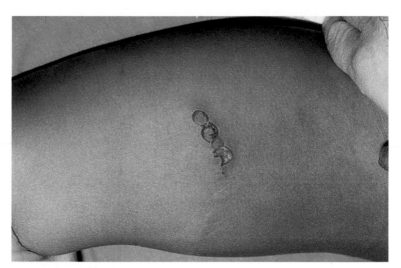

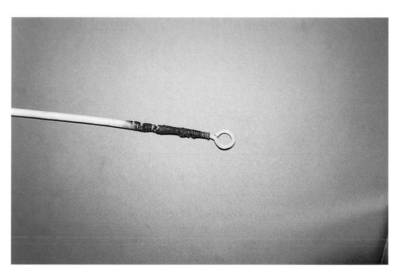

▲ 12.23, ▲ 12.24 Male aged 2 years
The curtain wire had been heated to cause the burns shown.

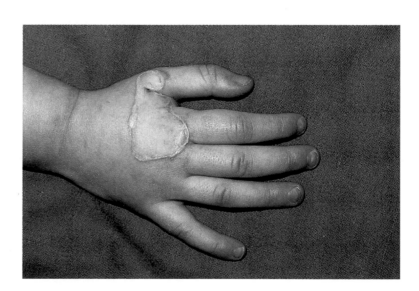

▶ 12.25 Aged 3 years
Contact burn on the back of the hand 'caused
by iron'. This was an unwitnessed and
unexplained injury in a 3 year old.

▶ 12.26 Female aged 15 months

Contact burn due to an iron. Presented late to the A&E Department with very angry, noisy parents. The history given was that the child had lifted her hand up and put it against the iron which the mother was holding. A further history was that the mother had been ironing and had put the hot iron at the back of the worktop but the child had reached up and burned her hand.

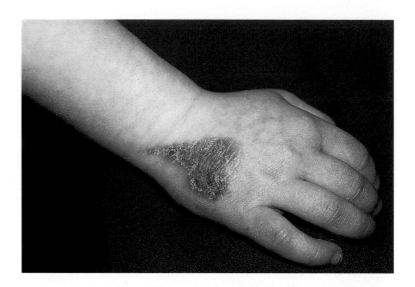

▶ 12.27 Female aged 10 months

Her 6-year-old brother was seen at his school for children with emotional difficulties with a burn on his back. A doctor diagnosed this as a burn; the mother then sought a second opinion and the further examination of the younger sibling showed unexplained burns on the baby too. The mother explained that the boy had burned himself on the washing line, and the baby had crawled backwards in to the radiator. She had not sought treatment for either child. The photograph shows an old, almost healed contact burn over the buttocks and left upper thigh. These were unexplained contact burns in both children. Further investigation was difficult but showed a severely dysfunctional family. The burns were thought to be inflicted but no further information was forthcoming.

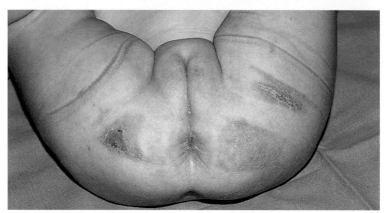

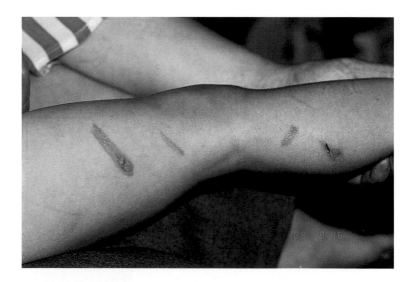

▲ 12.28, ▶ 12.29 Male aged 4 years

He was seen by a paediatrician as part of a planned follow-up following earlier neglect, and his mother mentioned that he had been sitting too close to the fire. Paired linear contact burns of the outer aspect of the thigh and lower leg are seen. Note that when the leg is flexed the pattern is seen clearly (Fig. 12.29). It is difficult to see how the injury was caused with the child's leg bent.

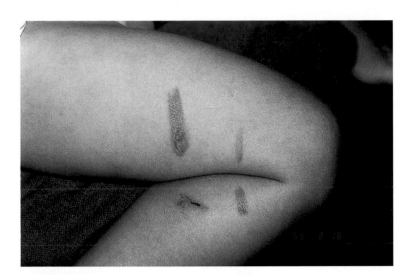

◀ **12.29**

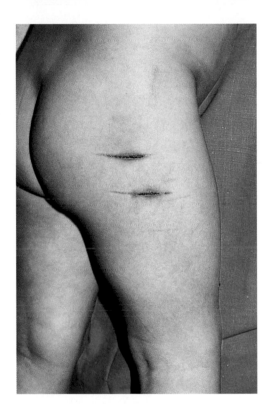

◀ **12.30–12.33 Male aged 4 years**
When the health visitor was visiting routinely she was shown a burn, and the child's father commented that he was always falling against the fire. Multiple linear burns are seen, both recent and well healed, on the outer aspect of the thigh. These were deliberately inflicted with a hot implement over a period of time (Note: accidental burns rarely occur more than once to the same child.)

◀ **12.31**

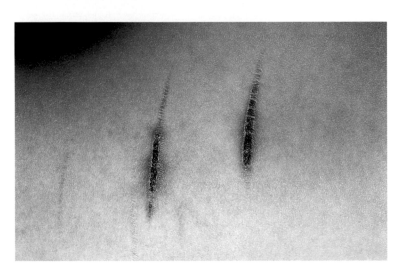

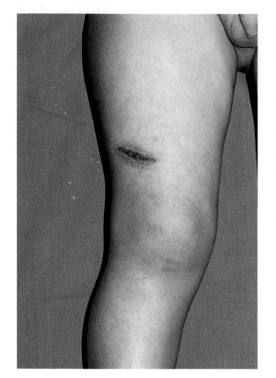

▲ 12.32

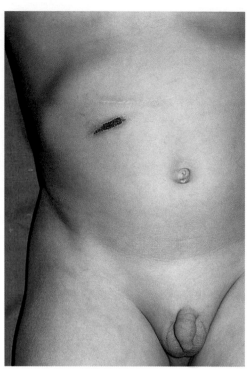

▲ 12.33

► **12.34 Male aged 5 years**
Contact burn due to edge of a hot iron on buttocks. The child said 'Mummy did it'.

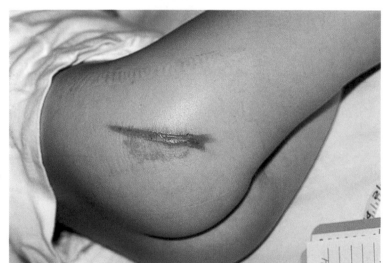

► **12.35 Aged 10 months**
Iron burn caused by infant 'crawling across the floor and bumped into the iron'. This history is clearly unacceptable.

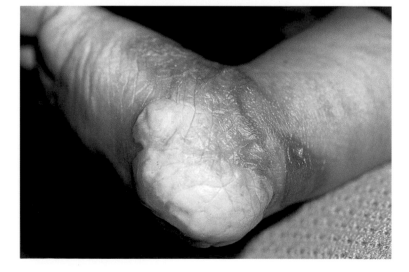

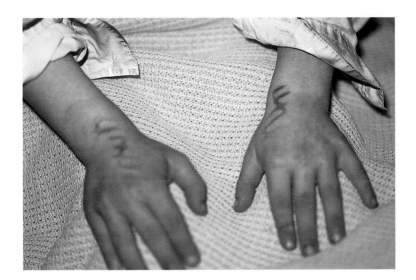

◀ **12.36 Male aged 7 years**
This child, with a long history of emotional and behavioural difficulties, was presented with contact burns. The parents gave the history that he had put his hand deliberately on the radiator. This injury clearly needs further investigation whether the injury was self-inflicted or inflicted by other(s).

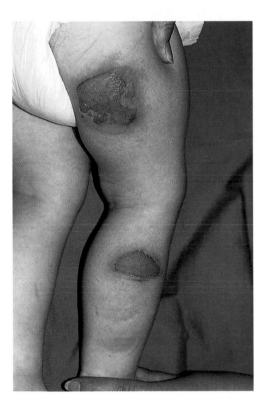

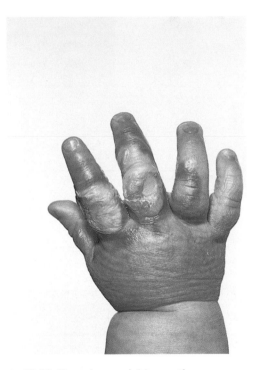

▲ **12.38 Female aged 11 months**
Presented at the A&E Department with a history of an unwitnessed incident. The mother speculated that the child had crawled across the floor, pulled the iron flex and the iron fell off the ironing table and landed on the child's hand. The burns were serious and full thickness on the second and third digits.

▲ **12.37 Female aged 17 months**
Child with contact burns on back of thigh. The child was presented when the burns had already started to heal with crust and erythema. The history given was that the child had climbed onto the cooker and burned herself. The mother was preoccupied with her own domestic violence. The child also had unexplained scratches and bruises to the face. The association between domestic violence and child abuse is now more recognized.

▶ **12.39,** ▶ **12.40,** ▶ **12.41 Female aged 11 years**

She attended a school for children with moderate learning problems and was already known because of emotional difficulties in relation to her stepmother. She presented in school with bruising to the face, burns on the back of the hand and neck, and signs of sexual abuse. Healing burns can be seen on the dorsum of the hand and back of the neck. The stepmother admitted burning the child with a spatula while frying eggs. Figure. 12.41 shows healed skin at the back of the neck with depigmentation, which ensures differentiation from superficial skin infection, e.g. impetigo.

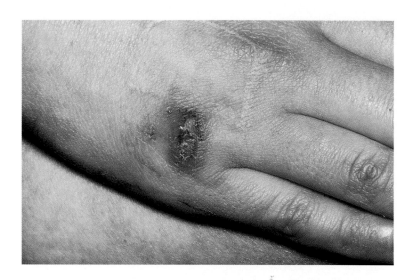

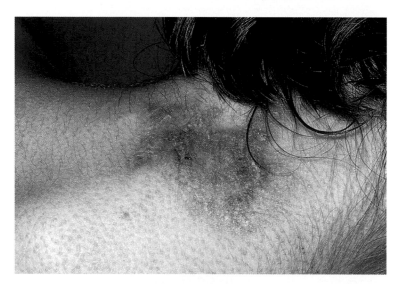

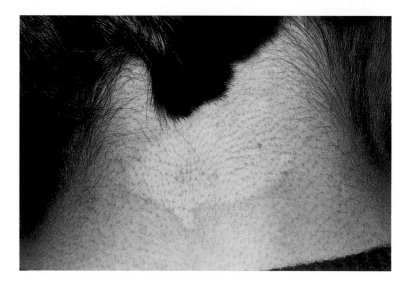

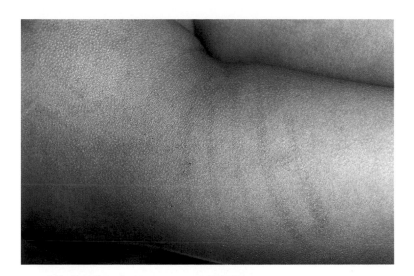

◀ **12.42 Female aged 7 years**
Burns were an incidental finding when she was being examined in the follow-up clinic because of a vaginal discharge. There was a past history of physical, sexual and emotional abuse and neglect. The photograph shows a burn from a grid mark which has healed with linear hyperpigmentation. This is a very worrying injury, especially in the context of the other abuses.

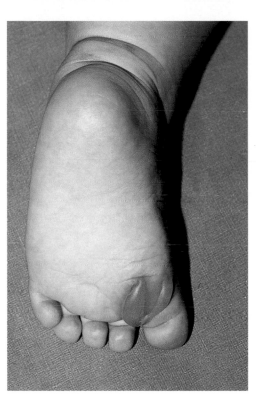

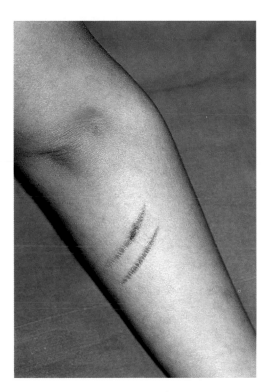

▲ **12.43 Male aged 12 months**
He was seen with his 2-year-old brother at the request of the social services after a convicted child abuser had become part of the household. The older brother was demonstrating disturbed behaviour including soiling. Examination of the older boy showed signs consistent with anal abuse and the baby had an unexplained burn. The photograph shows a superficial blistering burn on the sole of the foot, which was unexplained.

▲ **12.44 Female aged 6 years**
She was referred because of possible sexual abuse, and burns were an incidental finding. Parallel linear contact burns are seen on the outer aspect of the elbow, which were unexplained.

▶ **12.45 Male aged 5 years**

He had a history of being beaten by his father. Extensive bruising of both buttocks is seen, but also skin loss: on the left buttock, seen as linear healing marks, and on the right buttock a roughly rectangular area of skin loss without evident healing. This is a difficult case to interpret but there is a probability of a burn superimposed on a beating.

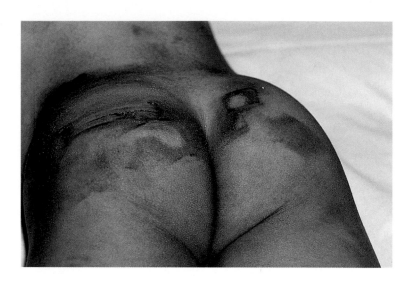

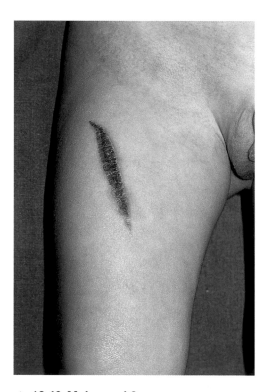

▲ **12.46 Male aged 2 years**

He was referred because of neglect and failure to thrive, along with his siblings. The parents said he had picked up a hot iron and burned himself, but they had not sought medical help. The photograph shows a long linear healing burn on the anterior aspect of the right thigh, of partial thickness. The burn is consistent with contact with the edge of a hot iron; the history however needs further investigation.

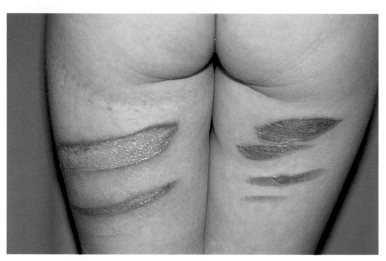

▲ **12.47 Female aged 6 years**

She was severely mentally handicapped. The history given was that she 'sat on the fire' but medical help was not sought. Linear contact burns are seen on the back of the thighs, of several days standing and of variable thickness. There was previous history of unexplained bruises and scratches. This is a significant injury in a vulnerable child who is not being protected.

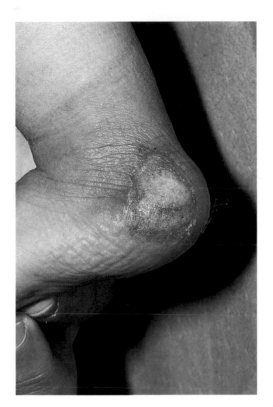

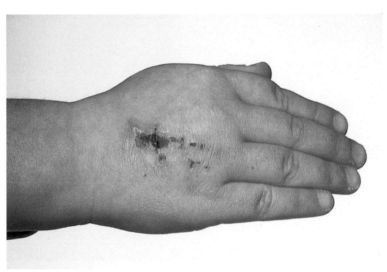

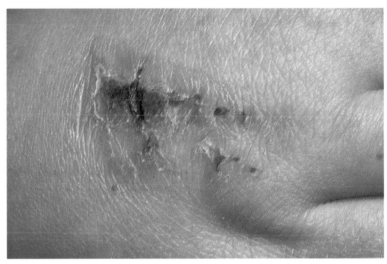

▲ **12.48 Male aged 8 months**

It was claimed that he had 'crawled against the fire'. The photograph shows a healing contact burn on the outer aspect of the left heel. Accidental contact burns are usually trivial as the child removes the limb quickly; this is a deep burn and of great concern.

▲ **12.49,** ▲ **12.50 Female aged 4 years**

She presented as having 'touched the fire with her hand'. A healing contact burn of the dorsum of the right hand is seen, of several days' duration. Contact burns of the hand are usually on the palmer aspect; therefore this is an usual site. There is also a past history of sexual abuse, physical abuse causing a fracture of the tibia and emotional abuse of this child.

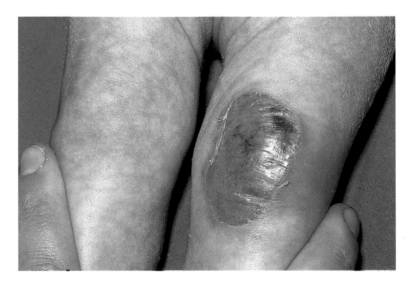

▶ **12.51 Female aged 3 months**

The burn was found by a health visitor on a routine visit. The parents speculated that they had perhaps put the baby's feeding bottle in the carrycot with the baby and this had caused the injury. An extensive healing contact burn is seen over the left lower thigh and knee, which is unexplained. It is also not clear if this a scald or a contact burn.

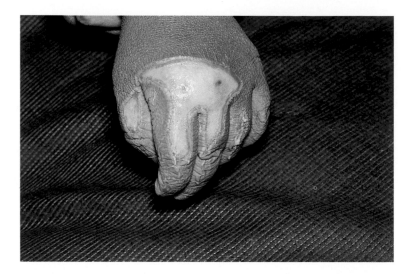

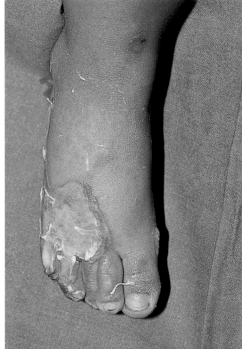

◀ **12.52 Male aged 18 months**
He was said to have touched the fire. There is an extensive irregular contact burn on the back of the left hand. The injury looked superficially like a scald, but note the burn is over bony prominences, and the alteration in skin texture due to treatment. The cause is unknown.

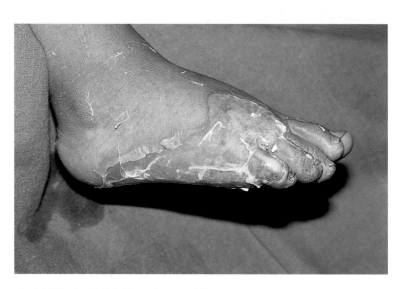

▲ **12.53,** ▲ **12.54 Female aged 2 years**
Her history, as given by teenage babysitters, was that the child had fallen asleep on a settee and slipped so that her foot touched the fireguard. An extensive burn with blistering of the outer aspect of the right forefoot with clearly demarcated edge is seen. This is a serious, unexplained injury possibly due to immersion in hot water.

▶ **12.55 Female aged 15 months**
She was taken to the hospital emergency department several hours after the parents said that she had been injured falling against a fire whilst left alone in a room. The photograph shows an irregular, roughly triangular scald to the front and side of the forehead. The history was inconsistent with a contact burn – later her parents said she had been eating very hot pizza. Additionally there was a fresh, unexplained burn on the child's arm and unusual bruises on the thighs and feet.

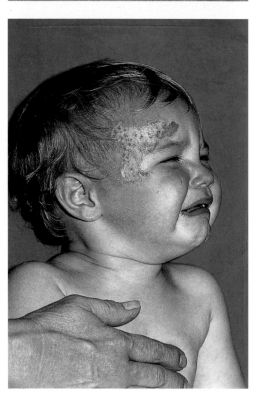

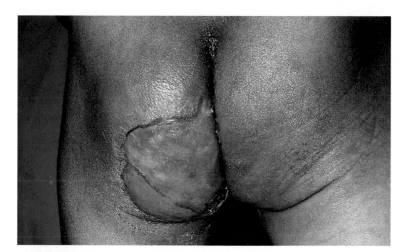

◀ 12.56 Male aged 6 years

He presented with a history of having 'leant against a convection heater'. The photograph shows an immersion scald primarily affecting the left buttock but extending into the natal cleft. The history is inconsistent with the injury, particularly as the child was already known to be failing to thrive and also suffering severe emotional abuse.

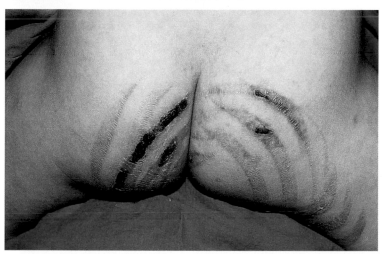

◀ 12.57 Female aged 13 months

She presented as having climbed onto the worktop and then sat on the cooker. Her father had heard her crying and had lifted her down. Concentric circular burns to both buttocks and to the top of the right thigh can be seen in the photograph. The injury is not consistent with the history given. More than one contact has occurred, and in a position not consistent with sitting. A serious and sadistic injury.

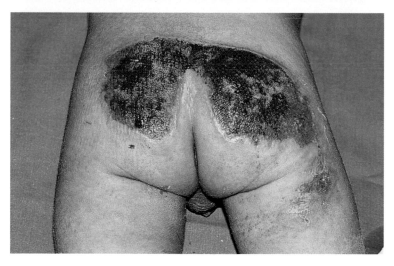

▲ 12.58 Male aged 4 years

The history given by his foster father was that the child was found in a bath of hot water, the father having left the room to get a towel. There is an extensive contact burn of the buttocks and right upper thigh with healing already apparent. This injury is not consistent with the history given, and this has the appearance of a contact burn, complicated by delayed presentation.

▲ 12.59 Male aged 14 months

He presented with a history of being 'wedged' between a storage heater and the back of a settee; however, on a visit to the home, a distance of 3 feet (0.9 m) was observed between the furniture and the heater. There is an extensive superficial contact burn on the back of the left thigh but sparing the back of the knee. This is an unsatisfactory history in a child who had previously had unexplained apnoeic attacks, failure to thrive, and at the age of four an unexplained fractured femur.

Chapter 13

Scald Injuries

Scalds are thermal injuries resulting from contact with hot fluids, usually water.

Characteristics of scalds

- variable thickness between and within different lesions;
- contouring of depth (tendency to be deepest in the middle);
- dip, splash or pour patterns;
- smooth curved edges;
- peeling and sloughing;
- skin loss in sheets;
- moist, macerated, soggy lesions spread into flexures, depressions, e.g. natal cleft;
- blisters pronounced.

Accidental scalds

- One of the commonest reasons for admission to hospital for a scald injury is the teacup or kettle scald.
- Caused when a toddler pulls a cup of hot tea or a kettle containing recently boiled water over themselves.
- Injuries can be severe and usually affect the upper part of the body, including chest, shoulders and sometimes back. The head and neck may be involved.

Bath scalds

Only children and impaired adults sustain bath scalds. Bath scalds in children should strongly suggest abuse or neglect.

How is the child scalded?

Explanations for domestic tap water scalds, which are often proposed, include:

- fall into an excessively hot bath (running of bath by sibling or inadequately supervised by adult);
- tap turned on by child or sibling when child in the bath;
- put hand into hot water in sink or bath (e.g. to retrieve toy or to prevent self from falling in);
- accidentally placed in a bath of too hot water by a carer;
- plastic/portable bath fell over on to child;
- water from hosepipe (draining washing machine) spilled onto child.

Injuries from tap water are serious because they are frequently extensive and severe, requiring the care of a special burns unit. Frequently a quarter or more of the body surface area may be involved.

A major factor contributing to these injuries is the high temperature of domestic hot water in many homes.

Dip scald or forced immersion injury

- Relatively common non-accidental injury.
- Affects hands, feet, buttocks/back or sometimes the whole child.
- Child is held in the hot water, unable to struggle, clear demarcation lines are found between scalded and spared skin (glove and stocking distribution, modified if the fist is clenched or if the sole of the foot presses against the cooler base of the bath). With the child's buttocks, the central area may be spared if pressed to the cool bath base, leaving the 'hole in the doughnut effect'.
- Children will not have the splash marks expected of children who accidentally fall into the bath.
- Water will find its way into hollows in the child's body but, where surfaces are opposed, the skin will be spared, e.g. if legs flexed and the child dunked, confluent areas of non-scalded skin in opposition will be seen.

Splashed, thrown or pour scald injury

- Unusual sites, e.g. genitalia.
- Pattern of separated areas, as when fluid is thrown, may suggest abuse.
- Back of the hand is uncommonly scalded in accidents but may be affected when the hand is held under a flow of hot water.

Time taken to scald (approximate time in adults − children scald more quickly)

49°C: 5−10 minutes
54°C: 30 seconds
60°C: 5 seconds
70°C: <1 second

▶ **13.1,** ▶ **13.2 Male aged 18 months**
Child who was said to have climbed in the bath when his mother's back was turned. She heard him shout and on turning found him on all fours kneeling in the bath. Both forearms burned for a distance of 4 in from the wrist. Circumferential scalds symmetrically to both arms; clear demarcation line without splash marks. No scalds elsewhere. Pattern of forced immersion scalds.

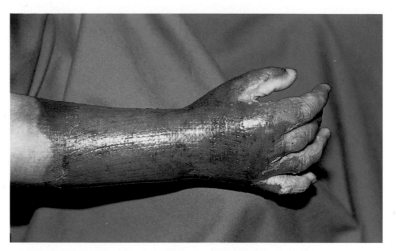

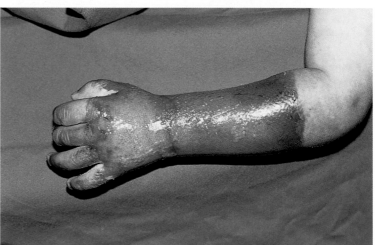

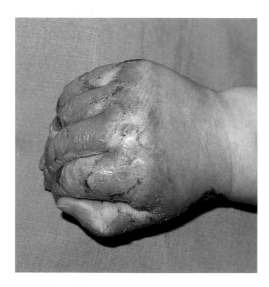

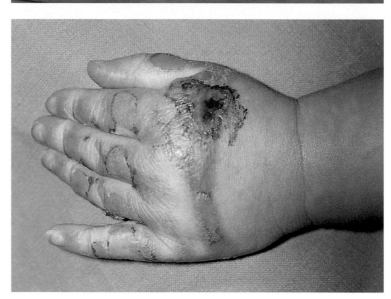

▲ **13.3,** ▲ **13.4 Female aged 3 years**
She was claimed by her mother to have climbed into a hot bath fully clothed, where she was found sitting upright with her hands immersed in the water. The photographs show immersion injury to the distal part of both hands only – a symmetrical injury with a clear tide mark. This is a typical forced immersion scald.

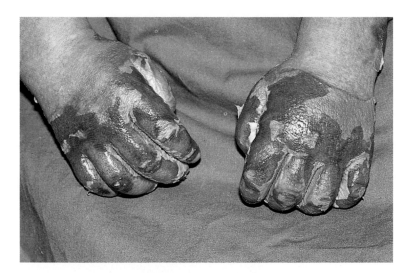

◀ 13.5 Male aged 21 months

The history given was that he fell forwards into the bath. He was treated at home by his mother, who was a nurse, for 4 days. He was also found to be failing to thrive. This is a typical forced immersion scald. (Note: bath scalds do not occur in non-impaired adults.)

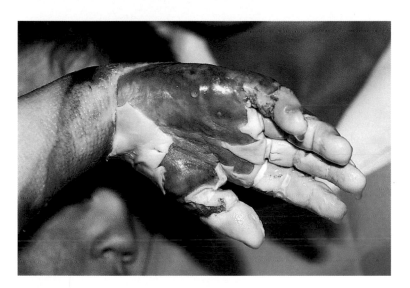

◀ 13.6 Male aged 3 years

He was said to have put his hand into a kettle of boiling water. An immersion scald of the hand and wrist is seen, with extensive skin loss. The history given is unacceptable.

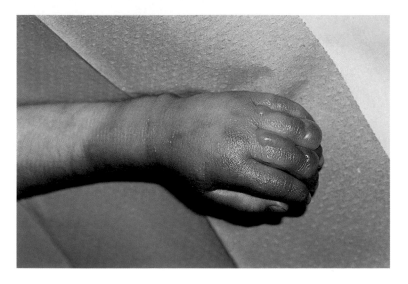

◀ 13.7 Male aged 3 years

The history given was that he fell into a hot bath. There is an immersion scald of the hand and wrist with blistering and swelling. A clear tide mark can be seen. This is an unacceptable history. Other members of the family have failed to thrive and there is also history of sexual abuse.

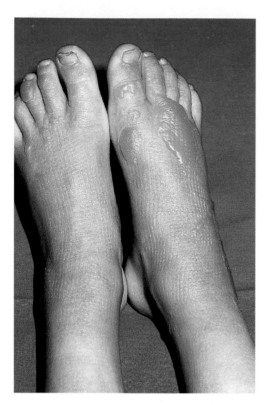

▲ **13.8 Male aged 5 years**
He was made to stand in a bath of hot water by his mother's partner. He had a long previous history of emotional abuse. An immersion scald of both feet is seen with a faint tide mark and blistering. The injury is consistent with the history given.

▶ **13.9 Male aged 4 years**
A changing history was given; initially the mother said she left him to play in the bath when she went to fetch the soap, and he must have turned on the hot tap and then got himself out of the bath. When she dried the child's foot the skin came off. The mother assaulted the policewoman during an interview and then admitted that she had put him into the hot bath to teach him a lesson. There is a typical immersion scald of both feet and the bottom (only the right foot is shown here). The injury was deep and the foot required grafting. The injury is consistent with the history, i.e. abuse.

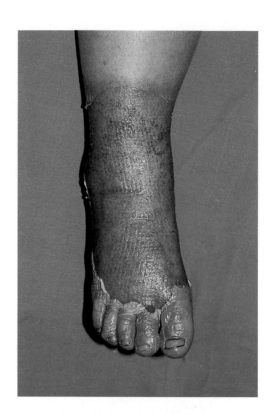

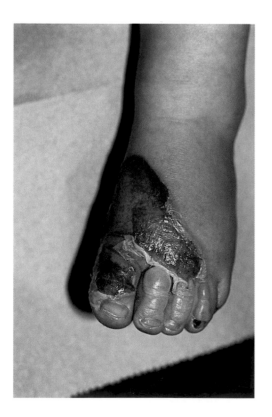

◀ **13.10 Male aged 18 months**
He was said to have put his foot in a bowl of porridge which was on the floor. There is a clear immersion injury of the left forefoot. No other features of the history suggest abuse, but this is a worrying injury and a preventable one. Adherent porridge caused an enhanced injury.

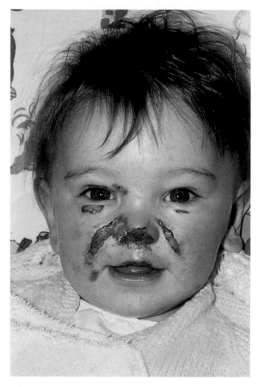

▲ **13.11 Male aged 1 year**
The history given was that he picked up a mug of hot soup and tipped it over himself. The child was failing to thrive and had feeding difficulties. His father initially refused admission to hospital. An extensive scald to the face is seen in an unusual pattern. The mechanism for this injury is not clear; the mug may have been pushed in his face, the soup thrown, or the child could have caused this injury to himself.

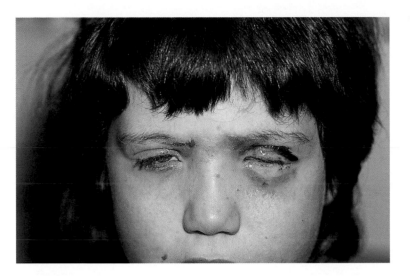

◀ 13.12 Female aged 6 years
The history given was that she 'looked into a kettle of boiling water'. There is a scald injury to both eyes, worse on the left, with early infection evident. This is an unusual and worrying history, not previously encountered.

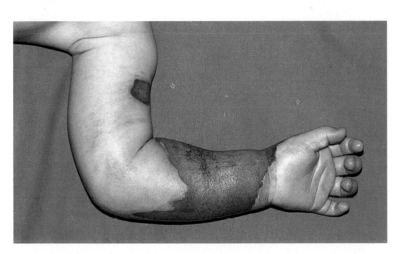

◀ 13.13–13.16 Female aged 2 years
These scalds to this child superficially resemble a forced immersion pattern. Although circumferential there are upper and lower 'tide marks', a separate upper circular lesion and hand sparing. It was felt more likely that water had been poured over the child.

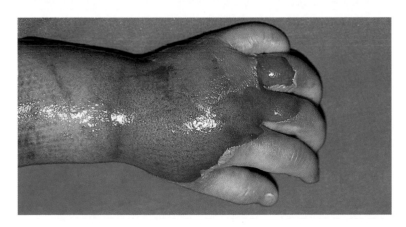

◀ 13.14

▷ **13.15**

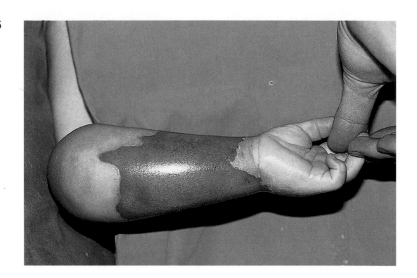

▷ **13.16**

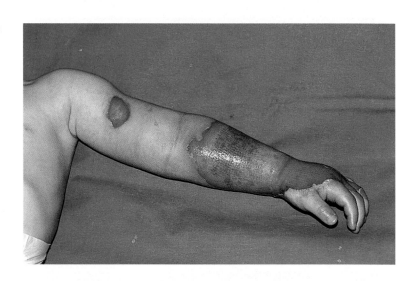

▷ **13.17,** ▷ **13.18**
Male aged 2 years
The history given
was that he pulled a
mug of hot tea over
himself. There is a
scald to the side of
the face, ear, left
shoulder and upper
arm. This is a typical
pour scald, though
more severe than
usual.

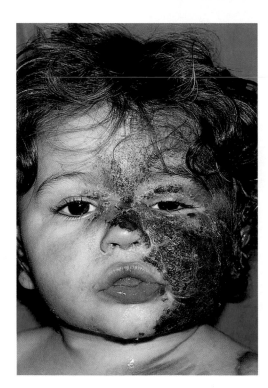

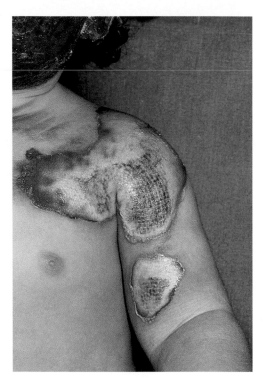

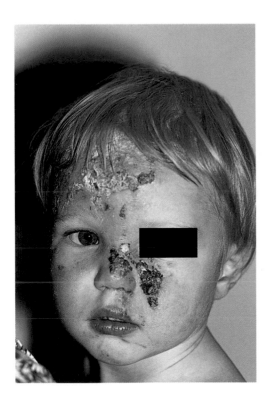

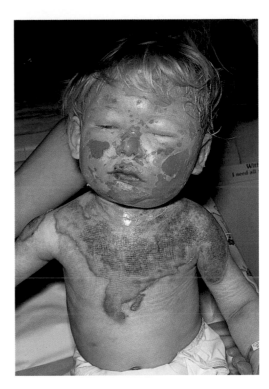

◀ **13.19 Male aged 18 months**
Old healing scald (? about 3 days) on a toddler. The injury was compatible with the history and that he pulled a cup of tea over himself was consistent. Concern was raised about delay in presentation. The presence of other bruises and old rib fractures confirmed physical abuse as well as neglect to seek treatment. Child was also failing to thrive.

▲ **13.20 Male aged 1 year**
He presented as having pulled a kettle of hot water over himself. There is an extensive scald of variable thickness with skin loss and swelling over the face, upper chest and upper arms. This is a common accidental injury, which should be preventable with coiled kettle flexes.

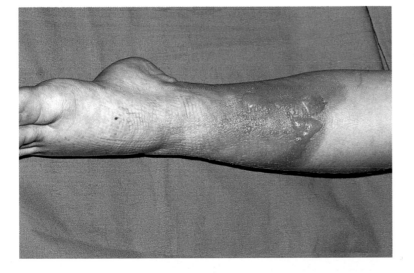

◀ **13.21** and ◀ **13.22 Male aged 4 years**
He was seen in the A&E Department with scalds on both lower legs. The child was said to have knocked over the kettle which had been placed on the floor. The extensive nature of these injuries, which were symmetrically placed on both legs, in a child with cerebral palsy was not consistent with the history. This boy had been shaken as an infant, resulting in cerebral diplegia.

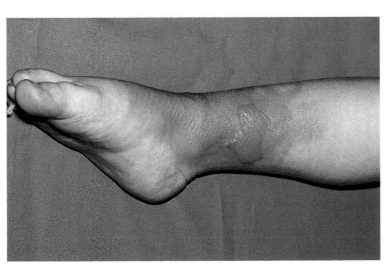

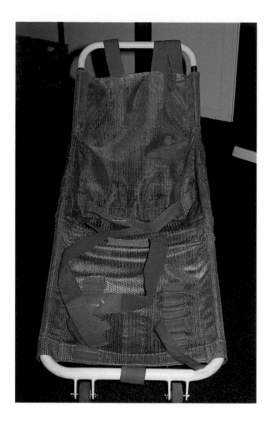

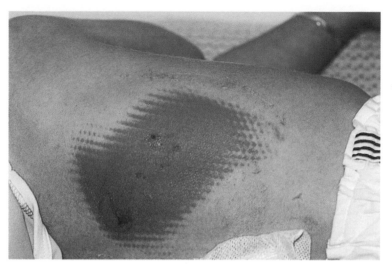

◀ 13.23, ▲ 13.24 Female aged 3 years
The child is severely mentally and physically handicapped. She was scalded while being bathed in a bath appliance (Fig. 13.23). Her family are known to have a history of child sexual abuse, physical abuse and murder. A patterned recent superficial scald is seen with blistering over the trunk. This is consistent with the history of being washed with excessively hot water.

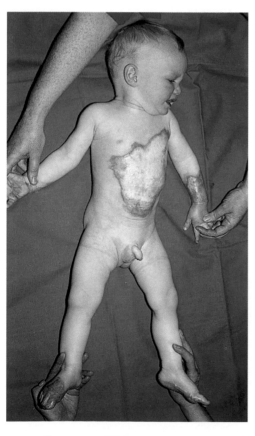

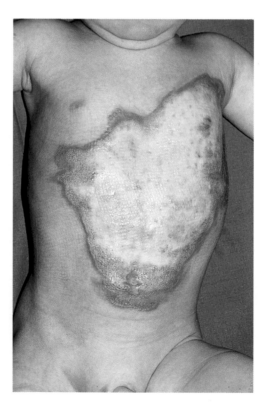

▲ 13.25, ▲ 13.26 Male aged 18 months
The child had a past history of severe failure to thrive. The history given was that he pulled a kettle of boiling water onto himself, with the water splashing his abdomen, foot and arm. There are widespread scalds to the abdomen, arms and foot, which are showing signs of healing. The accident was due to serious neglect.

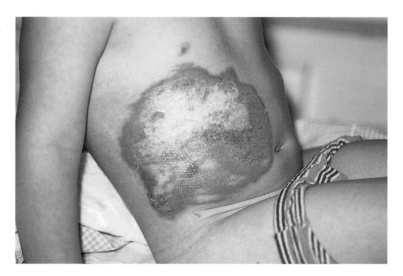

▲ **13.27 Male aged 4 years**
Extensive serious scald on abdomen is unexplained.

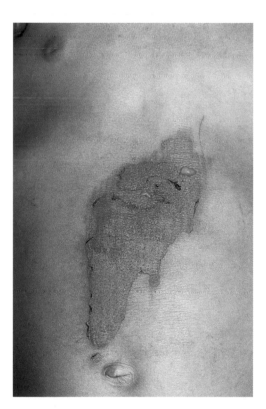 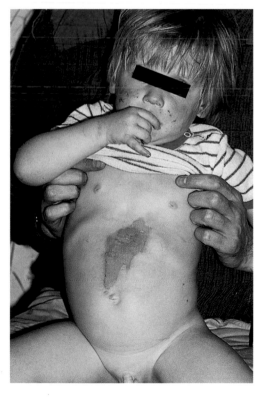

▲ **13.28,** ▲ **13.29 Male aged 2½ years**
He was seen to be scalded when attended by the health visitor on a routine visit. An older sibling
was said to have poured a mug of hot tea on her brother. A healing scald with blistering and healing
is seen on the upper abdomen. This is probably an accidental scald, but note the bite on the right
forearm, and a younger child in the same household died of bronchopneumonia following measles.
The care of this scald had been neglected.

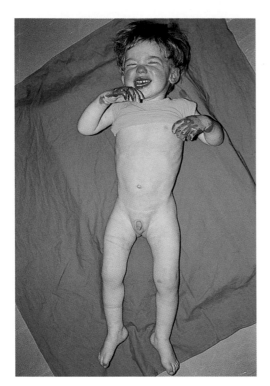

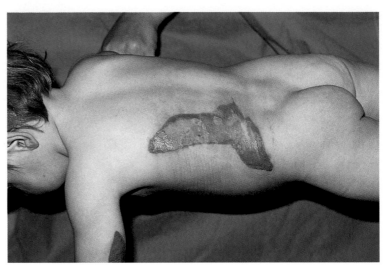

△ 13.31 Male aged 16 months

He was 'found screaming in the kitchen'. An extensive scald is seen over the back and left upper arm posteriorly. The distribution of the scald suggests a splash injury, but this is an unusual distribution and there is a worrying lack of history.

△ 13.30 Male aged 21 months

It was claimed that he had 'reached over the edge of the bath and fell forward with his hands in the hot water'. The mother, a nurse, pulled him out and treated him at home initially; then took him to the hospital emergency department. There is marked, previously unrecognized failure to thrive, as well as partial thickness bilateral immersion scalds in glove distribution. This is a forced immersion scald. (This is the same child as in Fig. 13.5).

▶ 13.32 Female aged 3 years

She was taken late at night to the hospital emergency department with a recent scald. It emerged that the drunken father had thrown a cup of coffee at the child because he felt 'she was up too late'. The photograph shows the splash effect with scattered, separate areas of superficial scalding.

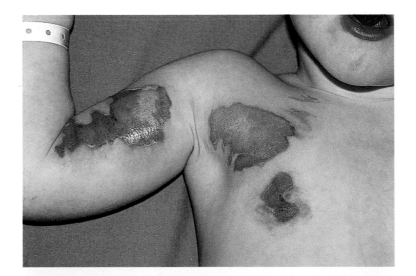

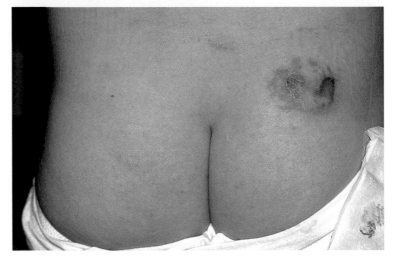

▶ 13.33 Male aged 6 years

Boy who laughed when his mother's partner bent over and his jeans slipped. The man took a teabag from his newly made cup of tea and placed it on the child's buttocks.

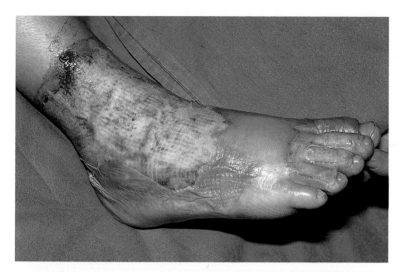

◄ 13.34

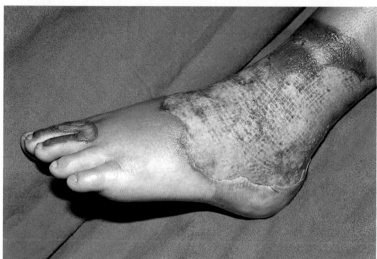

◄ 13.35

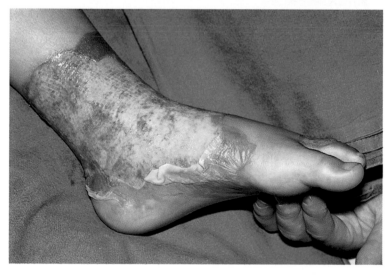

▲ 13.36

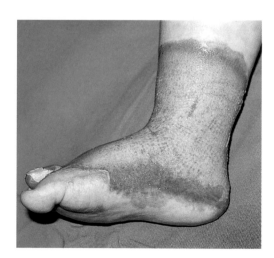

▲ 13.37

▲ **13.34–13.37 Male aged 3 years**

His father claimed that the child had fallen into the bath of hot water with his shoes and socks on. Bilateral, severe partial to full thickness scalds of both feet can be seen. There are no splash marks and the dorsum of the feet have been spared. All of this indicates a typical forced immersion injury.

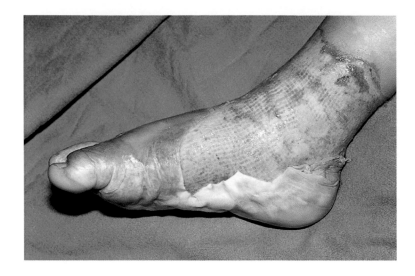

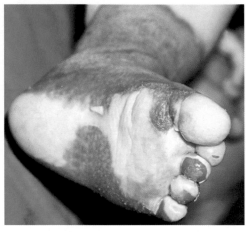

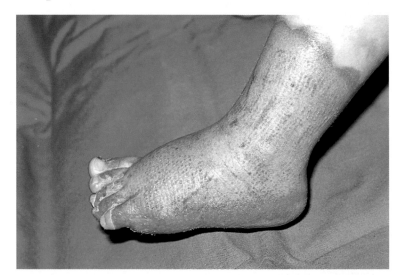

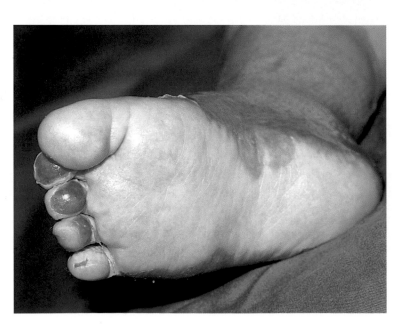

◁ **13.38,** ▲ **13.39,** ◁ **13.40,** ◁ **13.41**
Male aged 3 years

Characteristic scald of forced immersion burn in a child. There is a clear line of demarcation with sparing of the sole of the floor (placed against the cold bottom of the bath). There is an absence of splash marks above the demarcation line. The absence of splash marks and the clear line of demarcation indicate that the child has been forcibly held in the water.

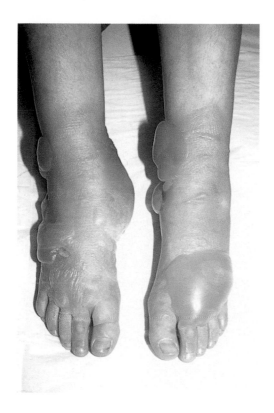

◀ 13.42 Female aged 4 years

Presented at the A&E Department with blistered feet. The mother described going up to the bathroom and finding her standing by the bath with scalded feet but not complaining of pain. This was a forced immersion scald with clearly demarcated areas. The scalds were superficial and the buttock was spared bar minimal erythema. The history is inadequate.

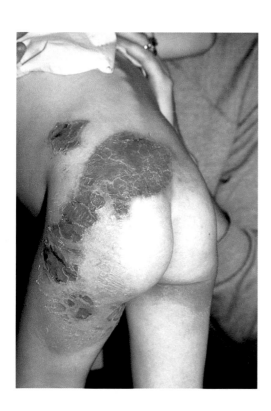

◀ 13.43 Female aged 3 years

Extensive bath scalds in a child who was also failing to thrive. Central part of buttocks spared where pressed onto cool base of bath – the hole in the doughnut effect.

Chapter 14

Other Burn Injuries

Causes and types

- conflagrations and flame burns;
- outdoor fires and house fires;
- flammable liquids;
- cigarettes or lighters, responsible in that order;
- paraffin heaters and liquid petroleum gas cylinders;
- faulty wiring, bare wires and faulty appliances – fires or electrocution;
- food burns;
- friction burns;
- chemical, including caustic burns;
- sunburn.

Characteristics of other burns

1. Cigarette – circular 0.5–1.0 cm diameter.
   - in abuse, often full thickness cratered, leaving circular, depressed, paper thin scars;
   - in accident, superficial, eccentric with tail from brushed contact.
2. Flame – tissue charred, hair singed.
3. Chemical, e.g. scald-like distribution, staining ±. May be caustic liquid – deep with underlying tissue destruction.
4. Friction – occurs over body points, e.g. nose, point of shoulder. Usually superficial. Intact blisters not seen. Child dragged across carpet; burns occur where ropes used to restrain a child.
5. Electrical – deep, small, localized. Exit and entry points. Common site – hands and fingers. Tissue charring and deeper necrosis.
6. Microwaves – unusual, sharply demarcated, full thickness burns widely distributed on body (opposite microwave emitting devices). Deeper burns to muscle described.
7. Food scalds – the lips and mouth common sites.
   - sticky foods such as hot porridge can concentrate heat and produce unpleasant scalds;
   - scalds in the groin, e.g. when a bowl was tipped into a child's lap; and a scalded foot, when a child put his foot in his bowl of porridge on the floor.
8. Sunburn/radiant burns – infants neglectfully left in the sun. Children forced to stand in front of a fire until their legs were burned from radiant heat. Erythema with or without blistering over exposed areas.

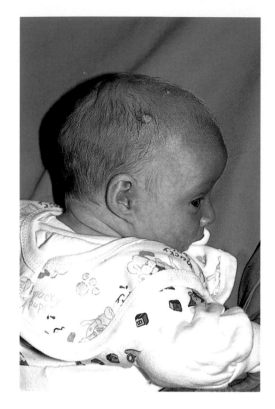

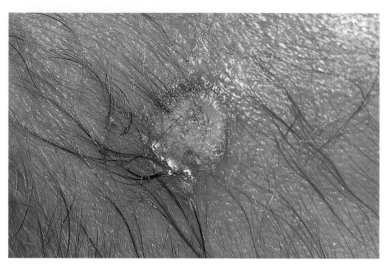

◄ 14.1 and ▲ 14.2 Male aged 8 weeks
Infant with cigarette burn on head. The father was wheeling the pram down the road when ash fell off his cigarette. This explanation was not acceptable. Figure 14.2, shows a close-up of the burn showing the typical rolled edge and deeper burn centrally.

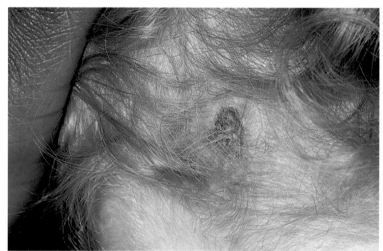

▶ 14.3 Female aged 10 years
Older child with healing cigarette burn on scalp. The burn had become infected and had been picked, which had delayed healing.

▶ 14.4 Male aged 6 months
He was referred because of unexplained lesions on the face. This is a typical cigarette burn: round with a punched out centre and showing early healing. The child had several similar burns on his face, all consistent with cigarette burns.

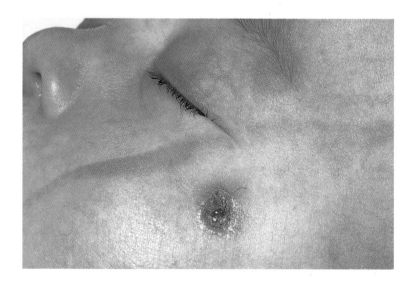

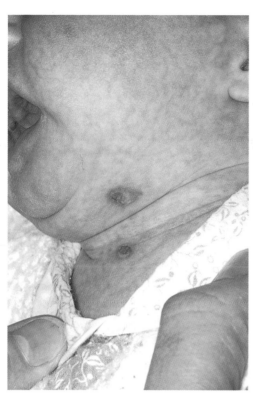

14.5 Female aged 6 weeks
She was with her mother in a child and mother's home. The mother said she dropped ash accidentally on the baby when she was smoking. A typical punched out cigarette burn can be seen on the lower jaw and neck. These two lesions are superimposable; the cigarette may have been held forcibly against the child while the neck was flexed.

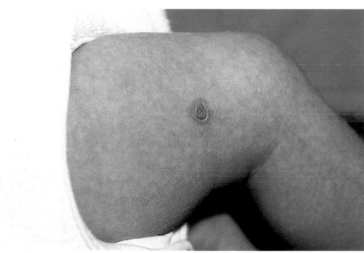

14.6 Female aged 6 weeks
The mother had initially wanted the child to be adopted. The mark was found incidentally by the midwife. A typical punched out cigarette mark is seen on the outer aspect of the right upper thigh.

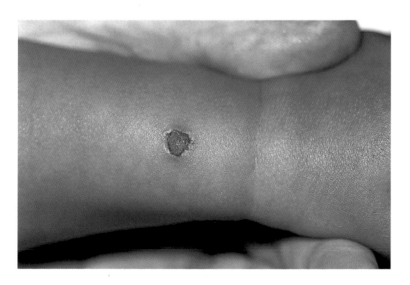

14.7 Female aged 2 years
Infant with probable cigarette burn. The mother was a heroin addict who left the child with various other substance abusers. She told her social worker that the injury had occurred when in the care of one of her friends.

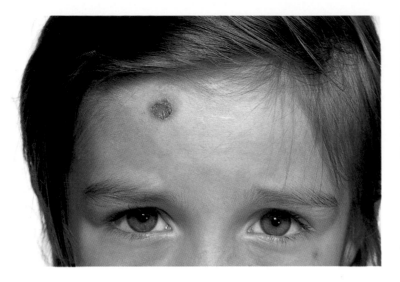

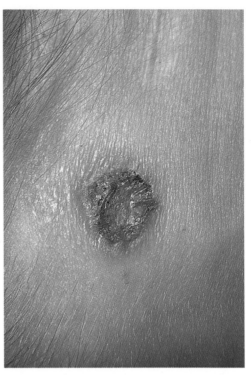

▲ **14.8,** ▶ **14.9 Female aged 7 years**
The child told her school teacher that her father had burned her with a cigarette. There is a typical cigarette burn on the forehead.

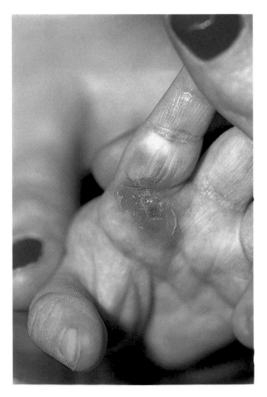

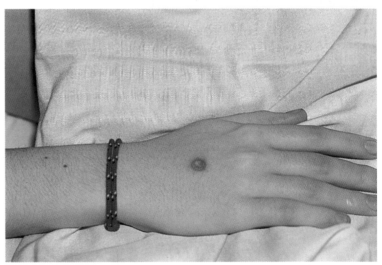

▲ **14.11 Female aged 16 years**
She had a long history of physical and sexual abuse at home. She refused to say who had caused the cigarette injury to the back of the hand as shown, and 16 other similar lesions found on limbs, breasts, back, thighs, etc. The lesions were seen when she returned to a safe house from home. This is a typical punched out cigarette burn.

▲ **14.10 Male aged 3 months**
The history was that the child grasped hold of a cigarette. There is a superficial burn with blistering over the metacarpophalangeal joint of the index finger. This is a very worrying injury in a young infant, consistent with a cigarette burn.

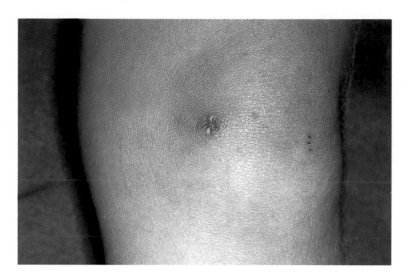

◀ 14.12 Male aged 2 years
He presented in the hospital emergency department with a metaphyseal fracture of the humerus. There was unexplained bruising of the face and ear, and the lesion as shown. There were also signs of sexual abuse. This is a typical healing cigarette burn with heaped up skin, over the front of the left knee. This was a multiply abused child.

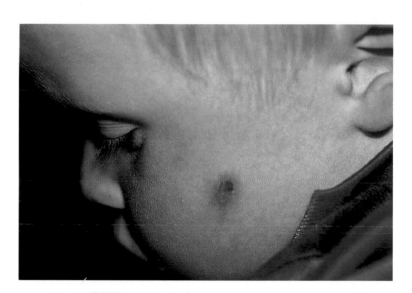

◀ 14.13 Male aged 2 years
He had a history of playing in the garden when he brushed against an adult neighbour's cigarette. An eccentric but moderately deep burn is seen on the left cheek, consistent with glancing contact with a cigarette.

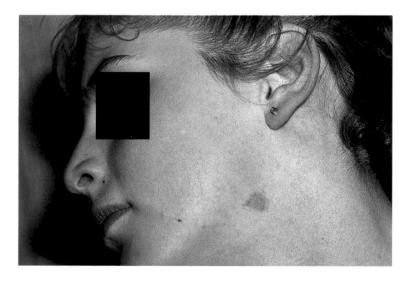

◀ 14.14 Female aged 15 years
She was deliberately burned by her older brother with a cigarette during 'horseplay'. The girl made a complaint at school about the injury. There is an asymmetrical burn below the lower jaw, showing healing, which is consistent with the history. This is abuse.

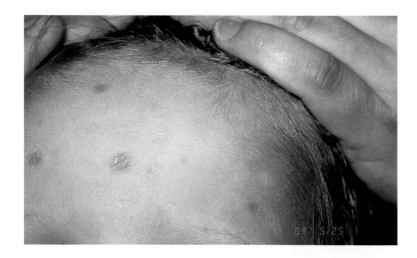

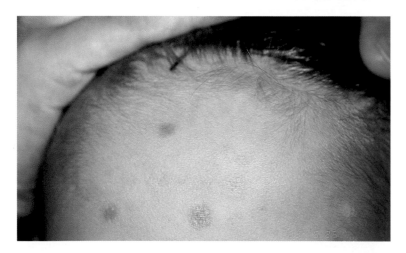

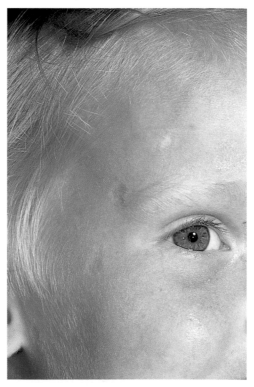

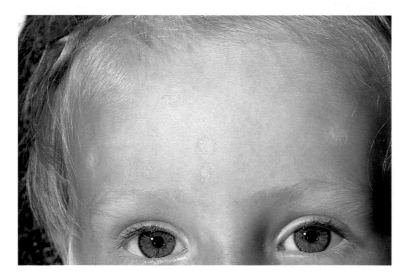

△ **14.15,** △ **14.16,** △ **14.17,** △ **14.18 Brothers aged 3 years and 5 years**
The boys presented to the paediatrician after the younger child was found wandering in the street and was referred by police. A doctor had been 'treating' the lesions on the boys for the previous 2 years. Multiple circular, punched out lesions are seen at various stages of healing, some with paper-thin scarring. The lesions are all on the upper half of the face. They are consistent with cigarette burns at various stages of healing. The mother had several cigarette burns on her forearms; she initially admitted to causing these lesions but then retracted. Several expert opinions were obtained; these included a diagnosis of chickenpox, acne excoriée and impetigo. The lesions all healed quickly in care, and the final diagnosis was cigarette burns.

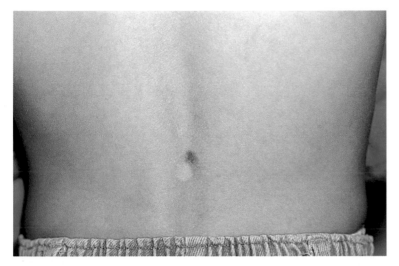

◄ 14.19 Male aged 8 years
The child was profoundly deaf. He presented saying he had been burned in the street by a stranger. There was a history of previous sexual abuse by an older brother. A circular scar is seen on the lower back with depigmented scar tissue. There is also a recent irregular burn just superior to the scar. These appear to be a healed and a recent cigarette burn. (Note: children with disability are at high risk of abuse.)

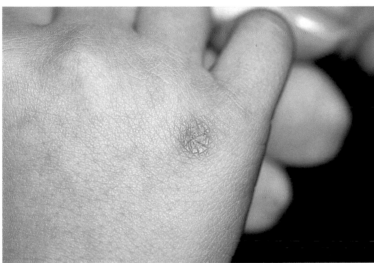

◄ 14.20 Male aged 4 years
He presented in the context of a custody dispute, where both parents made allegations of sexual abuse. The physical signs were consistent with anal abuse. There is a healed circular cigarette burn at the base of the fifth finger. Note the association with sexual abuse.

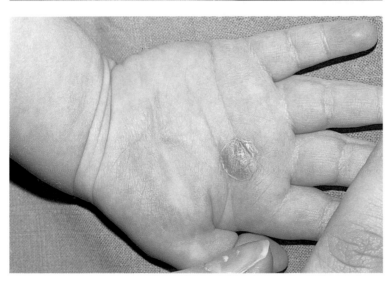

▲ 14.21 Female aged 10 months
The child was examined as part of an investigation in a family where older siblings were failing to thrive and had been severely abused. A healing circular scar is seen in the palm of the right hand, consistent with a cigarette burn. No history was available: this is an unacceptable injury.

▲ 14.22 Male aged 4 months
He was seen by a health visitor with unexplained marks on the face and ear. A cigarette burn is seen in the inner aspect of the left pinna. Two smaller burns, one partially healed, and a small laceration can also be seen. This is a non-accidental injury, and a serious sadistic repeated physical assault.

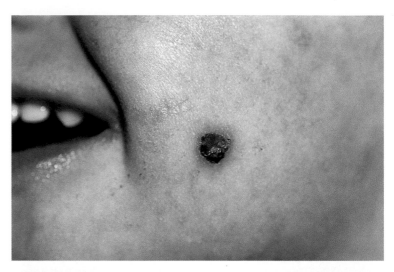

▶ **14.23,** ▶ **14.24 Male aged 5 years**

It was claimed that he had been burned with a match by an unknown assailant. There is a circular, deep burn in the left cheek with charring. This is consistent with a match burn, but it is not acceptable to have no named assailant.

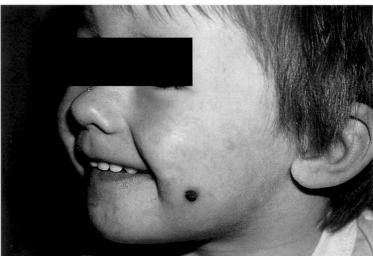

▶ **14.25 Male aged 5 years**

He presented a history that he had been playing out with older boys and he said they had burned him with matches. There are several small burns on the palmar aspect of hands. These injuries are consistent with burns from match ends. The child is from a large, extended, neglected family.

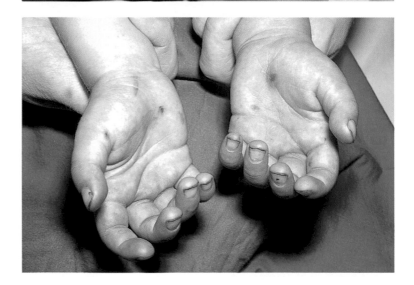

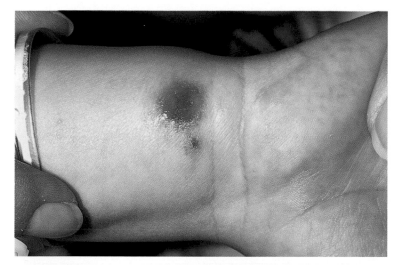

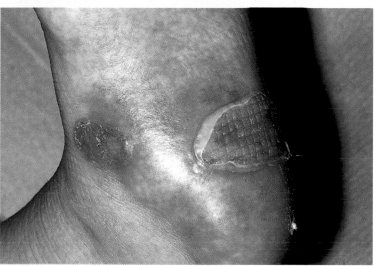

◄ 14.26 and ◄ 14.27 Male aged 5 months
Seen in the A&E Department after the police had raided a party in the parent's house. The child was found to have this old cigarette burn with secondary infection on the wrist and a scald on the foot. The scald was due to hot water; the mother said it had been an accident.

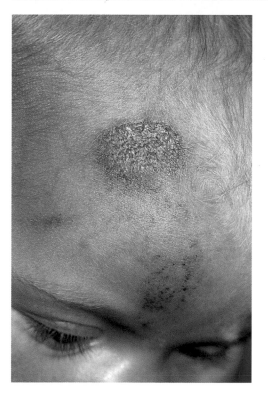

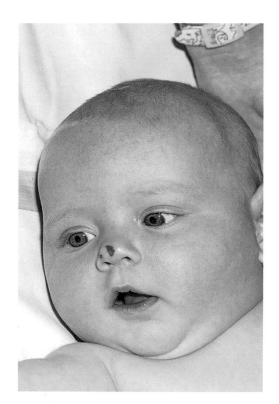

◄ 14.28 Female aged 6 months
She presented to the hospital emergency department with an unexplained lesion on her forehead. She was a healthy, well-nourished, thriving baby with a superficial, circular burn on the prominence of her forehead and a graze above the nose. There was also recent diffuse blue bruising of the buttocks. A carpet burn was diagnosed, and the mother subsequently gave a history of dragging the child across the floor by her feet.

▲ 14.29 Female aged 6 weeks
She had been pulled across the floor by an arm. Superficial skin loss of the nose can be seen. This is a carpet burn. The child also had a spiral fracture of the humerus.

▶ **14.30 Female aged 13 years**
She presented with a history of previous physical abuse by the mother. The girl recalled that her feet had been burned by her mother's partner with whom she had been left as a toddler. Extensive scarring of both feet can be seen, which was an incidental finding. This demonstrates how abuse by burning leaves life-long scars.

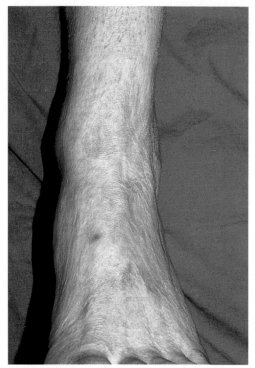

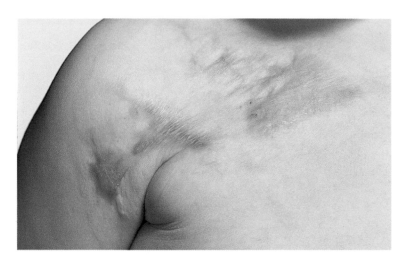

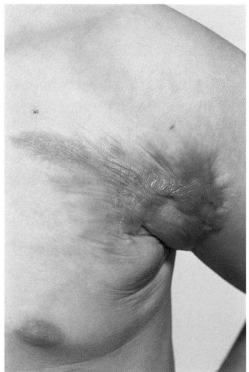

▲ **14.31,** ◀ **14.32 Male aged 4 years**
He was seen because of bruising to his face. Scarring was noted on the anterior chest, and he was claimed to have pulled a cup of hot fluid over himself. There was also a history of physical and sexual abuse involving his mother. The photographs show scarring on the anterior chest and right upper arm with keloid formation. Note the unusual distribution of the injury. Note: Burns are now well recognized to be part of the wider picture of child abuse, particularly child sexual abuse. Accidents also occur more commonly in abusing families.

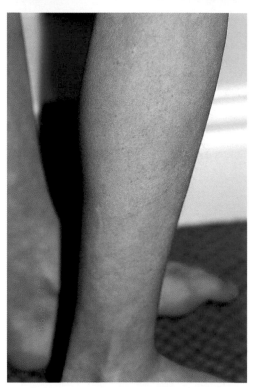

▲ **14.33 Male aged 10 years**
He was referred back for assessment of long-term damage. Scarring was noted.

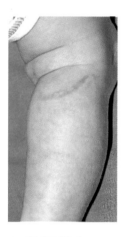

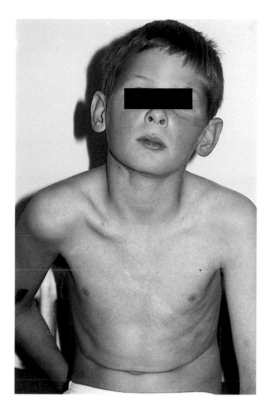

▲ 14.34 Male aged 4 months

This scar was found on the back of the leg of an infant who had presented with subdural haematoma and retinal haemorrhages. The mother said that she thought the injury had been caused by the hot buckle on the car seat although she had only realized that the child was burned later, when the lesion was pointed out to her by a friend. (See also Fig. 9.2.)

◄ 14.35 Male aged 11 years

Scarring was found incidentally after he had been referred because of emotional abuse and failure to thrive. Extensive old scarring can be seen over the centre of the chest. The mother recalled the history of scalding when the child was very young and pulled a cup of tea over himself

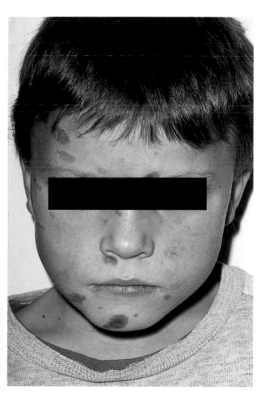

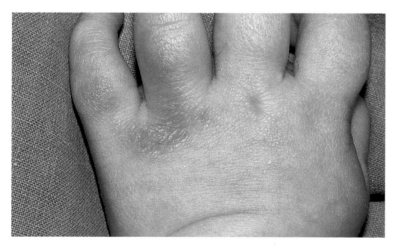

▲ 14.36 Female aged 18 months

She was examined with her siblings because of black eyes, failure to thrive and sexual abuse. A healed burn is seen on the dorsum of the fourth and fifth fingers of the left hand. The appearance is consistent with a healed burn. Note the unusual site for accidental injury. No explanation was offered.

▲ 14.37 Male aged 6 years

He was taken to the hospital emergency department with a history that he had been playing outside with older boys when a canister was thrown on the fire and exploded. There are multiple burns on the face with blistering and skin loss consistent with explosion injury. The child had had previous other minor injuries, and was poorly protected.

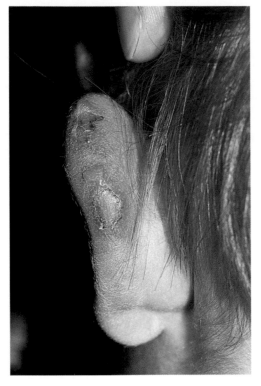

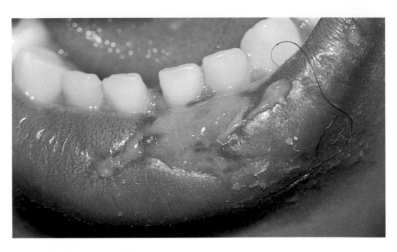

▲ **14.39 Male aged 3 years**

He was brought to the hospital emergency department with a history that he had fallen into the bath. However there were burns on four separate areas, i.e. lower lip, arm, foot and leg. There was previous history of a bilateral wrist drop from a suspension injury. The photograph shows a burn with skin loss and marked swelling of the lower lip. This injury is not explained by the given history. The mother later confirmed abuse by her partner.

▲ **14.38 Male aged 2 years**

The history given was that the child had poked a piece of paper in the fire and set himself on fire. The photograph shows a burn to the left upper ear with skin loss. Singed hair is also seen. These injuries are consistent with flame burn of the ear in a non-protected child.

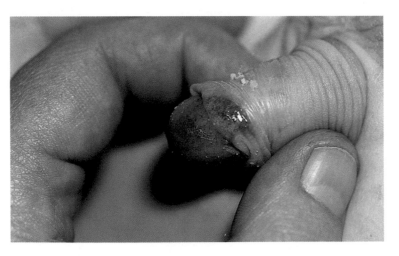

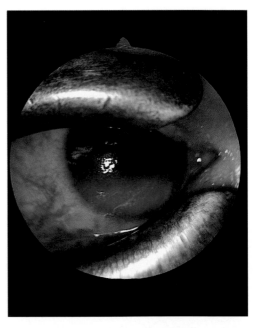

▲ **14.40 Male aged 2 years**

The child was taken to the hospital emergency department with an unexplained lesion on the penis. Recent superficial burn of the foreskin and glans penis can be seen, only visible with the foreskin retracted. This is a contact burn. The parents later said that he must have caught his penis on the radiator while standing micturating in the WC. The diagnosis is sadistic injury.

▲ **14.41 Female aged 2 months**

She was taken to the hospital emergency department with a history that the mother's partner had fallen on the stairs, banging the child's head. Examination showed severe facial bruising, a fractured skull and eye injury. The photograph shows clouding of the cornea and injected conjunctivae. This is an unexplained burn to the eye, in the context of severe physical abuse. The child lost sight in the eye.

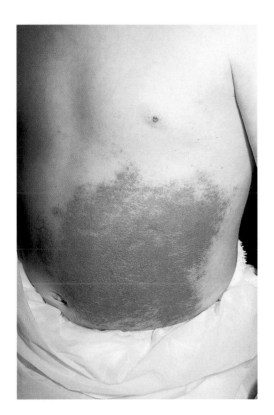

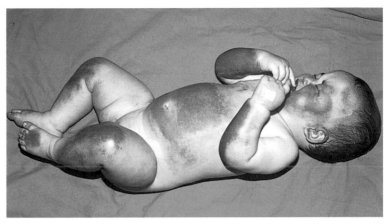

◀ **14.42 Female aged 1 year**

The mother admitted to putting bleach in the bath water. There are extensive superficial chemical burns over the abdomen. This is abuse.

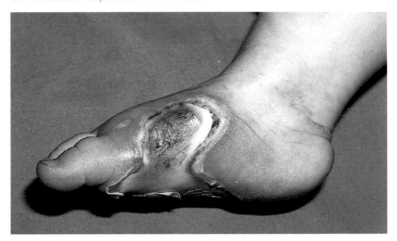

▲ **14.43 Female aged 6 months**

Mother found her 2-year-old child and this infant in the bathroom in the early hours of the morning. The baby was lying face down on the floor and suffered chemical burns due to bleach. The 2-year-old had taken the top off the bottle and poured it on the floor.

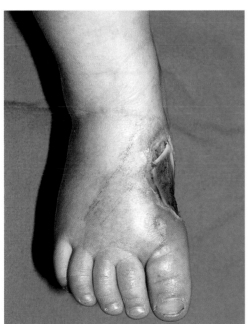

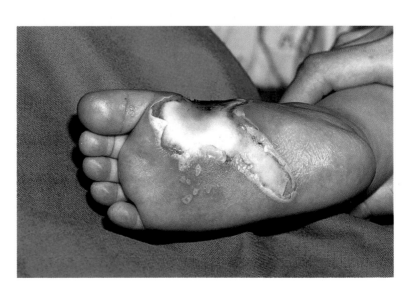

▲ **14.44,** ▲ **14.45,** ▶ **14.46**
Female aged 14 months

Her teenage parents, both heroin addicted, noticed 'smoke and the sound of frying bacon' when the child stood on a cool fire surround. The parents suggested a bare electrical wire had touched the surround and electrocuted the child. There was no evidence of this. There is an extensive, very deep burn of the sole and instep of the right foot. The injury was estimated to be 3–4 days old, and required a skin graft. This is a severe contact burn, not acquired as described.

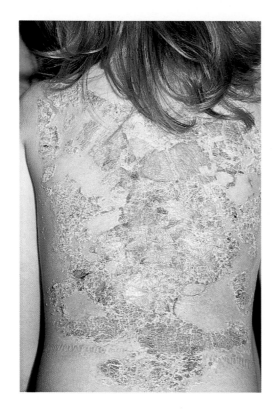

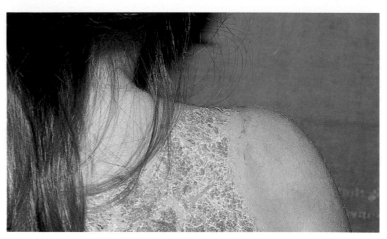

◄ **14.47,** ▲ **14.48 Female aged 3 years**
The child was burned after a family outing to the seaside, where she spent the whole of a sunny day on the beach. The child was taken to the hospital emergency department 1 week later. There is an extensive burn covering the entire back, with blistering and healing evident. The burn is limited to the area usually covered by clothing. The diagnosis of severe sunburn was made after considerable thought, with recognition that the skin underlying clothing had not received any previous tanning and therefore was susceptible to burn.

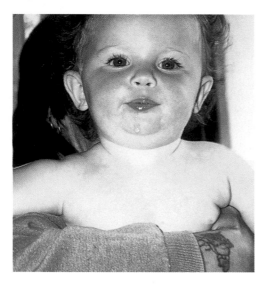

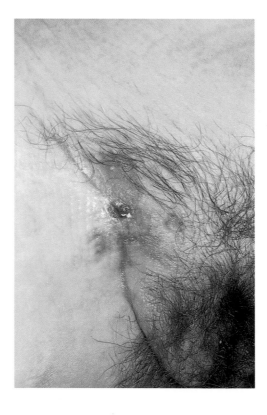

▲ **14.49 Female aged 15 months**
She was left in a buggy all day outside a public house. Police officers going on duty noticed her and saw her again as they went off duty. They were incensed at the poor care of this child, who had sunburn.

◄ **14.50 Female aged 13 years**
The child, with spina bifida and impaired sensation in lower limbs, presented with a sudden and unexplained breakdown of 'bedsore in right groin'. There is an area of ulceration resembling a burn in the middle of healed, reddened skin following an earlier bedsore. This is a chemical burn due to antiseptic cream on previously injured skin.

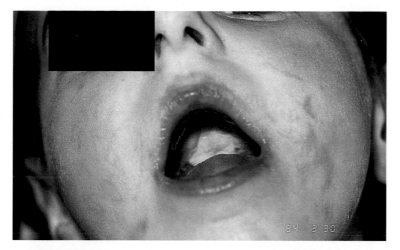

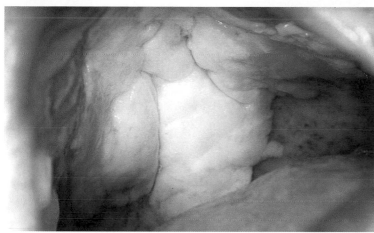

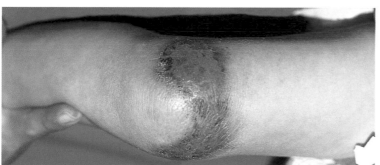

◀ 14.51, ◀ 14.52 Female aged 4 years

The child was in foster care because of a failure to thrive, emotional abuse and sexual abuse. The foster mother stated that the child had picked up a hot drink and had thus burned her mouth. Investigation revealed an extensive slough across the palate, and red marks on the cheek and above the upper lip. The indications are that the child has probably been forcibly fed hot food.

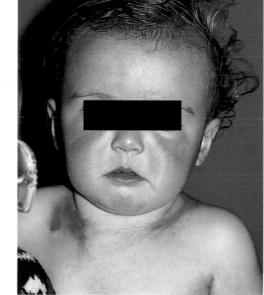

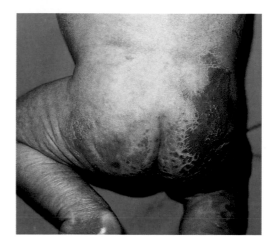

▲ 14.53, ▲ 14.54 Female aged 2 years

Child was referred to the A&E Department by the health visitor because of unexplained burns. The mother declared that the injuries were not burns but were totally unexplained. The lesion on the knee is an old healed burn, and the burn round the neck is more recent. These injuries were unexplained. The mother had mental health problems and the father was a Schedule 1 offender.

▶ 14.55 Male aged 1 month

He was referred because of poor weight gain and a skin rash. There is severe failure to thrive and an extensive ammoniacal burn. The diagnosis is a severe chemical burn due to neglect.

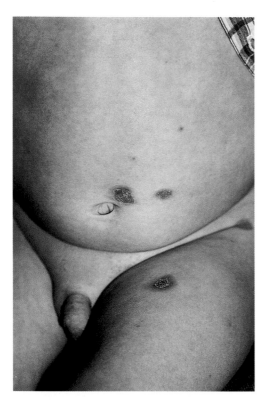

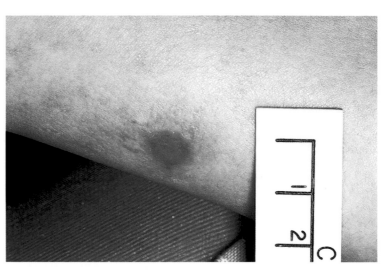

▲ **14.57 Male aged 4 years**
He was seen in nursery with an injury to the left forearm thought to be a cigarette burn. The photograph shows a circular lesion with skin loss and blistering (scale in centimetres). The diagnosis is impetigo. (Note: this was an early impetigenous lesion, which healed without scarring. If this lesion had been a cigarette burn it would have almost inevitably healed with scarring.)

▲ **14.56 Male aged 3 years**
He presented in day nursery with unexplained lesions on the abdomen and thigh. Circular red lesions with crusting can be seen, and small satellite lesions are visible. The diagnosis is impetigo.

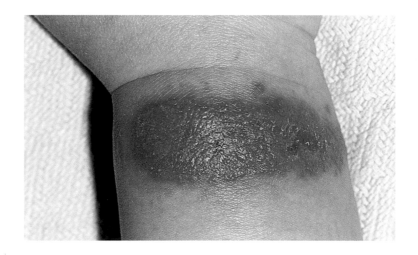

▶ **14.58 Male aged 6 months**
He had been wearing a hospital name band. A reddened swollen area with superficial skin loss is seen in an area in contact with the hand. Note the similarity to a contact burn.

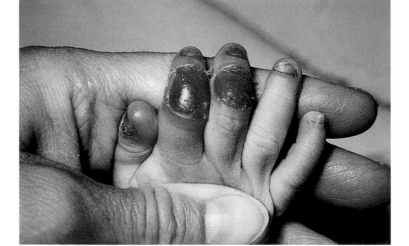

▶ **14.59 Neonates**
Presented with unexplained blistering of the skin. The diagnosis is epidermolysis bullosa.

Chapter 15

Differential Diagnosis of Physical Abuse

In lesions which appear to be injuries consider:
- abuse;
- accident;
- neglect;
- disease.

Conditions which may mimic physical abuse or injury
Bruises
- Bleeding disorders, e.g. ITP, haemophilia, haemorrhagic disease of newborn, platelet disorder infection, vasculitis, meningococcal septicaemia, disseminated intravascular coagulation, Henoch–Schönlein disease. See page 182 Dorlands Henoch–Schölein
- Skin conditions – Ehlers–Danlos syndrome, erythema nodosum, mongolian blue spots, capillary haemangioma, café au lait spots, prominent veins.
- Allergic periorbital swelling.
- Dye, ink or paint.

NB bleeding disorders and abuse may coexist.

Fractures
- Normal variant, pseudofracture, e.g. aberrant skull suture, symmetrical periosteal reaction.
- Birth trauma.
- Osteogenesis imperfecta.
- Osteoporosis.
- Copper deficiency.
- Osteomyelitis.
- Congenital syphilis.
- Caffey's disease.
- Rickets.
- Scurvy, vitamin A intoxication.

Osteogenesis imperfecta has several types
- Type I – autosomal dominant associated with blue sclerae.
- Type II – very severe, multiple fractures at birth and early death.
- Type III – similar to type II, but less severe. Cortical thickening, tendency to fracture. This is unlikely to cause confusion in terms of accident, abuse or organic disease.
- Type IV – Rare autosomal dominant with occasional mutations. Osteoporosis ±. Sclerae not blue.

Burns
- Infection – impetigo irregular, golden crusts, tend to spread, prompt response to antibiotics.
- Staphylococcal scalded skin syndrome – erythematous, painful lesions, positive Nikolsky's sign.
- Nappy rash, with or without infection.
- Photodermatitis – sensitization by contact with certain plant/fruit substances. Burn produced by light.
- Folk medicine practice – cupping, coin rubbing or rolling – red lesions, erythema, bruises. Middle East, Latin America, S.E. Asia, E. European.
- Fixed drug eruption – purple/red plaque clearly demarcated border in same site repeatedly follows drug ingestion.

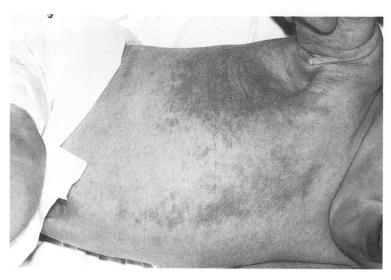

▲ **15.1 Neonate**
Purple discoloration on the chest was noted at birth. This is a port wine stain.

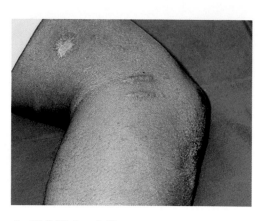

▲ **15.2 Male adult**
Incision inflicted on outer aspect of left forearm. These marks were inflicted to protect against hepatitis and resulted in the keloid scar. The patient was from North Africa.

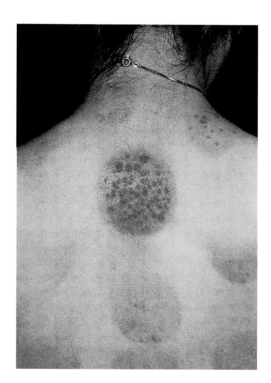

▲ **15.3 Female aged 16 years**
She was referred because of unusual lesions on her back. Circular lesions can be seen across the back with numerous purpura, due to cupping.

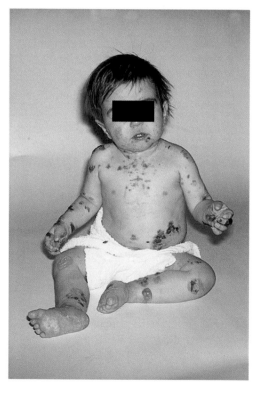

▲ **15.4 Male aged 18 months**
The child was anonymously reported to a child welfare charity as being battered. There are multiple bullous lesions in various stages of healing. This is a known case of epidermolysis bullosa.

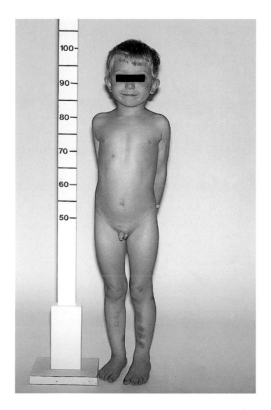
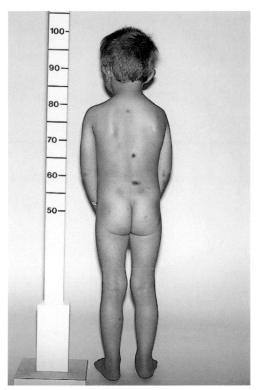
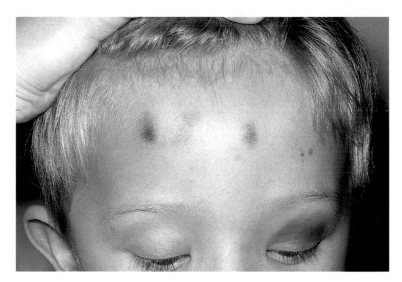
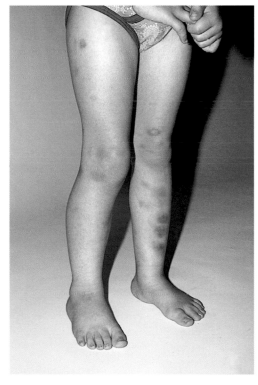

▲ **15.5,** ▲ **15.6,** ▲ **15.7,** ▶ **15.8 Male aged 5 years**
The child was referred by his doctor because of concern about physical abuse. There is extensive large purple bruising in a well-cared for child. The diagnosis is idiopathic thrombocytopenic purpura.

▶ **15.9 Male aged 2 years**
The child was referred to the paediatrician because of a swollen, bruised cheek. The photograph shows a very swollen left cheek with bruising at the corner of the mouth and a crusted lesion on the pinna. The medical opinion was haemophilia and impetigo. There was also physical abuse in this family and the children were all later put on the Child Protection Register.

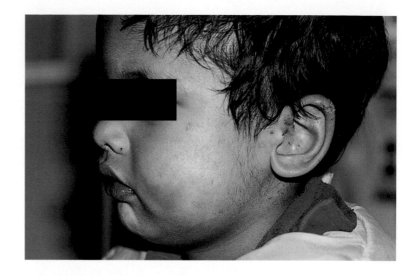

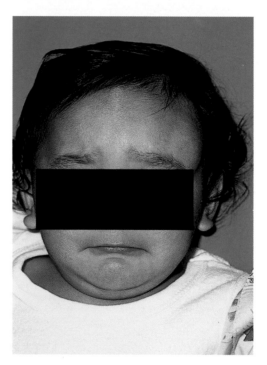

▶ **15.10 Female aged 9 months**
Infant presented with swelling on the left side of the forehead. On further investigation this had been present from birth.

▶ **15.11 Female aged 7 months**
Admitted after a severe shaking injury. Noted to have mongolian blue spots on the black.

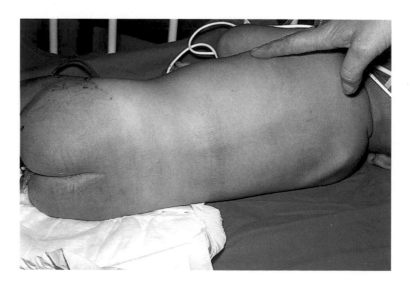

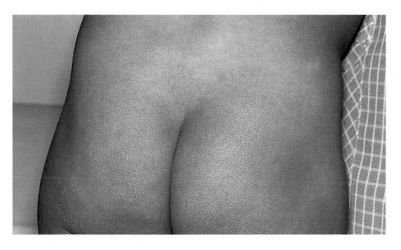

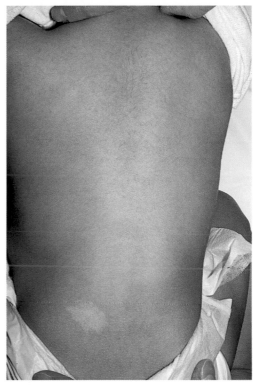

▲ **15.12,** ▶ **15.13 Female aged 2 years**
The child was referred from day nursery because of bruising on her back. Scattered mongolian blue spots are seen over the back and buttocks. A depigmented area is also seen on the lower back (Fig. 15.13).

▶ **15.14 Female aged 3 years**
Child was referred because of a burn on her hand. She has a white mother and Asian father. The photograph shows a mongolian blue spot.

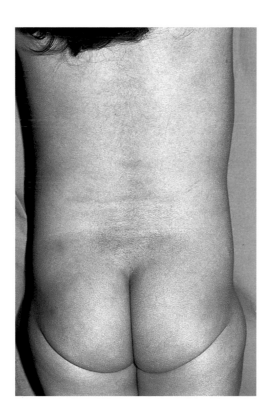

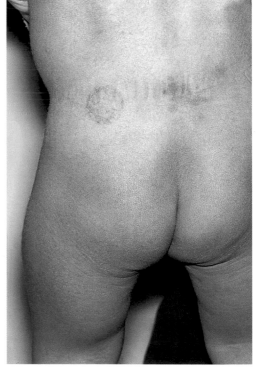

▲ **15.15 Male aged 5 years**
The child was referred after his foster mother said she had bitten him. A circular lesion is seen on the left lower back with flaking skin. A mongolian blue spot is also seen on the sacrum. The medical opinion was a fungal infection and mongolian blue spot.

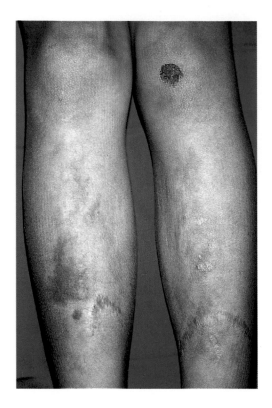

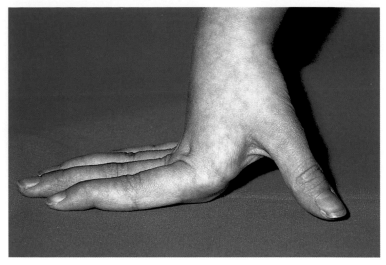

◀ 15.16, ▲ 15.17 Female aged 16 years
Ehlers–Danlos syndrome in a teenage girl showing characteristic scarring and bruising. This condition is also associated with marked hypotonia and hyperextensible joints. There may be some bone fragilitiy.

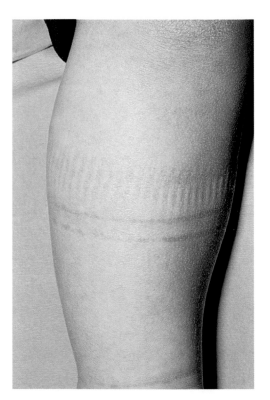

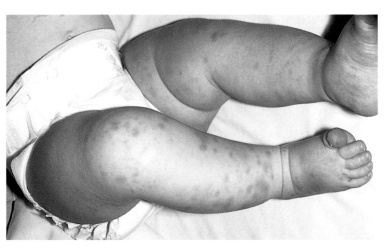

▲ 15.19 Female aged 6 months
Child was referred to hospital by her doctor because of febrile illness. The photograph shows extensive purpuric marks on the legs, due to meningococcal meningitis.

▲ 15.18 Male aged 7 years
The child was referred because of unexplained red marks around his lower leg. Linear erythematous parallel marks are seen below marks caused by elastic in socks. The marks were due to tapes applied too tightly to keep the socks up.

▶ **15.20 Female aged 3 months**
Child was seen in the clinic after she had become involved in a fight between her parents. The strawberry naevus shown was an incidental finding.

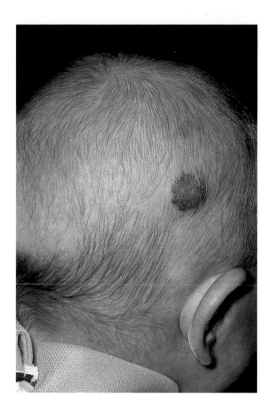

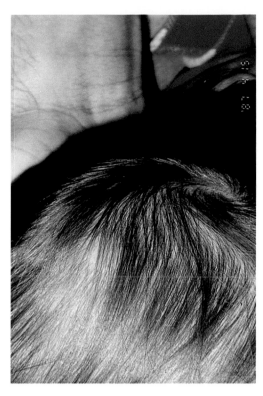

▲ **15.21 Male aged 2 years**
Raised lesion on scalp in infant, yellow in colour. Diagnosis: juvenile xanthogranuloma.

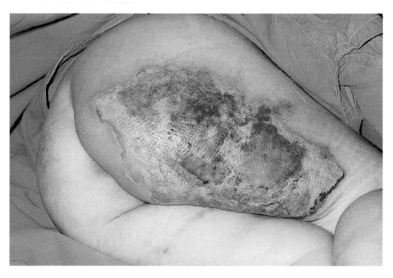

▲ **15.22 Female aged 4 years**
Child was referred by her doctor because of a rapidly spreading lesion on the buttock. This was diagnosed as a staphylococcal infection resembling a burn.

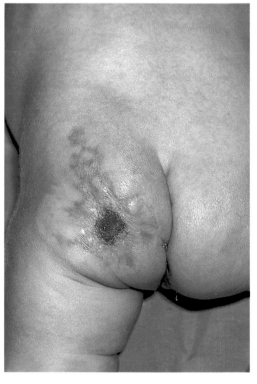

▲ **15.23 Female aged 2 months**
The photograph shows a healing lesion on the left buttock. This lesion had been present at birth and subsequently healed. It superficially looks like a healing burn. The diagnosis is congenital abnormality.

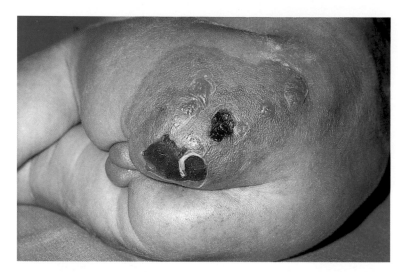

◄ 15.24 Female neonate
The photograph shows a lesion on the buttocks which was present at birth and resembles a burn. This is a congenital abnormality.

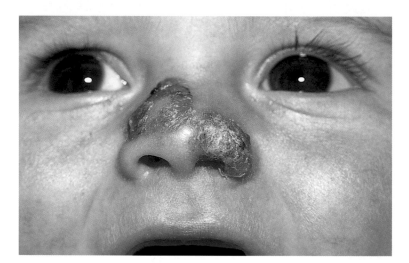

◄ 15.25 Male aged 6 months
Infant with severe and healing impetigo of nose.

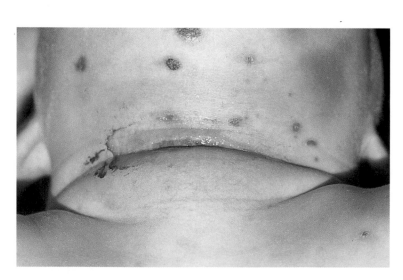

▲ 15.26 Male aged 12 months
Infant with infected skin in neck folds and circular lesions secondary to impetigo. Note bruise on left jaw in characteristic position for physical abuse.

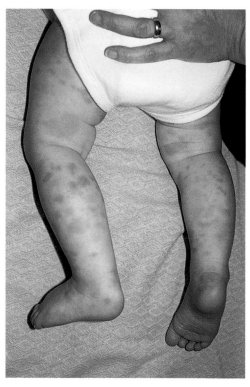

▲ 15.27 Female aged 10 months
Doctor referred child to hospital with extensive bruising on legs. The scattered bruises are due to Henoch–Schönlein purpura.

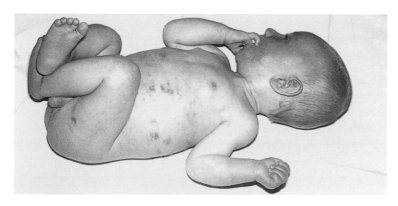

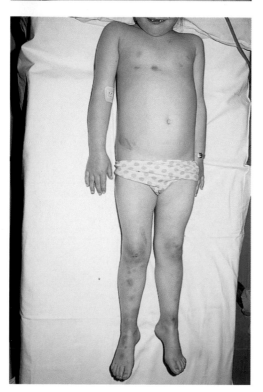

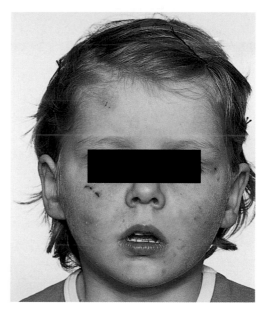

◀ 15.28 Male aged 6 weeks
Child was referred as a possible physical abuse victim. The diagnosis is extensive scabies.

▲ 15.29 Male aged 8 years
Child was referred by social services because of a number of bruises on his face and body. The diagnosis was idiopathic thrombocytopenic purpura. However, this boy also had scratch marks on his face allegedly because of fighting with his brothers. The whole family was neglected.

◀ 15.30, ◀ 15.31, ▶ 15.32 Female aged 5 years
Child was referred because of possible physical abuse in a family where the children were already on the Child Protection Register. The photographs show multiple bruises in unusual sites, and several bruises of unusual severity. The diagnosis is idiopathic thrombocytopenic purpura in a child known to have been previously physically abused.

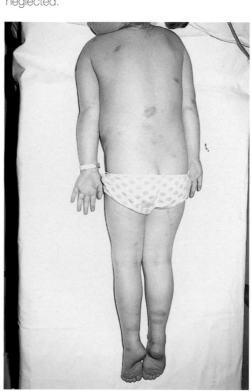

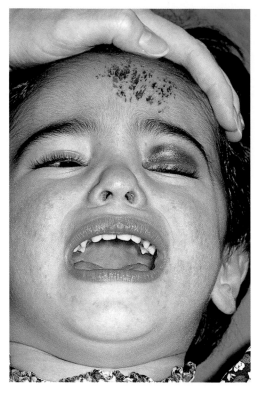

▲ 15.33 Female aged 3 years
Child presented in the A&E Department with an unexplained black eye and graze to the forehead. The graze was probably due to a simple fall but the penetrating injury of the orbit is unexplained.

▶ 15.34 Female aged 5 years
Bruising on shins of a pre-schooler. She claimed her older brother was kicking her.

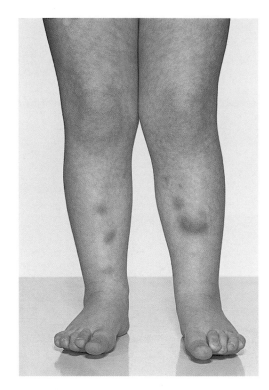

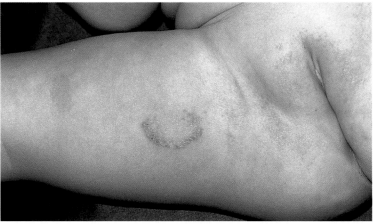

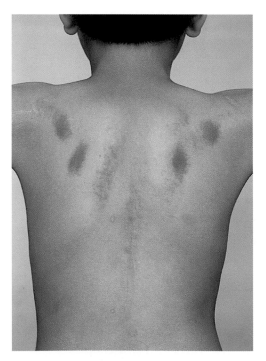

▲ 15.35 Male aged 8 years
Child was referred because of unusual markings on his back. Four roughly oval linear haemorrhagic areas are seen on the upper back. These lesions are due to coil rubbing.

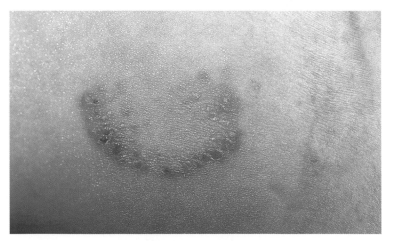

▲ 15.36, ▲ 15.37 Female aged 6 months
Child was referred by her nursery because of a possible bite. A semicircular raised lesion with some scaling is seen, caused by seborrhoeic eczema.

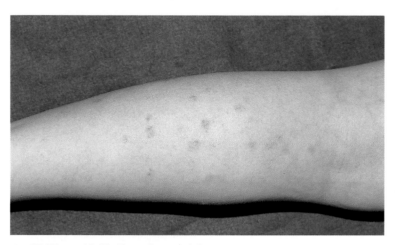
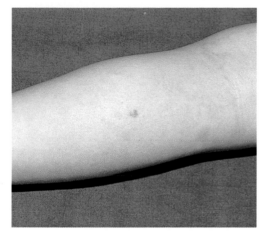

▲ **15.38,** ▲ **15.39 Female aged 6 years**
Child was referred by her doctor because of rectal bleeding. Crops of lesions are seen on the back of the lower leg and small irregular scaly lesions on the back of the leg. This is a fictitious rash caused by the mother scratching the skin in a child with mild eczema. The child was also sexually abused, probably by her mother.

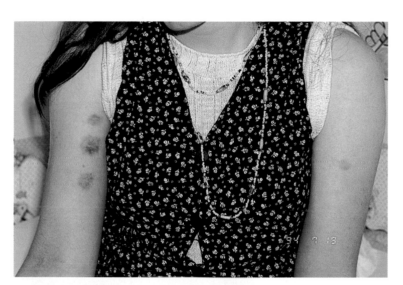

◄ **15.40 Female aged 12 years**
She was referred because of bruising on her upper arm. A vertical row of three bruises on the inner aspect of the right upper arm and one bruise on the anterior aspect of the left upper arm are seen. The diagnosis is self-inflicted bruises. This girl was being sexually abused.

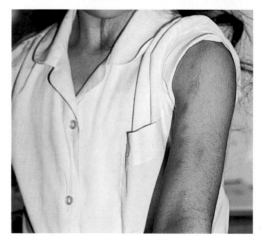

◄ **15.41,** ► **15.42 Female aged 9 years**
Child was referred because of unusual lesions on her left upper arm. There are several lesions on the inner and anterior aspect of the left upper arm and abrasions with some bruising. These are self-inflicted injuries. Figure 15.42 shows her drawings to be those of an emotionally disturbed child.

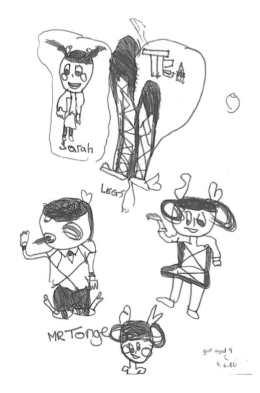

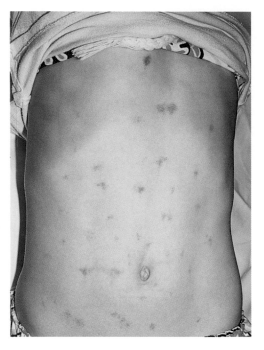

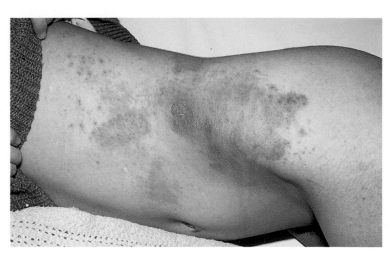

▲ 15.44 Female aged 13 years

She was referred because of an unexplained rash on her abdomen and upper thigh. The girl was known to have been sexually abused for several years previously. This is an extensive erythematous rash with some scaling, which is self-inflicted. This girl has become very distressed after recent further sexual assault at her special school.

▲ 15.43 Female aged 9 years

Child was referred because of a rash on her abdomen. There are paired and single lesions over the anterior chest and abdomen with the appearance of small abrasions. The diagnosis is self-inflicted injury. This child's father was a chronic alcoholic.

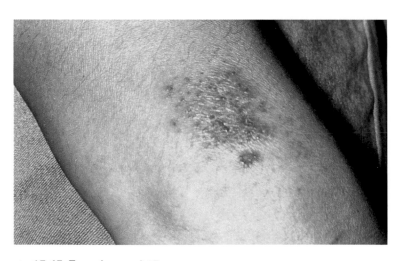

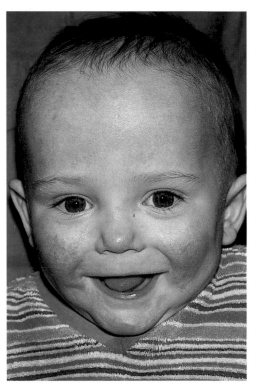

▲ 15.45 Female aged 15 years

Area of erythema and small vesicles secondary to nickel sensitivity in a teenage girl.

▲ 15.46 Male aged 1 year

He has an erythematous rash of the forehead and cheeks due to starch in hospital bedding.

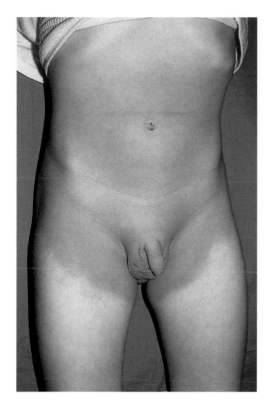

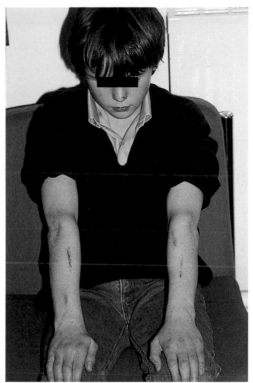

◀ **15.48 Male aged 13 years**
He was referred because of an unusual rash on his forearms, and because he was sexually abusing other children. Linear scratches are seen on the outer aspect of both forearms, which were self-inflicted. The boy was also being sexually abused by an uncle.

▲ **15.47 Male aged 8 years**
He was referred because of a rash possibly due to physical abuse. The photograph shows a generalized erythematous rash over the abdomen and upper thighs, which remains unexplained.

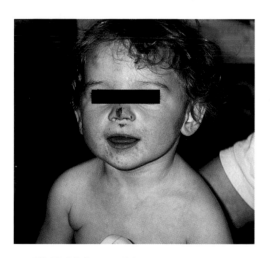

15.50 Male
Severely handicapped and hyperactive boy who jumped into his major buggy and caught his ear in the mechanism. Was this an accidental injury?

▲ **15.49 Male aged 2 years**
Child who fell on gravel path causing abrasion to nose.

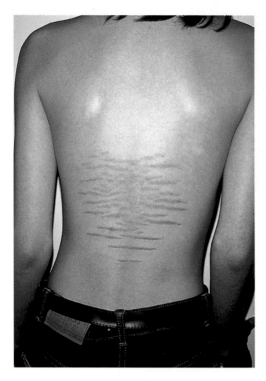

▲ **15.51 Female aged 14 years**
Teeange girl in growth spurt with horizontal striae densa. Confusion with scarring from beating with flex or whip.

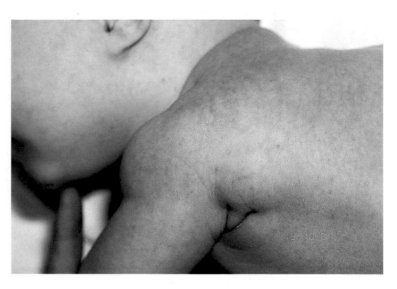

▲ **15.52 Female aged 5 months**
Child was referred from her nursery with a possible bruise in the left axilla. The diagnosis is haemangioma.

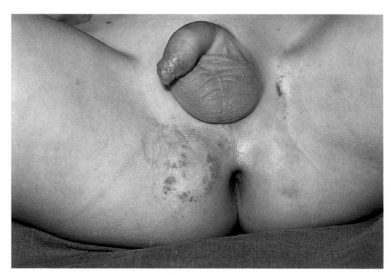

▲ **15.53 Male aged 15 months**
He was referred because of a 'bruise' seen at day nursery. The diagnosis is haemangioma.

SECTION 3

NEGLECT

Chapter 16

Neglect

Neglect is insidious. Recognition is a start.
Working Together 2000 defines neglect as:

> ...the persistent failure to meet a child's basic physical and/or psychological needs, likely to result in the serious impairment of the child's health or development. It may involve a parent or carer failing to provide adequate food, shelter and clothing, failing to protect the child from physical harm or danger, or the failure to ensure access to appropriate medical care or treatment. It may also include neglect of, or unresponsiveness to, a child's basic emotional needs.

Children at risk include:
1. Children with a disability – physical and sensory, learning problems.
2. Children who have parents with disability – learning, physical, sensory, psychiatric disorder.
3. Children who live in conditions of severe social disadvantage.
4. Children in large families with poor networks of support and poverty.

A paediatrician may assist in the multi-agency assessment by looking at the child in some detail (Fig. 16.1).

Physical appearance

◆ Dirty clothes, body, hair matted or thin, dirty nails, odour, dental caries, chronic infestation (head lice).
◆ Examination may reveal chronic nappy rash, infected sores (especially in skin folds), untreated squint, perforated eardrums, thin limbs, wasted buttocks, protruberant abdomen, cold injury (red, swollen extremities).
◆ Growth pattern is often of a long-term suboptimal pattern and assessment includes
  – a measure of the child's height, weight, mid-upper arm circumference, head circumference;
  – recording the measurements and plotting on standardized growth charts;
  – finding any previous measurements to assess growth rate.

Denial of problems by parents (may have learning problems)	History from child – bullied, no friends, aggressive	'Attention-seeking' Concern by nursery school of standard of care
Physical symptoms, e.g. pain from dental caries	Poor physical condition – dirty, thin hair, nappy rash	'Growth – stunted/ fails to reach potential height
Development delayed, e.g. language, social skills	Poor compliance with treatment, e.g. asthma	Increased risk of accidents: RTA, fire, drowning
Supportive network, i.e. with family and friends – little effect as share similar problems	Poverty with poor housing, diet, parents with poor health (physical and mental), little education	Large number of involved professionals – health visitor, school nurse, social worker, home care, housing, GP, paediatrician, etc.

◀ **Fig. 16.1**
The 'jigsaw' in the diagnosis of neglect

- There may be signs of physical and/or child sexual abuse
- Development may be globally delayed:
  - motor skills may be immature and the child is clumsy;
  - language is characteristically delayed;
  - social skills have not been acquired.
- Behaviour in the clinic may be quiet and apathetic (more usual in infancy) to the restless, flitting pre-schooler who is distractible, seeks attention and has frequent tantrums. Play is immature and lacks imagination, being typically more destructive than showing attention and perseverance to the task.

Information should be sought from the carers and nursery staff and others involved in the child's care.

Note: the severely neglected child may be clumsy, have a neglected squint, little language, few pencil skills, immature peer and adult relationships, visual and auditory attention poorly developed, distractible, over-active/apathetic, nursery/school attendance poor. Social skills like eating with implements, toilet training, dressing, nose-blowing may not have been taught.

- Medical surveillance – immunization, developmental checks, hearing and vision assessments: fails to attend.
- Medical appointments – asthma, convulsions missed – poor compliance with appointments and therapy.

The paediatrician should work closely with the primary care team, Social Services Department, and nursery, to minimize the consequences of the neglect but also have an opinion as to whether the parenting is 'good enough'.

The general characteristics of neglect

- A long history of intercurrent illness, accidents (in the home and on road/canal), ingestions, and repeated hospital admissions.
- Medical, education and social neglect.

Documentation of the effects of neglect

- on the physical appearance of the child;
- on growth;
- on development;
- on emotional and behavioural history – and observation in clinic.

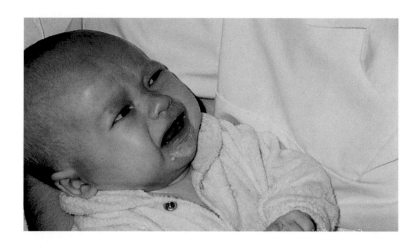

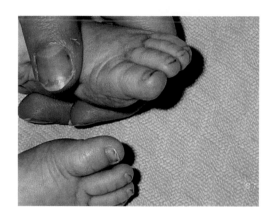

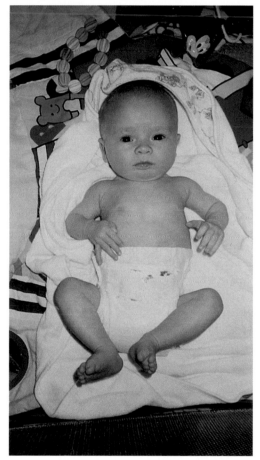

▲ **16.1,** ▲ **16.2,** ▶ **16.3 Female aged 4 months**

Infant with a very worried expression; pallid and hungry. Dirty toenails indicate poor grooming in infancy and are a good sign of neglect. Note improved condition during a brief admission to hospital but worried expression remains (Fig. 16.3).

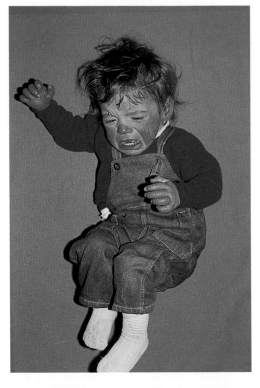
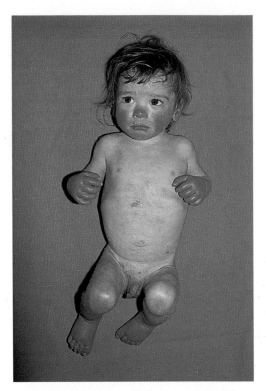
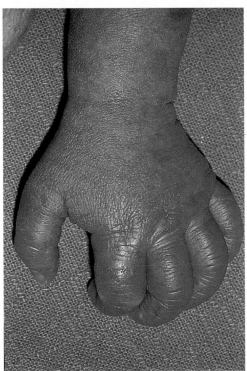
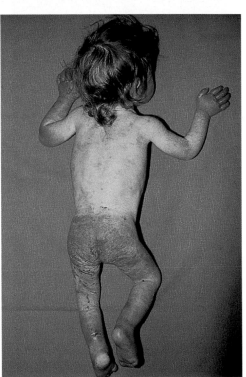

▲ ▲ ▲ ▲ **16.4–16.7 Male aged 22 months**

The social worker and paediatrician made a home visit after the family had failed to attend the clinic. The older child (see Figs 16.14–16.19) had been at nursery that day. Professional concern was around the failure to thrive and neglect. A previous child who was very underweight had died from sudden infant death syndrome at 6 months. The father had an addiction to gambling. Figure. 16.4 shows a small, unkempt child, in a flexed position, with red swollen hands and straggly hair. Note that the same posture is maintained when undressed (Fig. 16.5). Figure. 16.6 shows a swollen red oedematous hand, cold to the touch (deprivation hands and feet remain red and swollen even after heating up). Figure. 16.7 shows how the child is emaciated; note the wasted buttocks and severe chronic nappy rash extending down the posterior part of the leg. Swollen lower legs are also seen.

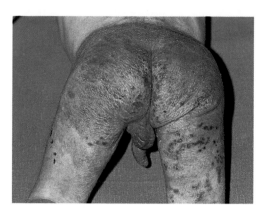

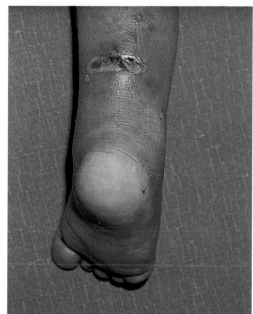

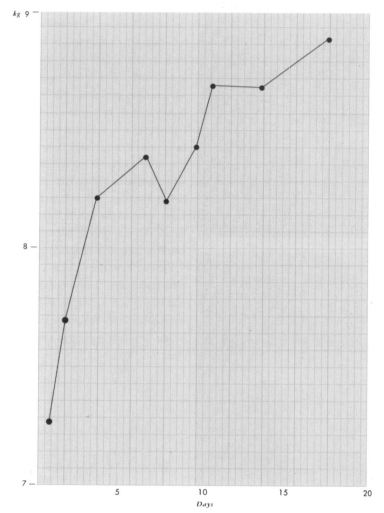

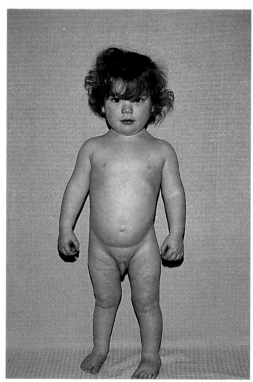

▲ **16.8,** ▲ **16.9,** ▲ **16.10,** ▲ **16.11 Male aged 22 months**

The same child as in Figs 16.4–16.7. Note the chronicity of the nappy rash (Fig. 16.8). An old ulcerated cold injury is seen in Fig. 16.9. Note the pallor of the heel, which was extremely cold to the touch. There was rapid weight gain in hospital over a period of 2–3 weeks (Fig. 16.10). Figure. 16.11 shows the same child a year later after being in foster care.

▶ **16.12 Male aged 22 months**
Growth chart (height) to 10 years of child in
Figs 16.4–16.11.

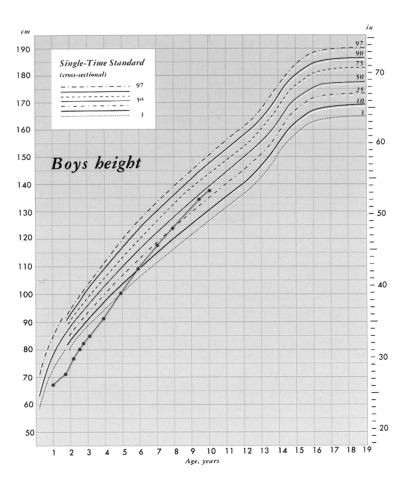

▶ **16.13 Male aged 22 months**
Growth chart (weight) to 10 years of child in
Figs 16.4–16.11.

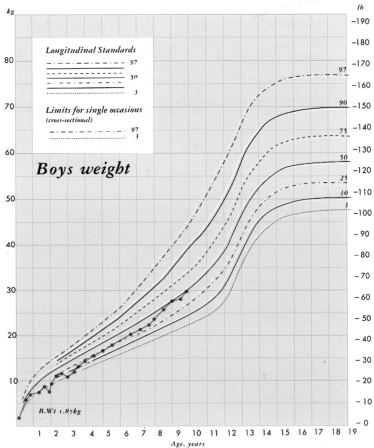

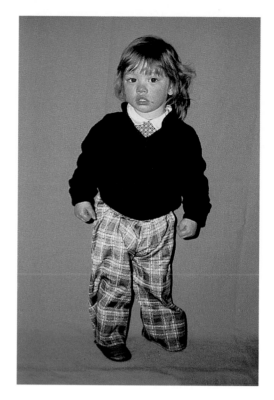
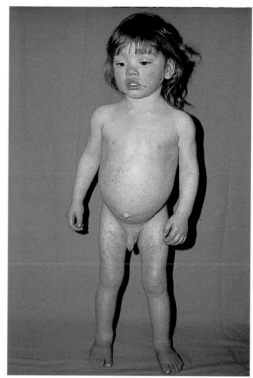
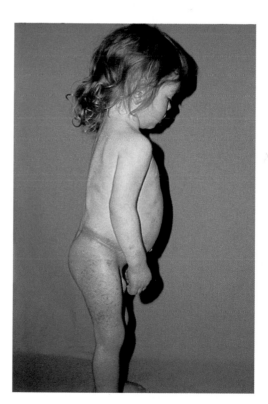
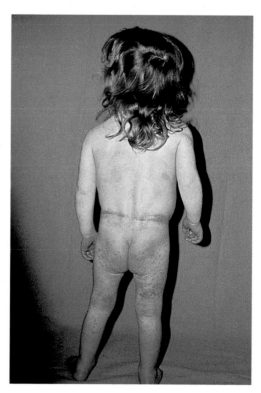

▲ **16.14–16.19 Male aged 2 years and 10 months (continued)**

The older sibling of the child in Figs 16.4–16.13. He had been at day nursery the day these pictures were taken. The photographs show a scruffy child with long hair, and over-size clothes concealing malnutrition. He has frozen body posture with watchfulness and clenched hands. There is gaze avoidance, and a swollen abdomen with very thin arms and legs. Note the passivity, and gross malnutrition. Nappy rash is evident, and red swollen feet are seen with early ulceration (p.198, Fig. 16.18). There was no weight gain during 3 weeks in hospital (p.198, Fig. 16.19).

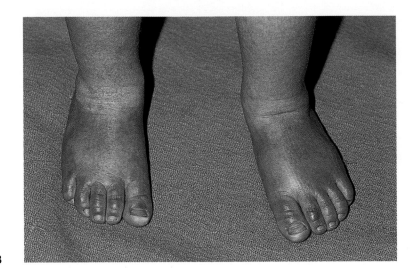

▶ **16.18**

▶ **16.19**

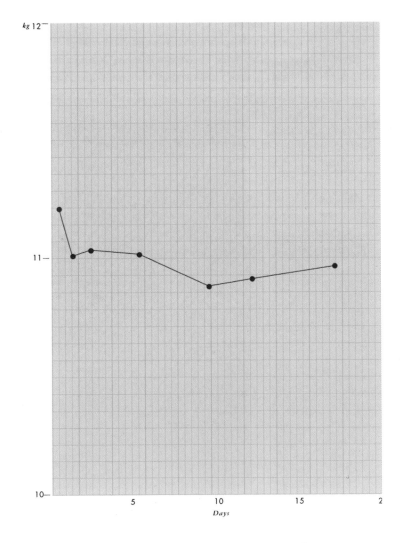

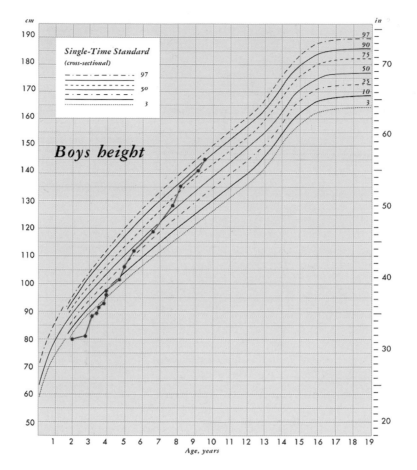

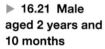

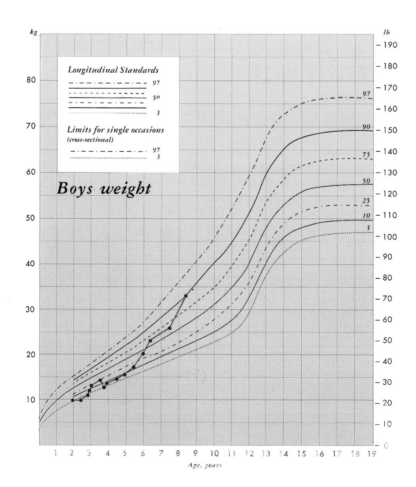

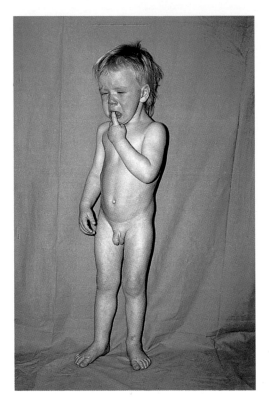

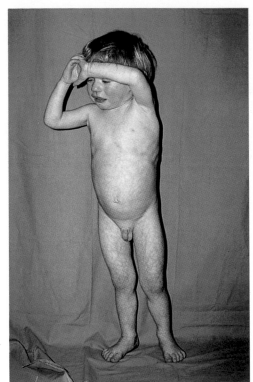

▲ 16.22, ▲ 16.23, ▶ 16.24 **Three brothers aged 2 years 4 months, 3 years 5 months and 4 years 8 months (a further two siblings were not photographed)**

There was longstanding concern about neglect and failure to thrive. All five children were found in the house alone, the house was extremely dirty and the children were playing in dog excrement. These photographs were taken a week after admission to foster care. Younger children were unhappy and fearful in the clinic, and sat crying, refusing to play. The youngest child (top left) is stunted with infantile proportions, masking a degree of malnutrition. The middle child adopted a fearful posture (top right). He has thin arms, protuberant abdomen and a reticular skin pattern on the legs. The oldest child is smiling, passive and wishing to please (bottom right). He is seen to be thin. All the children in this family had developmental delay and in particular poor language development.

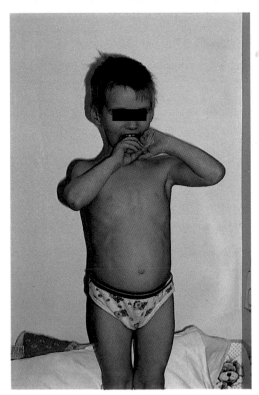

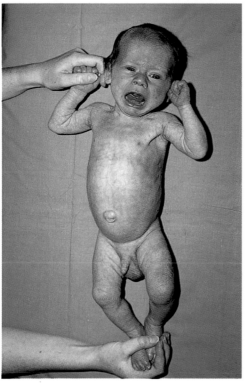
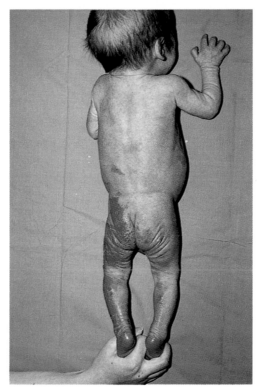
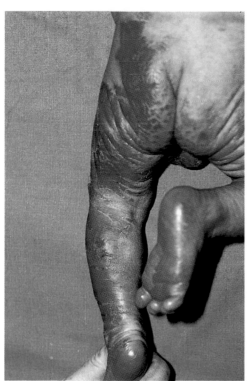
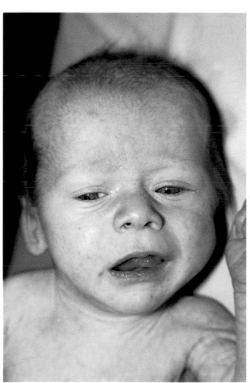

▲ 16.25, ▲ 16.26, ▲ 16.27, ▲ 16.28 **Male aged 4 weeks**
He was the fifth child in a family living in a house without gas or electricity in extreme poverty.
The mother who was aged 22 years had been refused a termination. The photographs show a pale,
emaciated, worried baby giving an appearance of rooting. Loose skin folds around the neck and
upper arm are seen. There is a distended abdomen, extensive nappy rash and deprivation hands
and feet. This baby put on weight very rapidly in hospital. (Note: infants who are failing to thrive and
have not yet given up the attempt to find food will usually put on weight very rapidly in hospital. The
older the child the less certain that the weight gain will be rapid in the early stages. If the child does
receive good care almost all children will then grow in spite of severe emotional deprivation in the
longer term.)

▶ **16.29 Male aged 3 years**
The brother of the child in Figs 16.25–16.28. A large head and short limbs of stunted growth are seen. He is emaciated, and has flexed posture. He was also developmentally delayed.

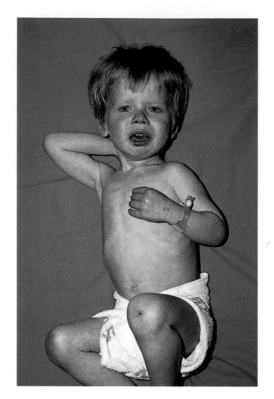

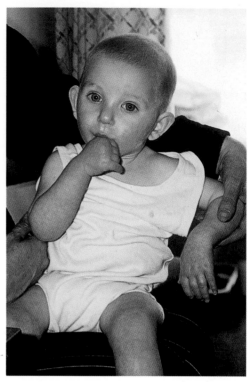

▲ **16.30 Male aged 2 years**
Apathetic day-dreaming boy. He is disinterested in his surroundings with very sad expression, and note the mottled arms and legs associated with cold and inactivity. His mother had recently begun to take heroin regularly.

▶ **16.31 Male aged 10 months**
He was followed up following skull fracture aged 3 months, having missed several appointments. The photograph shows a watchful, emaciated baby. Note the flexed posture and immobility. He gained weight rapidly in hospital.

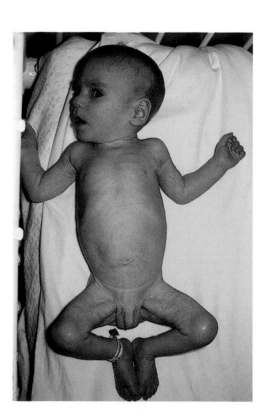

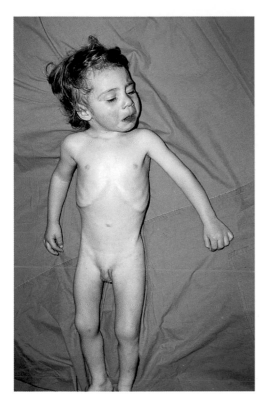 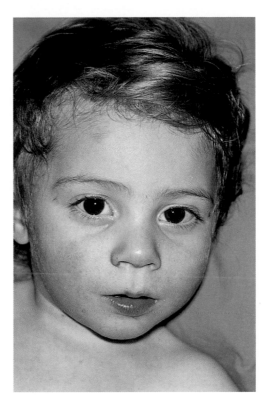

▲ 16.32, ▲ 16.33 Male aged 2 years
Child was referred by his doctor because of poor growth. The family was known to be impoverished and the mother had poorly controlled epilepsy. The photographs show a passive, emaciated child with anxious facies. Note that unless this child were to be undressed he does not look particularly thin.

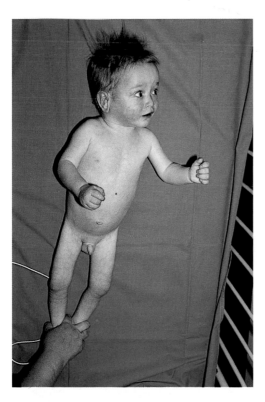 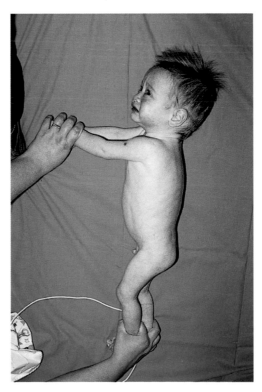

▲ 16.34, ▲ 16.35 Male aged 9 months
He was referred to hospital because of bronchiolitis. His mother said that she did not like this child who was one of twins. The photographs show a watchful, interested child, but with a distended abdomen. This child had also been previously physically abused, and his older siblings had been sexually abused.

▶ **16.36,** ▶ **16.37**
Male aged 2 years
His older siblings were found to have been sexually abused and taken into care. This child remained with his emotionally disturbed mother while his father was in prison. His nutrition was adequate but note the flexed posture. He also had severe bleeding nappy rash, and was developmentally delayed.

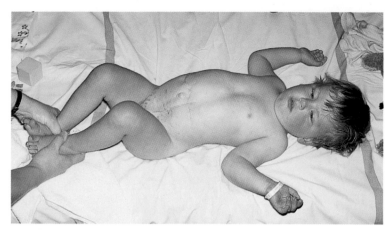

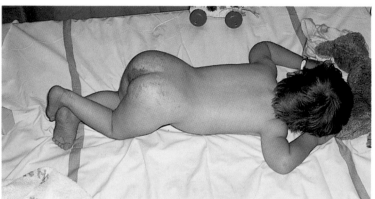

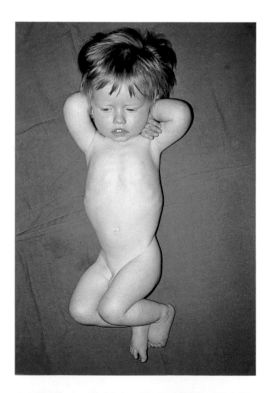
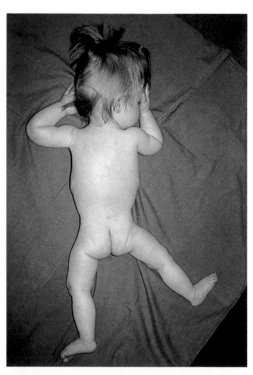

▲ **16.38,** ▲ **16.39,** ▶ **16.40 Male aged 15 months**
The child was referred by the health visitor because of concern about poor weight gain. He had very uncooperative parents, and in particular an angry father who was threatening towards all professionals. The child was very passive and still. The photographs show a stunted child, malnourished with wasted buttocks. A bald patch is seen on the occiput (Fig. 16.40), caused by being left for long periods alone in his cot. The child was fostered for several months before being returned home. He subsequently had language delay and behavioural difficulties.

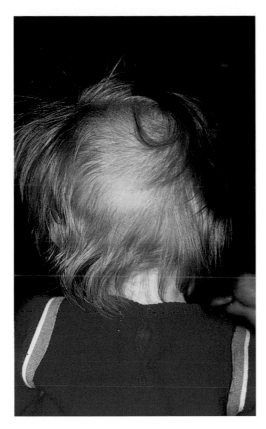

▲ 16.40

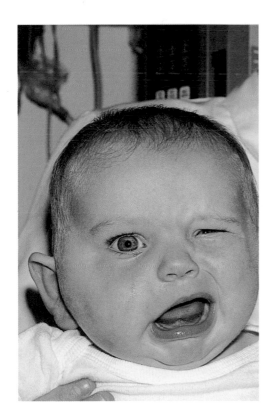

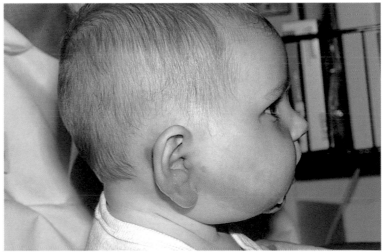

◀ 16.41, ▲ 16.42 Female aged 5 months

Infant found face down with her head trapped between the cot sides and mattress. Note marked swelling of the face and linear marks extending from behind the ear to the lower jaw. Temporary facial palsy from pressure on the 7th nerve (Fig.16.41). This otherwise well cared for infant had not been supervised adequately on the evening of the accident. Was this neglect?

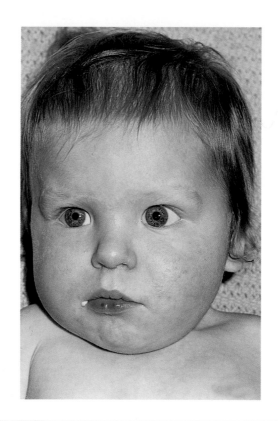

▶ **16.43,** ▼ **16.44 Male aged 15 months**
The younger of two brothers under social services supervision because of concern about neglect. He failed to thrive in spite of a 5-day placement at day nursery. He had a violent, threatening father who appeared on the ward with a knife when the child had been admitted for investigation. The photograph shows a watchful, anxious expression. Nutrition looks adequate but the growth chart (Fig. 16.44) shows growth failure.

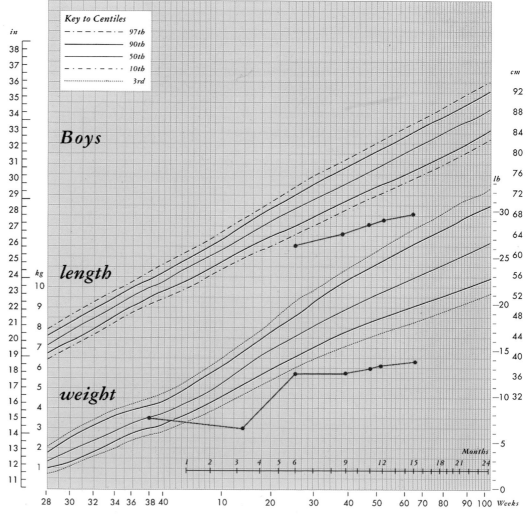

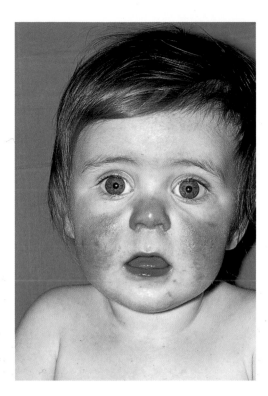 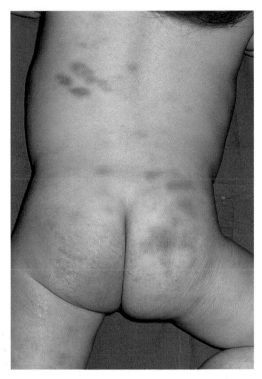

▲ **16.45,** ▲ **16.46 Male aged 2 years**

He was referred from a battered wives hostel with his older sister after bruising had been noticed on both children. The photographs show a tiny child with a worried expression and stunted growth. There is extensive bruising on the back of the buttocks consistent with hand marks. (Note: neglected children may be short and appear adequately nourished. This child demonstrated rapid catch-up growth in care. Children adapt to their circumstances, and may appear to have deceptively good nutrition.)

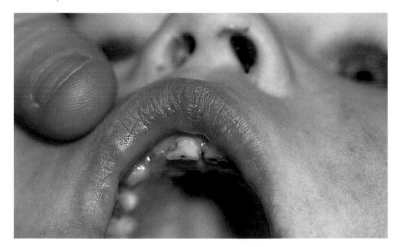

◄ **16.47 Male aged 5 years**

Child who was obese and had severe caries related to neglect and faulty diet.

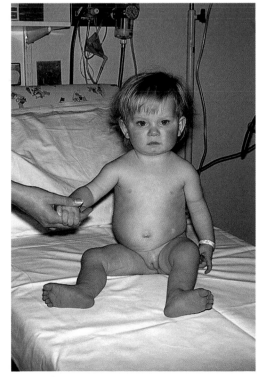

► **16.48 Female aged 18 months**

She was referred from a child welfare charity special unit where a family assessment was being undertaken. She was the middle one of three; the other siblings were thriving. She was a quiet, passive, undemanding child with marked developmental delay. Note the appearance of a large head and thin arms. The mother had a very poor emotional relationship with this child who was neglected and emotionally deprived.

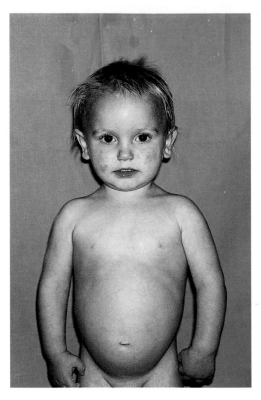

▲ **16.49 Male aged 3 years**
Child was seen in a follow-up clinic because of
previous non-accidental injury. His weight gain
at home was poor. He is seen to have a
challenging expression, distended abdomen,
thin arms and poor height. This child was failing
to thrive, but his mother's main complaints were
of his hyperactive, destructive behaviour.

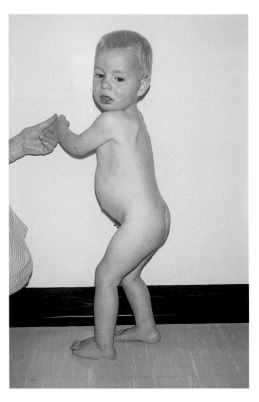

▲ **16.50 Male aged 3 years**
Apathetic neglected child who was taken into
care because of gross neglect and emotional
deprivation. Over the next few months he
became hyperactive but grew much more
quickly. At the age of 10 he showed
hyperactivity, was growing well but had
emotional and learning difficulties.

▶ **16.51 Male aged 2 years**
He was referred by the health visitor to the local
clinic because of poor weight gain. He was one
of three; the mother described the older brother
as being 'the devil'. These three boys were later
taken into care and described a lot of cruelty
including being tied to the bed at night. The
photograph shows a smiling, friendly boy with
thin limbs and protuberant abdomen. All three
boys subsequently had serious behaviour
problems. One was sent to a residential
school, and another to a day school for
children with emotional problems.

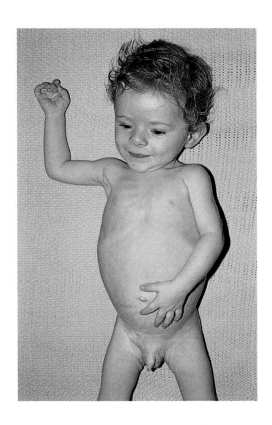

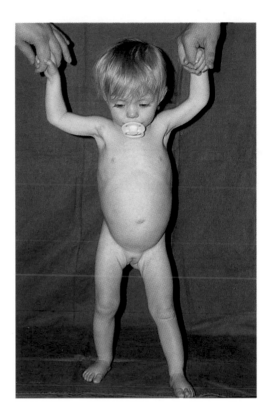

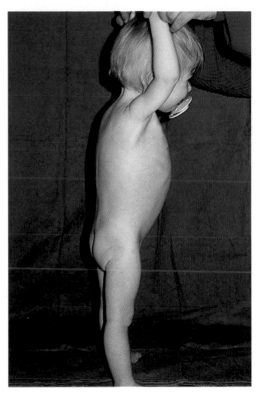

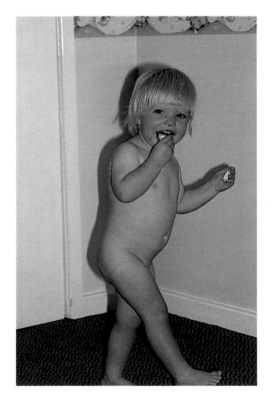

▲ **16.52,** ▲ **16.53,** ◄ **16.54 Female aged 14 months**

Child had been admitted to hospital several times with intercurrent illness, but no intervention was planned with reference to the failure to thrive. She was referred by the community health doctor to the community paediatrician. She had a history of difficult feeding and vomiting during and after meals. She was a passive child, and distressed with eye avoidance. She made attempts at indiscriminate attachment to all staff working on the ward. The photographs show a thin child with grossly distended abdomen, wasted buttocks and thin hair. There was also developmental delay. Her follow-up growth in foster care was good, and Fig. 16.54 shows a lively, friendly child. She still had difficult feeding patterns, but was interested and alert and much more confident.

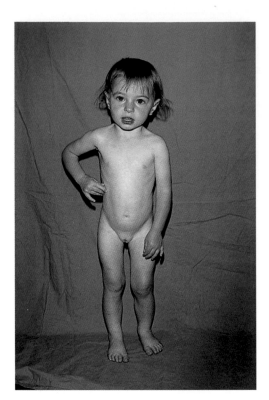 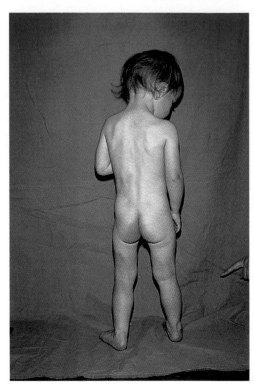

▲ **16.55, ▲ 16.56 Female aged 2 years**

At 10 months this child was sexually abused by her father. She remained in the care of her mother with whom she had a very poor relationship, and was repeatedly bruised and shouted at. She is an alert, thin child with fine hair, and indiscriminately friendly. Bruises are seen on the back of the left thigh. She was eventually taken into care by the local authority at the age of 4 years. She did not thrive in care, and further assessment showed her to be very emotionally disturbed following prolonged emotional abuse at home. At the age of 5 years plans for adoption have not yet succeeded. (Note: it is becoming evident that the damage caused by early maltreatment is not all reversible, and children may have persisting emotional difficulties.)

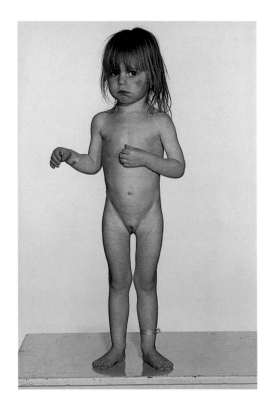

▶ **16.57 Female aged 2 years**

Child was referred by the health visitor after the mother had asked for help because the child refused to feed. The parents had recently split up, and the father had taken over the care of the baby. The mother was force feeding the child, who responded by biting. The photograph shows a flexed, frozen, wasted child. Note wasting of the upper arms and thighs.

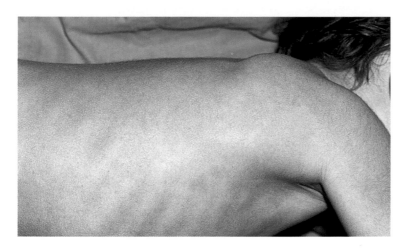 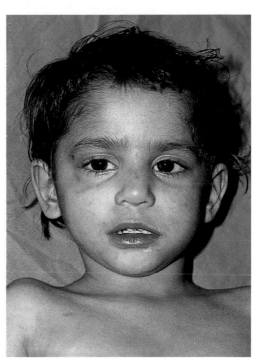

▲ **16.58,** ▶ **16.59 Female aged 3 years**

The family was known to social services because of previous physical abuse and failure to thrive. The child was referred back to the paediatrician when the black eye was seen in school. It was also known that this girl gained weight when cared for by the extended family but failed to gain weight when at home with her mother. Note the lack of subcutaneous fat and prominent rib cage (Fig. 16.58). Figure. 16.59 shows a thin, watchful child, with a peri-orbital bruise.

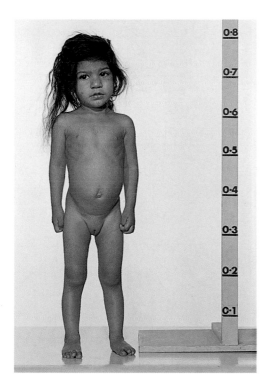 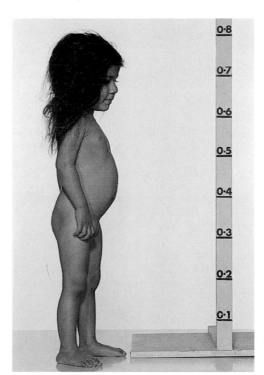

▲ **16.60,** ▲ **16.61,** ▶ **16.62,** ▶ **16.63 Female aged 2½ years**

She was referred by the health visitor to the paediatrician because of concern about poor weight gain. An older sibling was found to be stealing food in school. She is seen to be a silent, watchful, apathetic, passive child with long straggly hair. She also had delayed development. Note the stunting with infantile proportions, and distended abdomen. She is thin, with prominent ribs. This child and her older sister put on weight and grew rapidly in care (Figs 16.62–16.65).

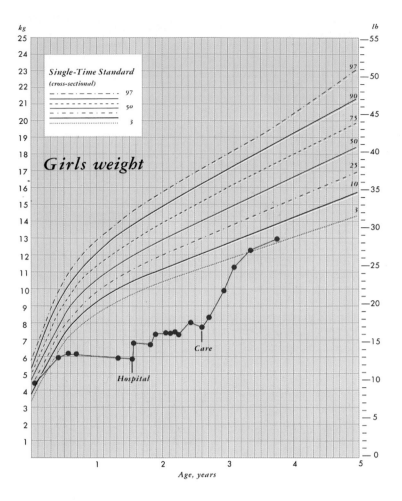

▶ **16.62,** (continued from page 211)

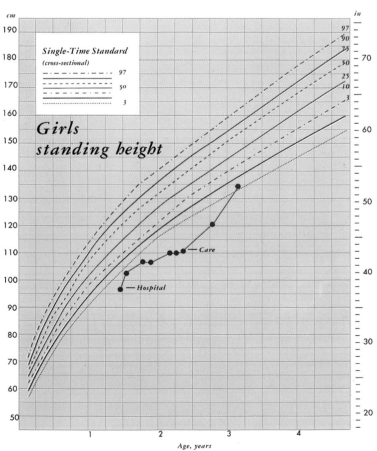

▶ **16.63**

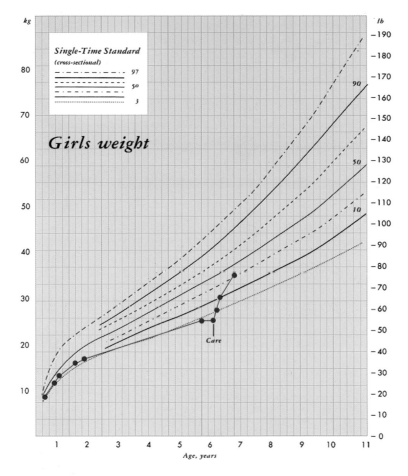

► **16.64**
Growth chart
(weight) of older
sibling of child in Figs
16.60 and 16.61.

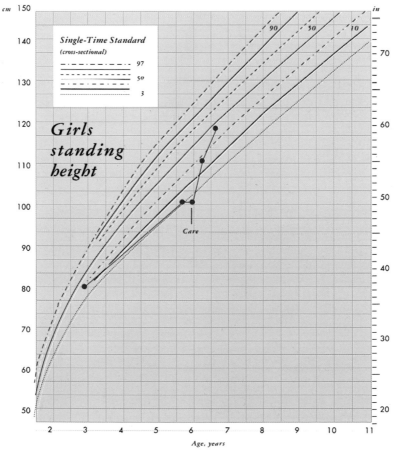

◄ **16.65**
Growth chart (height)
of older sibling of
child in Figs 16.60
and 16.61.

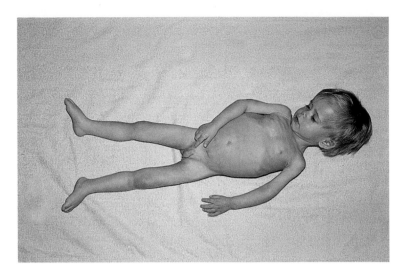

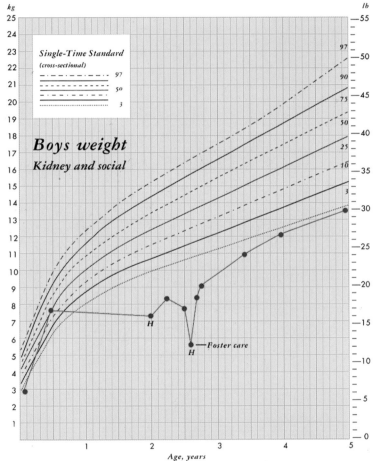

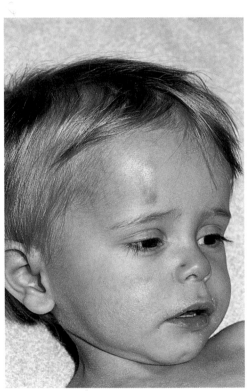

▲ **16.66,** ▲ **16.67,** ▲ **16.68 Male aged 2 years**

Child was referred by the paediatric nephrologist who was caring for the boy because of renal insufficiency. A child welfare charity was also involved because of concerns about neglect at home. He was admitted to hospital after weight loss accelerated by dehydration. He was a passive child with gaze avoidance. A bruise is seen on his right forehead. He is seen to be emaciated with thin arms and legs, a protuberant abdomen, and unkempt hair. This child did well in alternative care, but initially had a very difficult feeding problem. The anorexia had been put down to renal disease; in reality this child failed to grow because of organic and non-organic causes. (Note: organic disease and child maltreatment may coexist.)

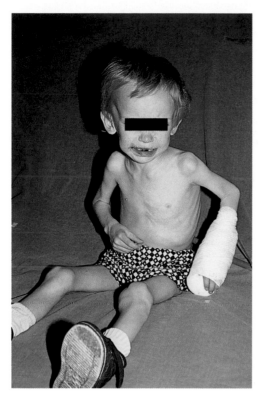

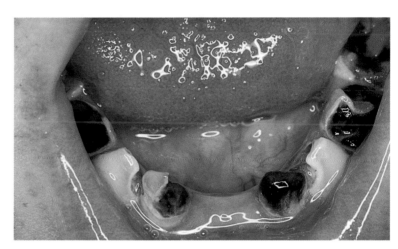

▲ **16.69,** ▲ **16.70 Male aged 4 years**

Child was referred to the paediatric out-patients by his doctor because of a cough, pallor and low weight. He was an emaciated pale child, with grossly carious teeth (Fig. 16.70) and a chest drain (he had a pneumococcal empyema secondary to pneumonia). He also had untreated hypospadias. This boy had been grossly neglected, and in spite of regular visits by the health visitor who said they were 'a nice family', this child's parlous state was not detected.

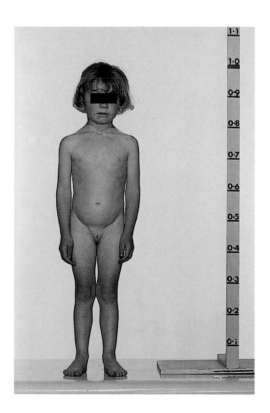

◀ **16.71 Female aged 5 years**

She was known to the paediatrician over a long period whilst social services supported the family. The photograph shows a thin, watchful child with thin arms and legs. She showed repeated catch-up growth when with alternative carers. When she was allowed to remain in foster care for a longer period her growth rate accelerated and she reached the 50th centile (growth chart in Fig. 16.72, p.216). There was severe emotional abuse in this family, and as a teenager the girl showed severe emotional damage.

▶ **Fig 16.72 Female aged 5 years**
Growth chart to 7 years of child in Fig 16.71.

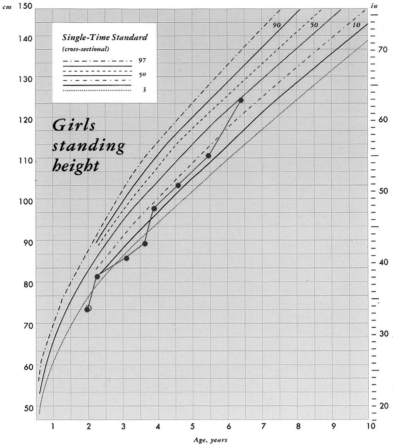

▶ **16.73 Female aged 3 years**
Growth chart of a child who was referred initially because of failure to thrive, but was subsequently overfed and became obese. Failure to thrive and obesity may be part of the same attachment difficulty, which amounts to emotional abuse.

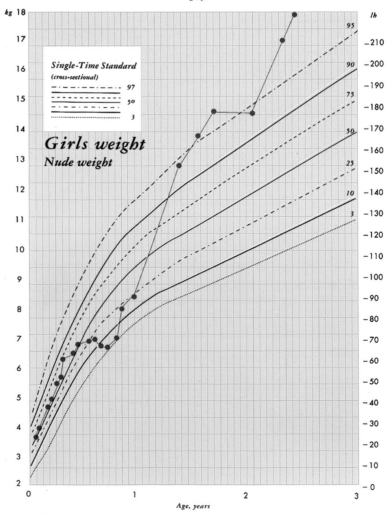

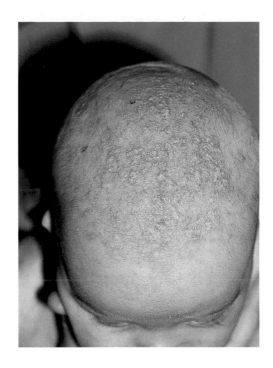

◀ **16.74 Male aged 6 months**
He was referred from the infant welfare clinic because of a rash on the scalp, which was due to neglected seborrhoeic dermatitis. This is a treatable disorder; the mother's failure to gain medical advice and treatment reflects her lack of care.

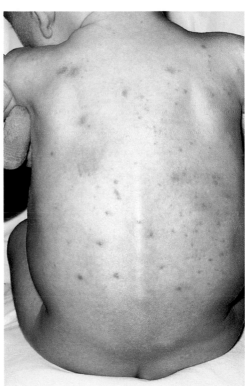

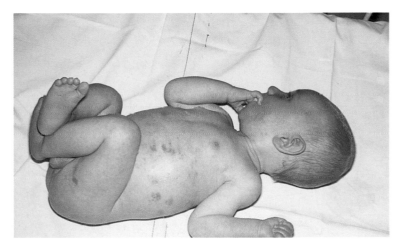

◀ **16.75,** ▲ **16.76 Male aged 6 months**
He was seen in the paediatric outpatient clinic for possible physical abuse and this rash was noted. This is a typical rash of scabies.

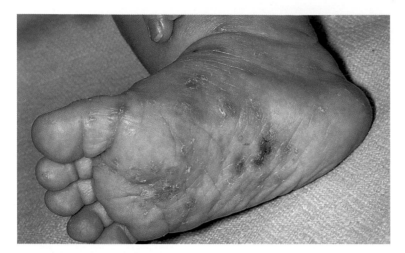

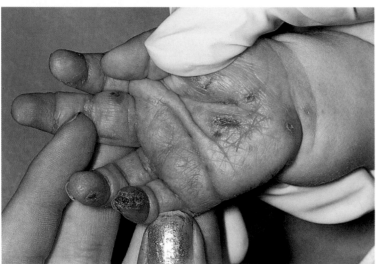

◄ **16.77,** ◄ **16.78 Male aged 4 months**
Infant with chronic scabies.

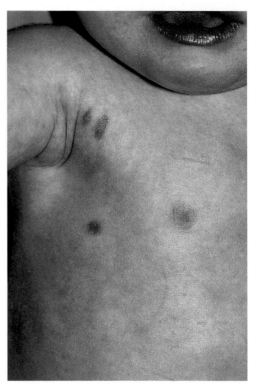

▲ **16.79 Infant aged 8 months**
Infant with chronic scabetic burrows on anterior chest.

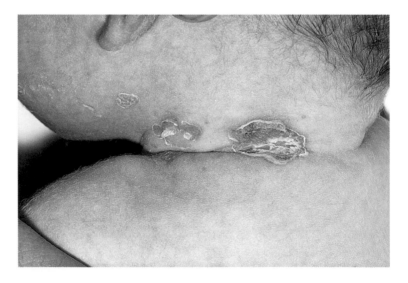

16.80 Male aged 6 weeks
Infant with infected skin in the skin creases round the neck. This child was subsequently killed by his mother.

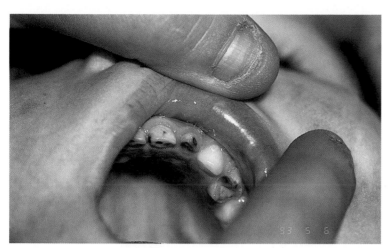

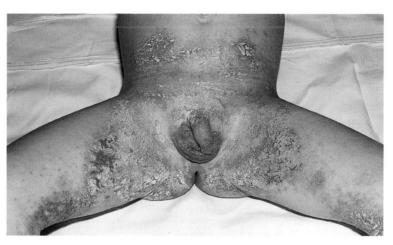

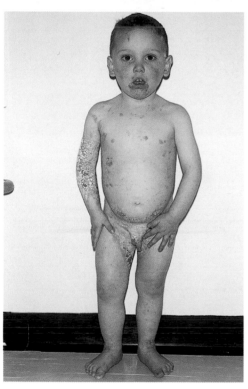

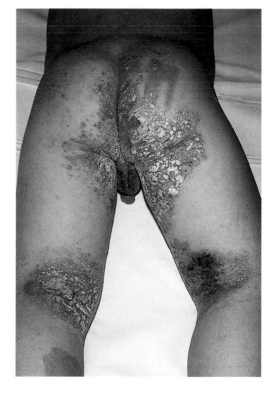

◄ **16.81 Male aged 4 years**
He was referred by social services because of extensive bruising and was found to have 60 separate areas of bruising and scratches, and carious teeth. Untreated caries such as these are part of the picture of neglect.

▲ **16.82,** ▲ **16.83,** ► **16.84 Male aged 3 years**
The child was referred by the dermatology department to the paediatrician because of concerns about neglect. The mother was known to be a binge drinker and four older siblings were on the Child Protection Register because of neglect and emotional abuse. The photographs show a stunted boy with a healing scald of the right arm and extensive eczema affecting the face, nappy area and back of the knees. The skin lesions were inappropriately treated by the mother with calamine. Note the unusual shape on the right buttock, possibly another burn. This child's skin healed up completely within a week on the ward, but deteriorated again rapidly at home. This child had been neglected, which led to the accidental scald. He had eczema, but this was made much worse by being left in wet nappies, and his mother in spite of being given appropriate treatment used calamine.

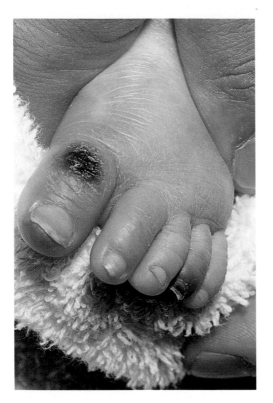

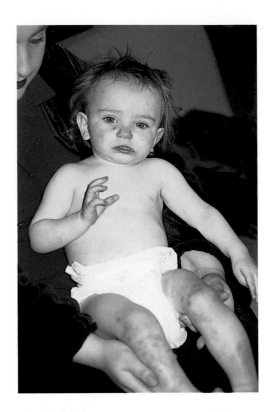

▶ 16.86 Male aged 16 months
This child presented with thin wispy hair, markedly underweight with cold injury of the legs and resolving cold injury of the hands and nose.

▲ 16.85 Male aged 3 months
Child was referred by his doctor because of worries about neglect. The child was suffering from frostbite. Note the gangrenous area on the great toe and fourth toe. Cold injuries of this degree only occur after prolonged periods of neglect.

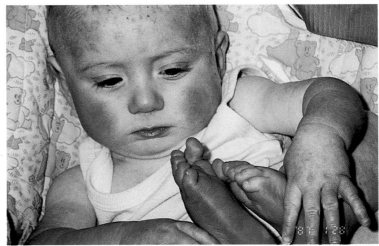

▲ 16.87 Male aged 6 months
Infant with severe cold injury.

▶ 16.88 Female aged 6 weeks
The parents took the baby to the hospital emergency department complaining about her 'black toes'. This is a cold injury, including frostbite of both feet. This child has been submitted to prolonged neglect.

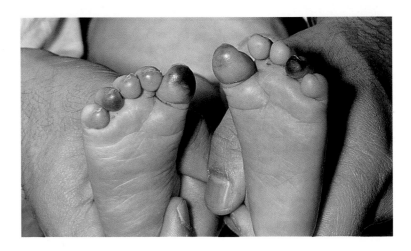

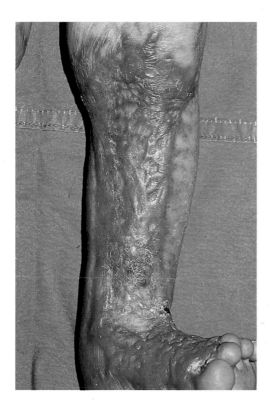
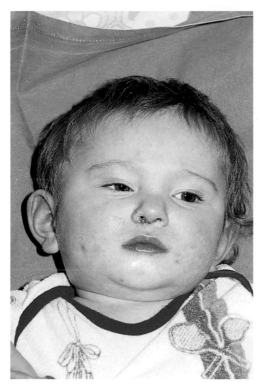

▲ **16.89,** ▲ **16.90 Male aged 18 months**

Child was left in the care of his 5-year-old sister, who tried to give him a bath, which resulted in severe scalds to both lower legs and feet. The child was in hospital for a long time, and the plastic surgeons referred the child to the paediatrician when the mother failed to visit the boy for weeks on end. It is very worrying, neglectful behaviour when adults leave children in the care of other young children.

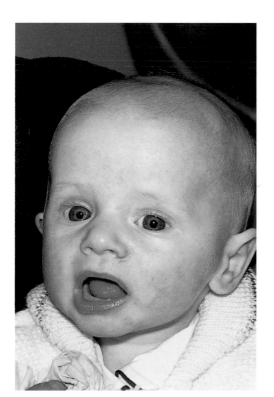

◄ **16.91 Male aged 8 months**

Infant seen in the clinic because of failure to thrive and admitted because of dehydration (depressed fontanelle, sunken eyes and dry mouth).

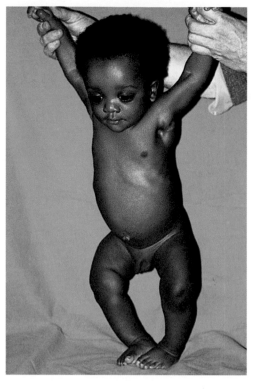
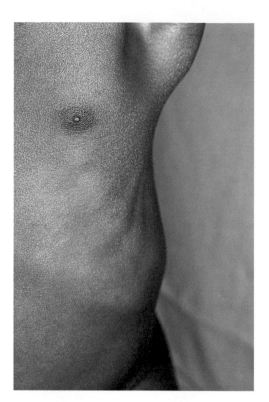
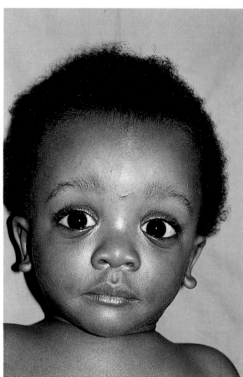
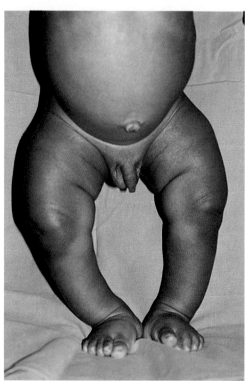

▲ 16.92, ▲ 16.93, ▲ 16.94, ▲ 16.95, ▶ 16.96, ▶ 16.97 **Male aged 12 months**
Child was referred to the paediatrician by his doctor because of poor growth. He was stunted, with weight and height under the 3rd centile, and florid rickets. Rickety rosary is seen, with frontal bossing (Fig. 16.95) and swollen wrists (Fig. 16.96). The X-ray (Fig. 16.97) confirms the diagnosis of rickets. This boy and his two older siblings were taken into care after they had been left alone in the house, which caught fire. They thrived in care.

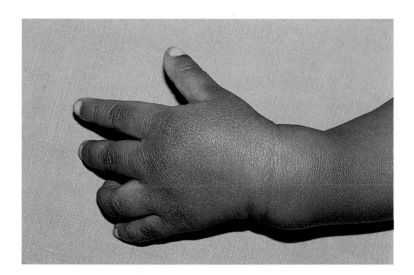

◄ **16.96**

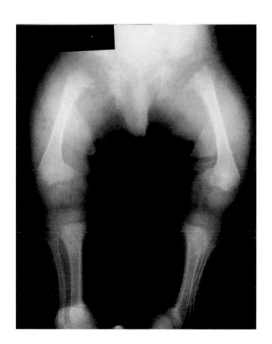

◄ **16.97**

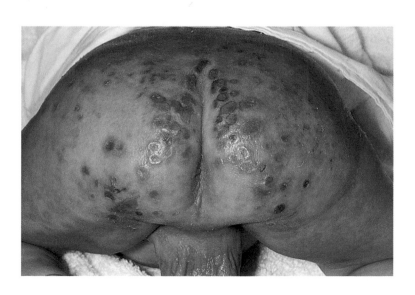

◄ **16.98 Male aged 6 months**
He was referred by the health visitor because of concern about neglect and poor weight gain. Severe chronic ulcerated nappy rash is seen, with wasted buttocks. Nappy rash of this order is a consequence of prolonged poor physical care.

▶ **16.99 Female aged 1 week**
Infant with severe nappy rash involving blistering. This infant was only a week old and clearly care was poor.

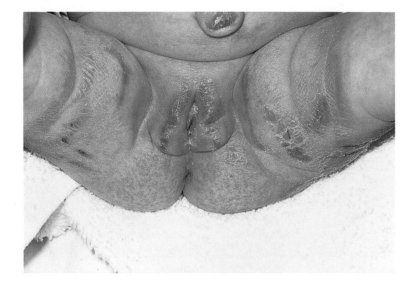

▶ **16.100 Female aged 3 years**
She was known to the paediatrician because of a long history of neglect within the family. She has a left convergent squint. The family repeatedly failed to attend for appointments in the eye department. Non-attendance for necessary hospital treatment, commonly squints and hearing difficulty, are part of the wider picture of neglect

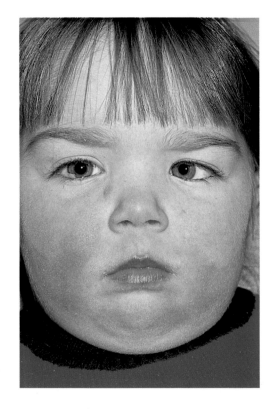

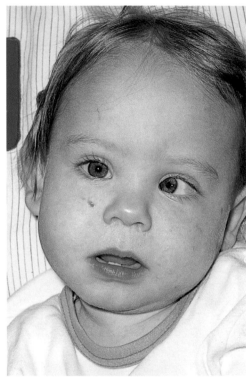

▲ **16.101 Male aged 9 months**
Infant stunted and failing to thrive with untreated squint, apathetic and neglected.

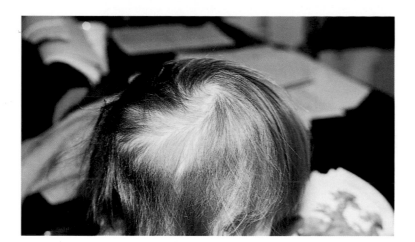

◀ **16.102 Female aged 4 years**

Child was referred to the paediatrician by her doctor because her 'hair was falling out in lumps'. Very thin, sparse hair is seen over the crown. Thin, sparse hair is commonly seen in children who are neglected and emotionally deprived.

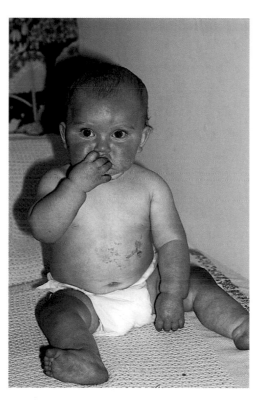

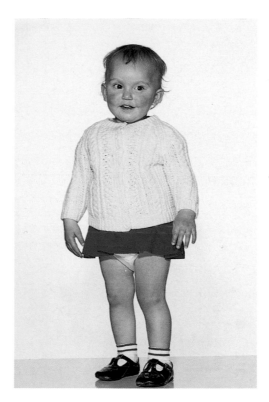

▲ **16.103 Female aged 12 months and** ▲ **16.104 aged 21 months**

Child was referred by social services after she was found to be living in a house with several convicted child abusers. She is seen to be an alert child, with ingrained dirt particularly on the lower limbs. She giggled when her nappy was changed and the paediatrician then found signs consistent with sexual abuse. Figure. 16.104 shows a follow-up photograph taken 9 months later when the child had been in foster care. The child's whole demeanour has changed.

Chapter 17

Non-organic Failure to Thrive

General characteristics of non-organic failure to thrive (NOFT)

NOFT is the failure of an infant or child to achieve his expected growth in the absence of an organic disorder. He may also fail to achieve his full potential in other parameters of development.

Documentation of failure to thrive (FTT)

- Requires serial measurement of height, weight, mid-upper arm circumference (Fig. 17.1) and head circumference.
- The measurements must be plotted on appropriate growth charts.
- Physical examination:
  - exclude organic causes of FTT: signs will depend on the disorder;
  - the child may appear well cared for or have a neglected appearance;
  - the associated signs seen in NOFT include wasting, protuberant abdomen, thin hair, signs of neglect (see Chapter 16);
  - behaviours observed include apathy, attention-seeking, over-activity and flitting from toy to toy;
  - development is variably delayed with language and social skills most affected.

The interpretation of growth charts in NOFT: there are several patterns including:
- falling centiles;
- parallel poor centiles;
- markedly discrepant height and weight centiles;
- discrepant family pattern;
- retrospective rise;
- saw-tooth – erratic, fluctuating pattern.

The differential diagnosis of failure to thrive

- Adequate intake with poor weight gain – malabsorption, e.g. coeliac disease.
- Inadequate intake due to swallowing difficulty – cerebral palsy.
- Poor appetite – renal failure.

The selection of laboratory investigations to elucidate the aetiology of the observed FTT depends upon the clinical assessment and the majority will require a haemoglobin check or no tests at all. The observation of improved growth as a consequence of an increased food intake renders further laboratory tests unnecessary.

Mid-upper arm circumference (MUAC) – where child is 12–60 months old	
Child older than 12 months and MUAC less than 14 cm	Likely to be significantly malnourished – warrants referral to a paediatrian
MUAC is 14–15 cm	If older, i.e. 4–5 years, likely to be malnourished, refer to paediatrician. Younger child – monitor carefully and assess in detail
MUAC is greater than 15 cm	Nutrition is likely to be adequate
MUAC at school entry, 5–6 years, 16–17 cm	Likely to be adequately nourished

▲ Fig. 17.1 Mid-upper arm circumference – where child is 12–60 months old

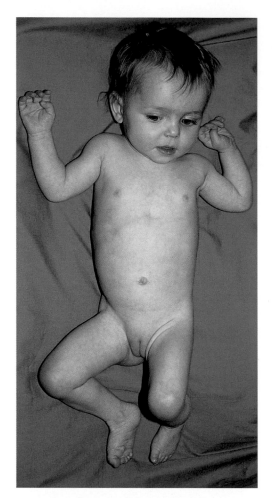

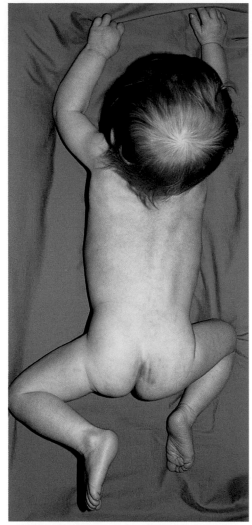

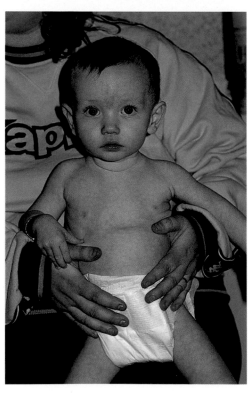

◀ **17.1,** ◀ **17.2**
**Female aged
12 months**
Infant in a flexed
posture lying very
still. She is also
stunted. Fig. 17.2
shows wasting of
the buttocks and
thighs. This child
also had delayed
development.

◀ **17.4 Female
aged 3 years**
Sister of child in
Fig. 7.3 also failure
to thrive. Note
protruberant
abdomen.

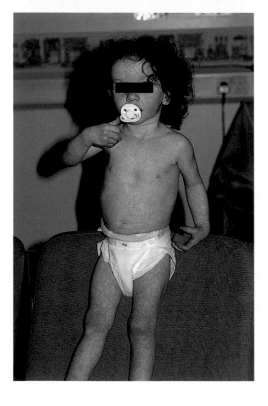

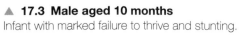

▲ **17.3 Male aged 10 months**
Infant with marked failure to thrive and stunting.

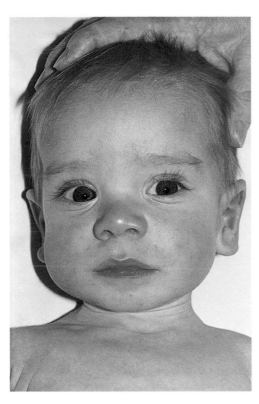
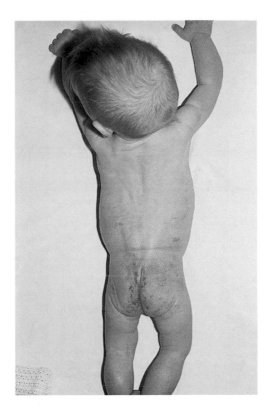

▲ 17.5, ▲ 17.6 Male aged 7 months

He was referred from the infant welfare clinic because of poor weight gain. A thin, watchful baby is seen, with wasted buttocks and chronic nappy rash. There is minimal subcutaneous fat, allowing the muscle pattern to be seen.

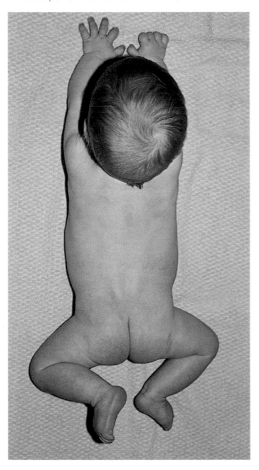
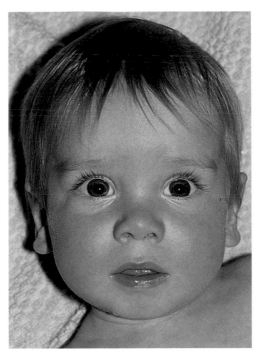

◀ 17.7, ▲ 17.8, ▶ 17.9, ▶ 17.10 Male aged 1 year

The same child as in Figs 17.5 and 17.6. He is visibly fatter with much thicker hair. He has an alert interested expression. Note the increase of subcutaneous fat. The growth chart (Fig. 17.10) shows falling away across the centiles during the first months of infancy, followed by dramatic acceleration in weight gain first in hospital and then foster care. Subsequently the weight gain begins to level off until reaching a position above the 25th centile.

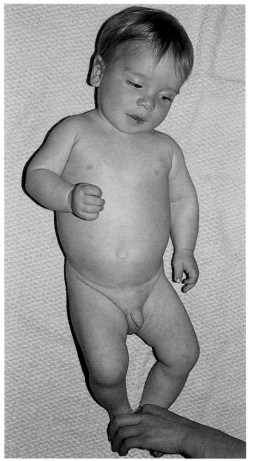

▲ 17.9

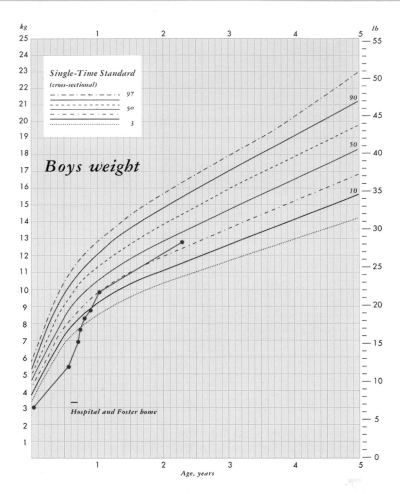

▲ 17.10

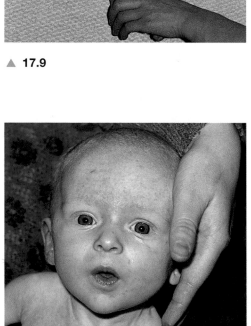

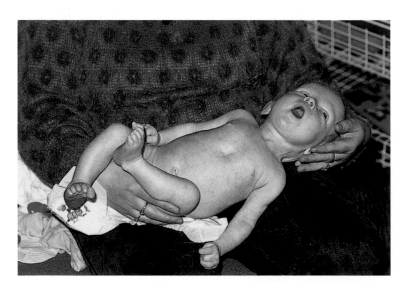

▲ 17.11, ▶ 17.12 **Male aged 5 months**
Poorly cared for, neglected and emaciated
infant with worried expression. He was failing
to thrive.

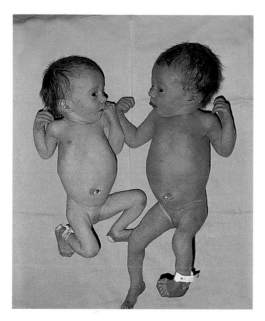

▲ **17.13 Females twins**
Differences in growth during intrauterine life reflect the state of nutrition of the fetus. This is well demonstrated in this slide of twins.

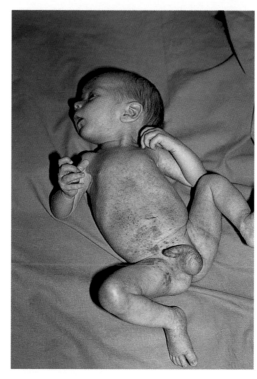

◀ **17.14 Male aged 3 months**
He had previously been seen because of a painful swollen leg due to a fracture of the fibula. He was seen again because of severe failure to thrive, with marked passivity, flexed posture, and signs of malnutrition.

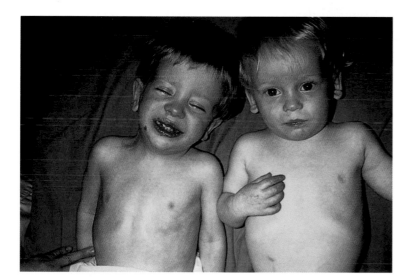

▲ **17.15 Male twins aged 18 months**
They were referred because both children were failing to thrive. One twin was markedly thinner than the other but both were underweight. In this case both twins grew much better in alternative care. This was post-natal non-organic failure to thrive.

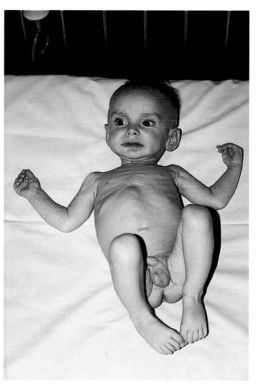

▲ **17.16 Male aged 8 months**
He was referred because of persistent vomiting. He was an alert, watchful baby, seen to be emaciated with a flexed posture. Rumination was diagnosed on admission to hospital. There was a very poor interaction with his mother. Rumination is a rare manifestation of severe emotional deprivation.

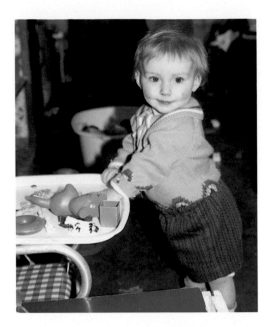

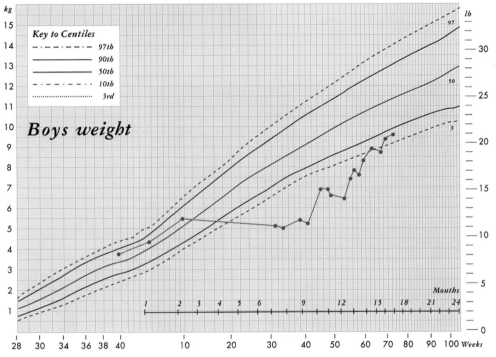

▲ **17.17,** ▲ **17.18 Male aged 15 months**

The same child as in Fig. 17.16, in a child welfare charity nursery where his mother was receiving intensive help. The growth chart (Fig. 17.18) shows that the child grew along the 50th centile for the first couple of months of life before progressively falling across the centiles. It was difficult working with this child and his mother and it was not until he was around 1 year old that he began to thrive consistently.

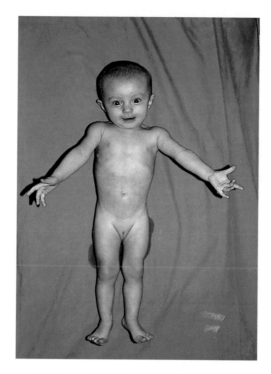

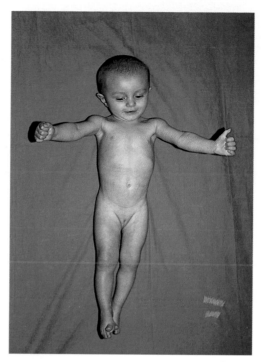

▲ **17.19,** ▲ **17.20 Female aged 12 months**
Infant with marked failure to thrive. Note posture with extension of all four limbs and adduction of hips. 'Soft neurological signs' are commonly seen in severely neglected children who fail to thrive.

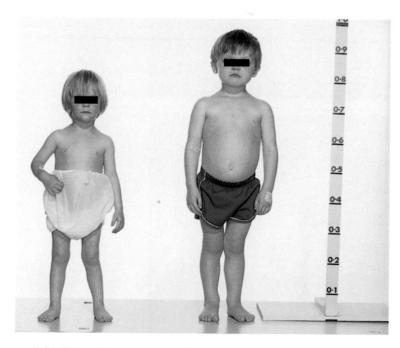

▲ **7.21 Two males both aged 4 years**
The child on the left has severe growth retardation and malnutrition, and is not yet toilet trained. Severe emotional abuse has an association with failure to thrive and leads to stunting which may be permanent. (Note: late development of social skills and language are also seen in cases of emotional abuse.)

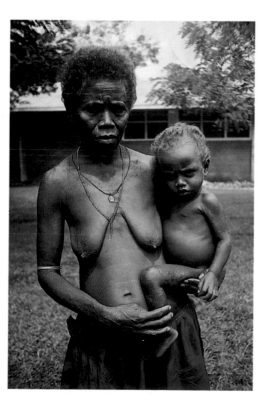

▲ **17.22 Male aged 2 years**
He is an anxious-looking child with patchy depigmentation, and is grossly emaciated with a pot belly. The grandmother was caring for the child after his mother was murdered. She too is malnourished. This child was thin due to emotional deprivation and inadequate diet.

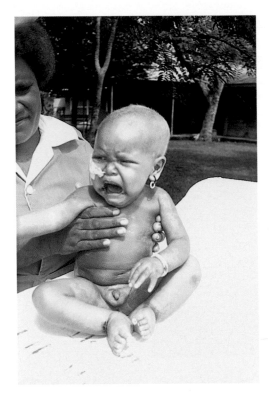

◀ **17.23 Male aged 12 months**

He was referred because he was irritable and not growing. He has thin arms and swollen legs, sparse, pale hair, angular cheilosis and flexural dermatitis painted with gentian violet. The pattern of malnutrition here is of nutritional oedema (kwashiorkor). The aetiology of kwashiorkor is complex.

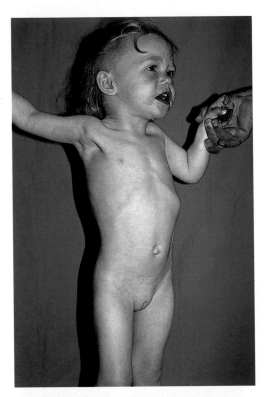

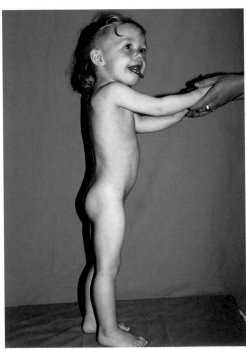

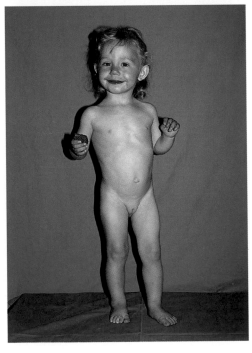

▲ **17.24,** ▶ **17.25,** ▶ **17.26 Female aged 2 years**

Severely emaciated girl. This child remained at home with inadequate caretakers and her failing to thrive siblings. She also had long straggly poorly cared for hair. She had marked language delay. This child was hungry in the clinic and enjoyed eating the biscuits.

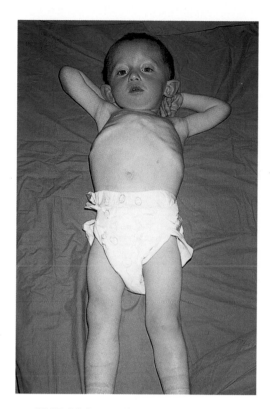

▲ **17.27 Male aged 15 months**

Infant who was severely failing to thrive. He was always infested with nits. His development was delayed with minimal language and little ability to play.

▲ **17.28 Male aged 15 months**

Same infant as Fig. 17.27. Mid-upper arm circumference (MUAC) measured about 13.7 cm. This is an indicator of malnutrition.

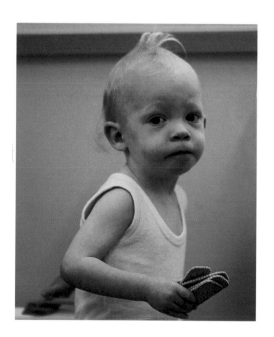

◄ **17.29 Male aged 18 months**

A useful adjunct to the assessment of failure to thrive is a supply of biscuits in the outpatient clinic. This child, who was failing to thrive, demonstrated an increased appetite by taking a handful of biscuits and eating them. Note the biscuit test has been shown to be a useful tool in the assessment of children, who are described as non-eaters, eat everything in sight, or who even hoard the biscuits in the clinic to take home.

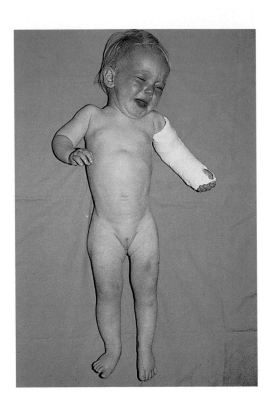

◀ **17.30,** ▼ **17.31**
**Female aged
14 months**

She was taken to the hospital emergency department because she was not moving her left arm. The history given was that she had fallen out of a highchair. She is a thin child, with bruises on the left outer thigh, and a treated fracture of the radius and ulna. The growth chart shows that this child thrived well in the care of her grandmother, less well when looked after by her aunt and badly when she was returned to her mother's care. She then showed catch-up growth in foster care. Although initially it was thought that the child had fallen out of the highchair her father subsequently admitted to swinging her round holding her by the wrist.

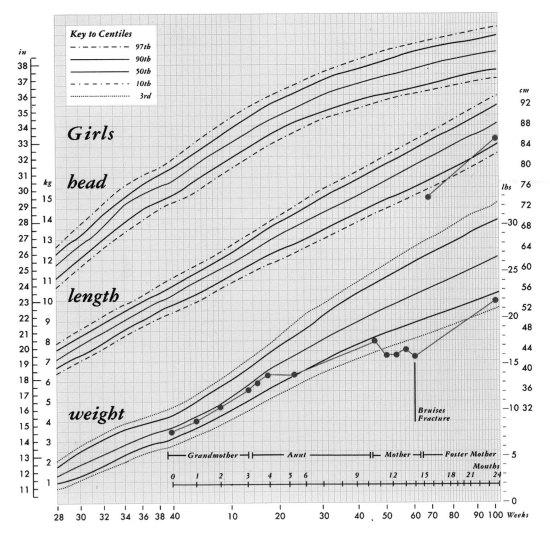

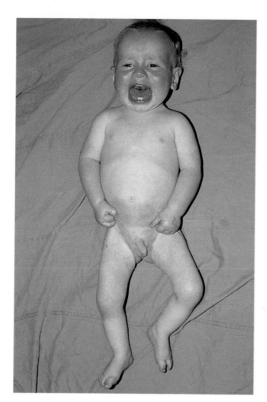

17.32 Male aged 15 months
He was referred because of poor weight gain.
The child does not look badly nourished,
although his thighs are thin. He weighed
6.6 kg (14.5 lbs), i.e. the weight of a child of
6 months, and had the body proportions of a
child of this age.

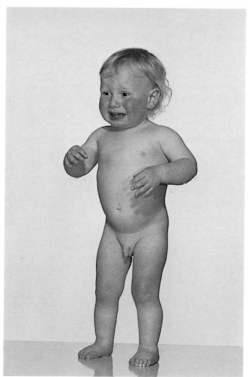

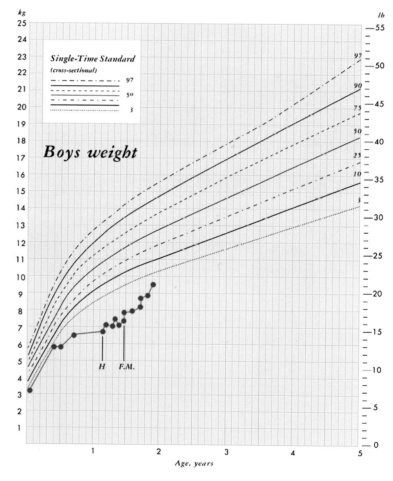

▲ **17.33,** ▶ **17.34 Male aged 2 years**
The same child as in Fig. 17.32. He still has
infantile proportions but is better nourished.
The growth chart (Fig. 17.34) shows that the
failure to thrive started early on in infancy and
the child did not start to thrive until in alternative
care. (H = admission to hospital,
FM = admission to foster care.)

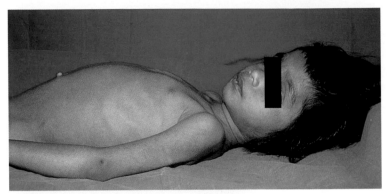

◀ **17.35 Female aged 6 years**
The child was referred from a district general hospital where she had been admitted with a swollen abdomen. The photograph shows a watchful, thin child with wasted upper arms and protuberant upper abdomen. Investigation showed pancreatitis and a pseudopancreatic cyst. Skeletal survey showed fractures of the spine, and a healing fracture of the humerus. The pancreatitis was thought to be secondary to a forceful blow in the abdomen, the spinal fractures due to a forced flexion injury and the fracture of the humerus was unexplained. This child was thin and part of her malnutrition was probably due to her intercurrent illness but she also had a history of failure to thrive. This therefore was a multiply abused child.

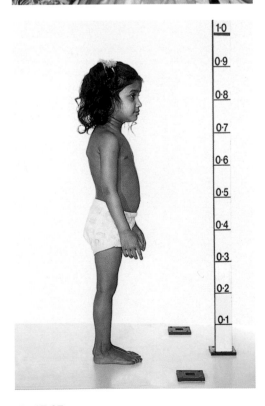

◀ **17.36–17.40 Female aged 3 years**
When fully dressed in baggy clothing she does not look unduly thin although she does have a pointed chin (Fig. 17.36). The same child unclothed with protuberant abdomen and thin limbs is shown in Figs 17.37 and 17.38.
Note: 'fresh air sign' when the child is standing. It is possible to see clearly the light between her thighs. There was medical disagreement about the cause of this child's failure to thrive, i.e. was this constitutional short stature? In fact the child began to thrive when taken into care. (See Fig. 17.40 where she began to gain weight.)

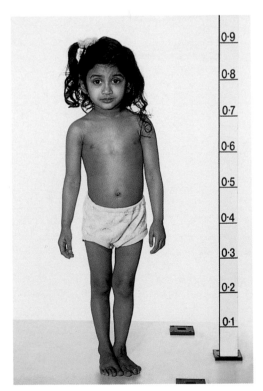

▲ **17.37**   ▲ **17.38**

▶ **17.39**

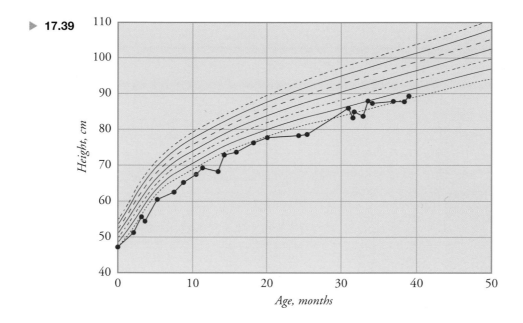

▶ **17.40**

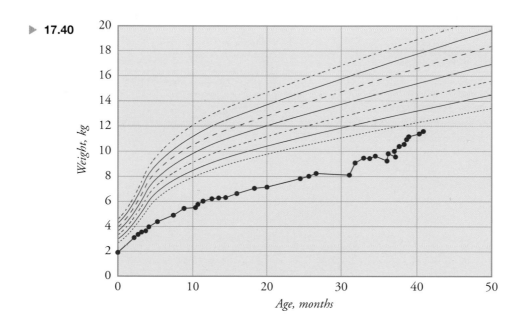

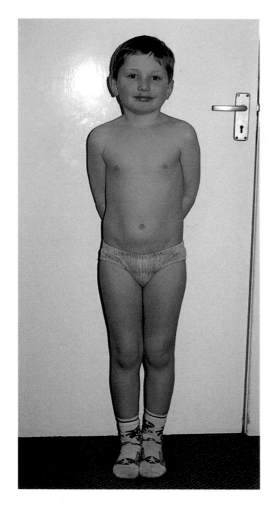

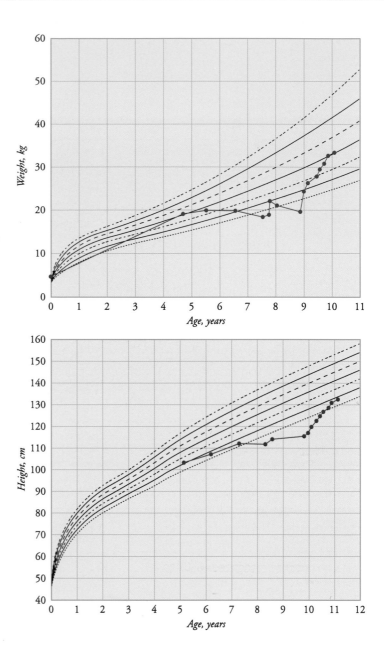

▲ **17.41,** ▶ **17.42 Male aged 10 years**

Boy who was emotionally and physically abused from early childhood. He did not grow in stature and his weight gain was minimal. When admitted to hospital he put on 3 kg in 9 days. At that stage there was no follow-up and the gravity of the situation was only acknowledged when he came back with bruising due to physical assault. On discharge to a different relative he gained weight and height very rapidly.

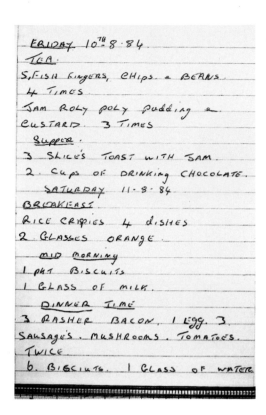

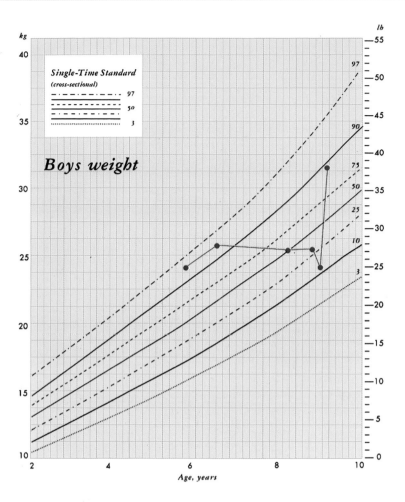

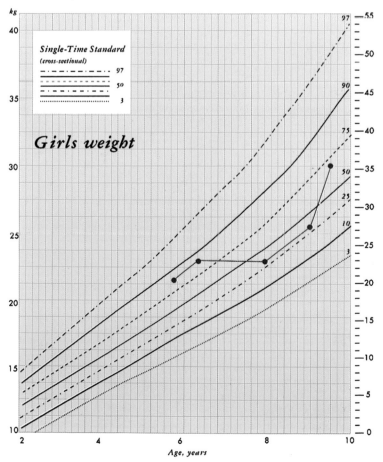

▲ 17.43, ▶ 17.44, ▶ 17.45

When children are failing to thrive it is often useful to ask the carer to write down the food consumed over a 2- or 3-day period, i.e. keep a food diary. The foster mother who filled in this diary (Fig. 17.43) for a child of 3 years describes a diet adequate for two or three children. The growth chart (Fig. 17.44) shows the weight gain of another child in the foster home who had not been recognized as failing to thrive. He had put on weight well until the age of 6 years and then failed to thrive over the next 3 years because of emotional abuse and food deprivation. Figure. 17.45 is a growth chart for the twin sister of the previous child who has a similar growth pattern to her brother, in the same foster home. It is important to assess all children in a family for failure to thrive if this condition has been recognized in one child.

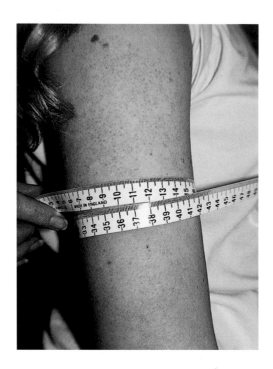

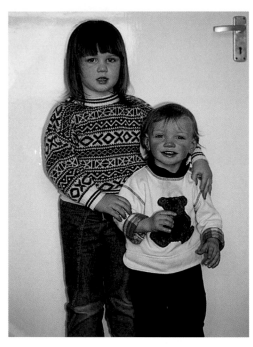

◀ **17.47 Female aged 3 years 2 months and her brother aged 1 year 9 months.** The boy had repeated admissions to hospital because of poor weight gain. Children in a family may show different growth patterns. This boy was emotionally deprived and failed to thrive.

▲ **17.46**

Mid-upper arm circumference (MUAC) is a useful measurement in the assessment of nutrition. A non-stretch tape measure is looped around the arm firmly opposed to the skin without causing compression and measurement is taken from the 10 cm mark. In the example shown the arm circumference is 26 cm. This measurement is sensitive to changes in nutrition in terms of weeks, compared with, for example, height, which often only accelerates slowly over months.

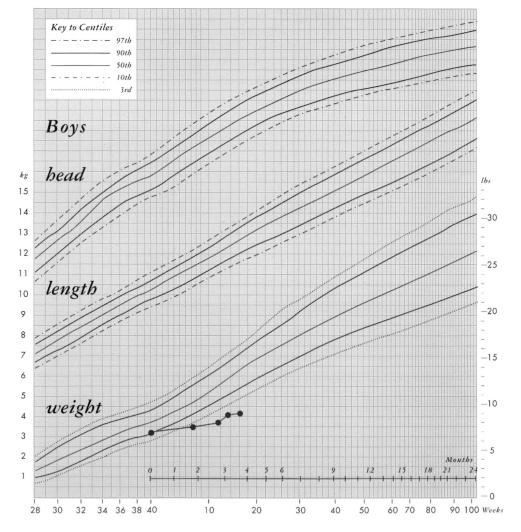

▲ **17.48 Male aged 3 months**

The growth chart of an infant who died at 3 months. The diagnosis was sudden infant death syndrome and a fractured rib. There is an increased mortality in children who fail to thrive.

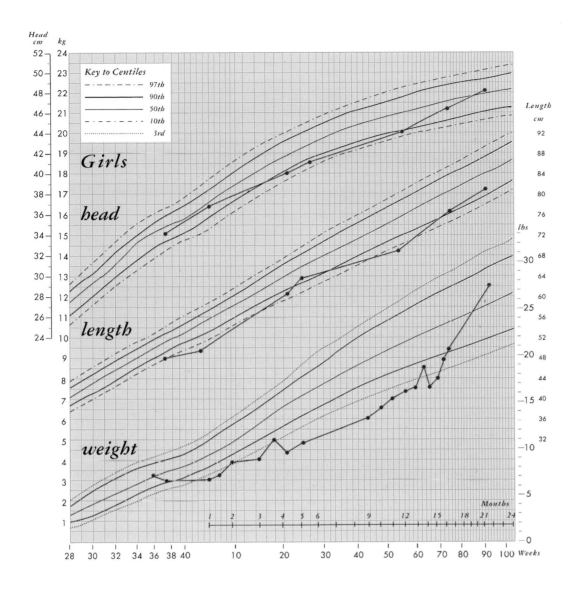

▲ 17.49

This growth chart shows measurements for a child from birth until 2 years. Early on in life she was repeatedly admitted to hospital with chest infections but also failed to thrive. Her head circumference did not grow optimally and neither did her length. She was admitted to the child welfare charity day nursery where she initially began to thrive but then lost weight and was admitted to foster care. This child has been followed up in the paediatric clinic and now has a height measurement on the 25th centile, which is matched with her weight.

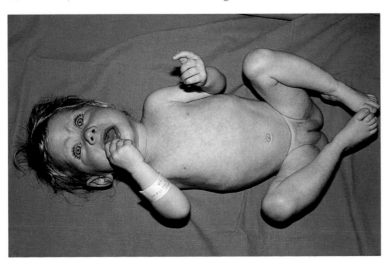

◄ 17.50 Female aged 10 months

She was referred to the clinic because of failure to thrive. The photograph shows a miserable, wasted, thin child.

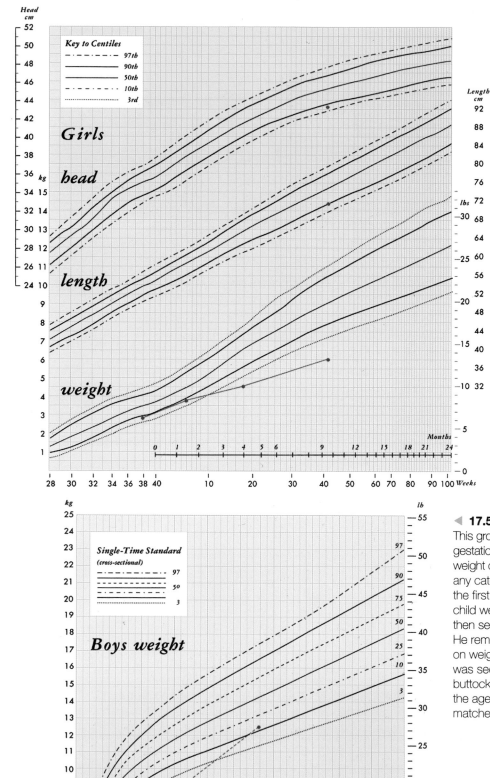

Girls head length weight

Boys weight

◀ **17.51 Female aged 10 months**
Same child as in Fig. 17.50. The growth chart shows marked discrepancy between length and weight. Her weight gain was acceptable in the first 6 weeks of life but then fell.

◀ **17.52**
This growth chart shows a boy born at 39 weeks gestation who was light for dates with a birth weight of 2.16 kg (4.76 lbs). He did not show any catch-up growth and failed to thrive over the first months of life. He was referred to a child welfare charity and gained weight but was then seen with a small facial bruise at 5 months. He remained at home with his parents and put on weight rapidly but at the age of 7 months was seen with severe bruising on his face and buttocks. The child went into foster care and at the age of almost 2 had a height and weight matched on the 10th centile.

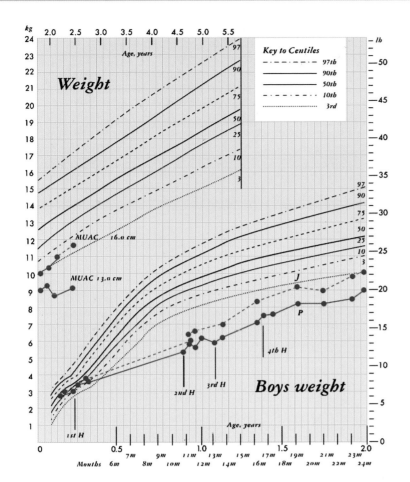

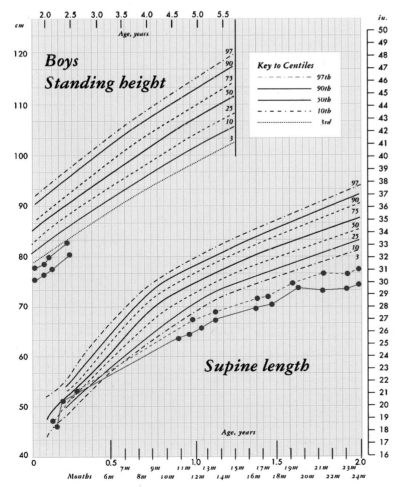

◀ 17.53, ◀ 17.54
These growth charts shows the weight and height gain of pre-term twins. Both twins severely failed to thrive, but showed they were able to put on weight more rapidly on admission to hospital. From the age of 21 months Twin J put on weight steadily and by the age of 2½ had a weight just below the 10th centile with a mid-upper arm circumference (MUAC) of 16 cm. Twin P continued to fail to thrive. The chart recording the height measurements shows the same disparity, and Twin J has failed to catch up in terms of his height compared with his weight gain. (H = hospital admission.)

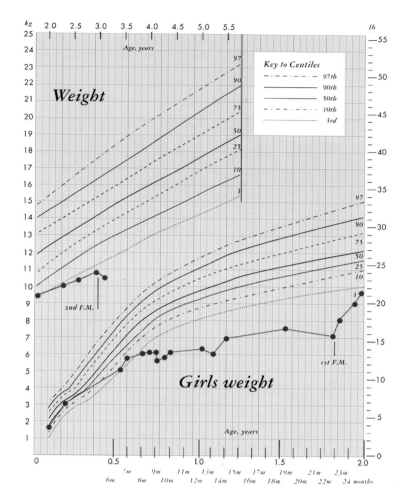

◄ **17.55**
This growth chart shows a child who failed to thrive from the age of about 3 months until she was taken into foster care and then put on weight very rapidly. Unfortunately she then had to change foster placement at about 3 years and immediately lost weight. The child was attached to the first foster mother and grieved on placement. Children who have failed to thrive previously tend to respond to stress by losing weight. (FM = admission to foster care.)

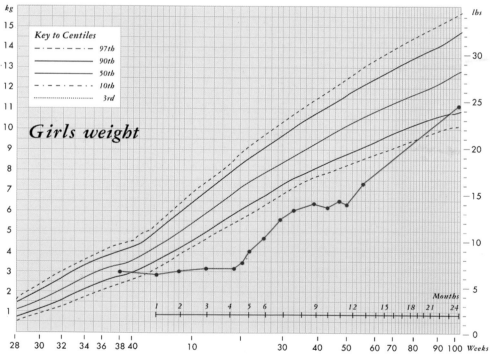

▲ **17.56**
This girl weighed 3 kg (6.6 lbs) at birth at 42 weeks' gestation. She failed to thrive very early on and was admitted to hospital at 9 weeks, 11 weeks and 3½ months with bruising to the face. From 9 months to a year she lost weight and was placed with her grandparents on an interim care order. Once with her grandparents she began to thrive very quickly. When the child was 21 months old her grandmother broke a leg and the child went home rather precipitously. However, she continued to thrive and at the age of 2 had a weight on the 25th centile.

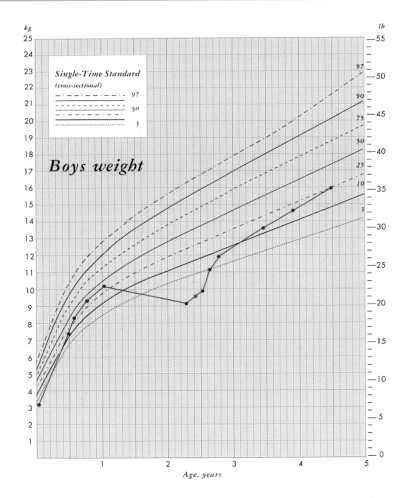

◀ **17.57**

This boy grew well at home but his mother asked for him to be received into care when he was around 6 months old. He continued to thrive until he moved to second foster parents at the age of 12 months. When he was having a medical before adoption it was realized that he had lost weight from the age of 1 until 2½. He had never been seen in the infant welfare clinic as the foster mother was very busy looking after 12 children. He was moved immediately to a third set of foster parents where he thrived well. He was subsequently adopted and at the age of 10 had a weight and height on the 50th centile.

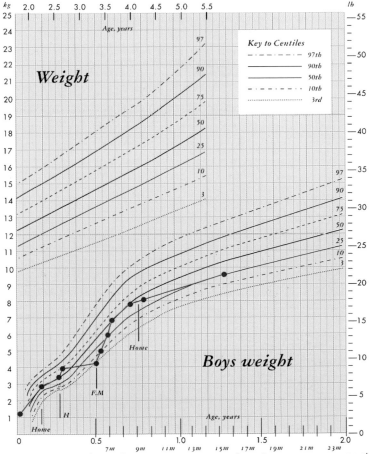

◀ **17.58**

This boy had a weight appropriate for his gestation at 30 weeks. He thrived initially in hospital but his weight gain at home was always poor. He was fostered from the age of 6 months until he was rehabilitated with his mother after a period of 3 months in foster care. He then continued to thrive in his mother's care. (H = hospital admission, FM = admission to foster care.)

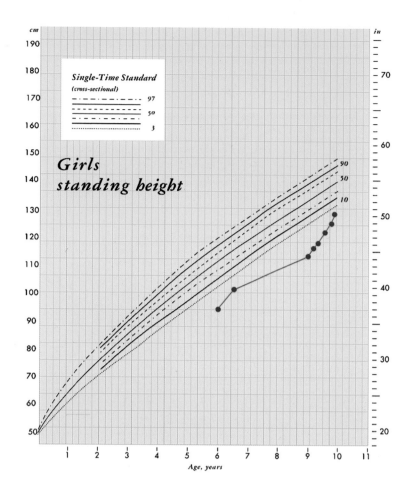

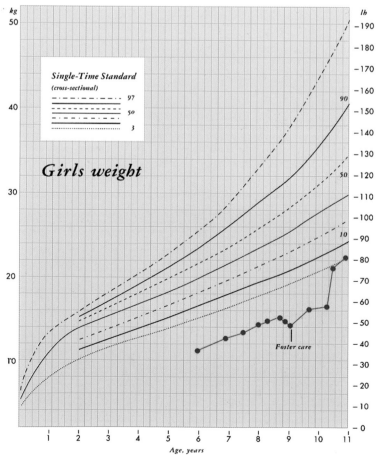

◄ **17.59**

This girl of 9 years was known to be very small and underweight from the age of 5 years. At 9 years she was referred because of education failure; she was also wetting in the day and was mute. She was fostered and began to put on weight quite rapidly although her linear growth acceleration took longer. Although her growth pattern improved and she began to talk and stopped wetting, she did not catch up developmentally.

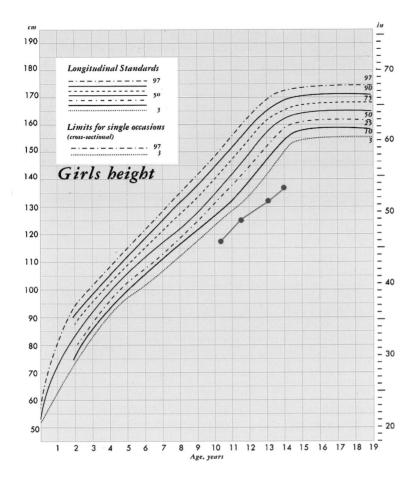

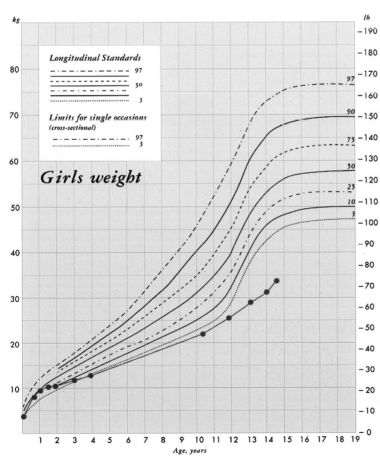

◀ **17.60**
When the child in Fig. 17.59 presented it was also realized that her sister was small and underweight and growth charts were constructed for her.

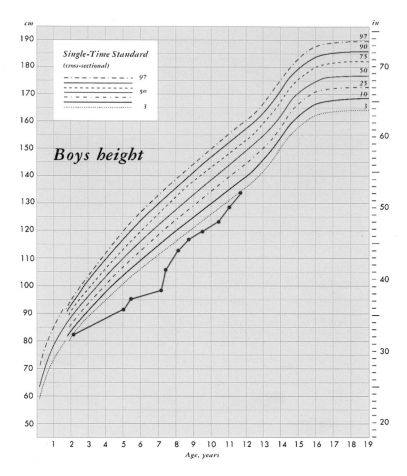

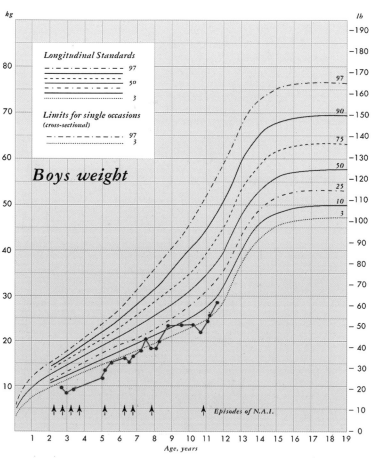

◀ 17.61, ▼ 17.62

This boy failed to thrive from early childhood and his weight gain was never really satisfactory, showing a saw-tooth pattern before having a sustained weight gain when he was taken into care. He was emotionally abused and intermittently physically abused throughout this period. This child came from an ethnic minority group and alternative appropriate care was not available. After the supervision order was made there was improvement, which was not sustained.

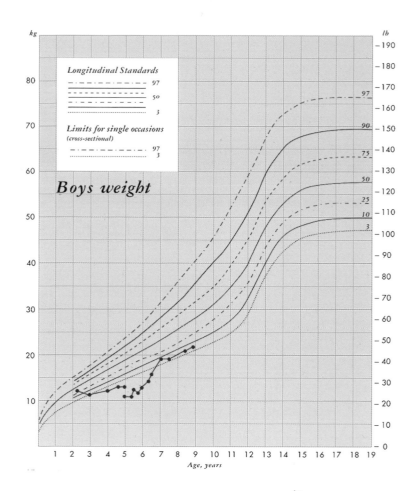

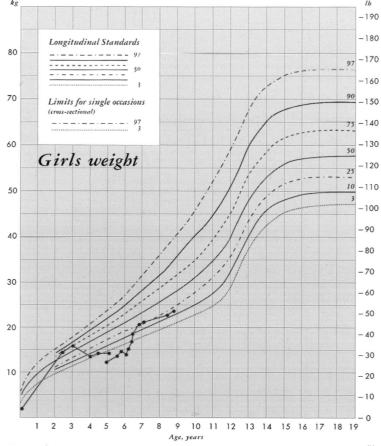

◀ **17.63,** ▼ **17.64**

The boy whose growth is shown in Fig. 17.63 was a twin born at 35 weeks', gestation weighing 2 kg (4.4 lbs). He did well early in life but was then received into care at the age of 2. His carers had 'healthy eating practices'. His failure to thrive was severe and by the age of 5 years he weighed less than he had done when he was 2½ years. The foster parents were very angry when asked to change his diet but the child did put on weight initially. After a further weight loss he was transferred to a children's home. He gained weight very rapidly and started to grow. His sister showed a similar growth pattern (Fig. 17.64). The two children were adopted.

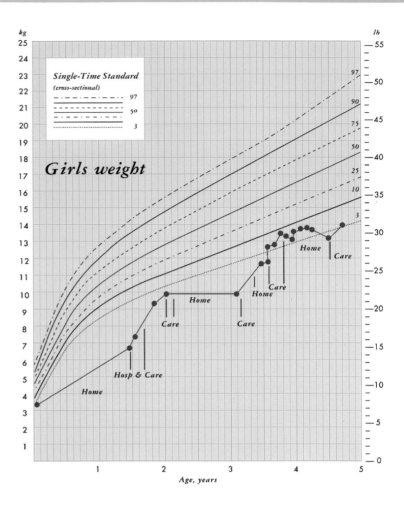

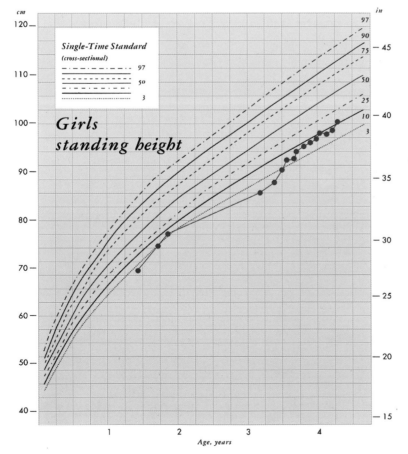

▲ **17.65,** ◀ **17.66**

This girl presented at the age of 18 months with physical injury (bites and bruises), failure to thrive and emotional deprivation. She showed catch-up growth in hospital and care and three attempts at rehabilitation were associated with failure to gain weight. The courts finally accepted that rehabilitation was not possible. As a teenager this girl has severe emotional problems.

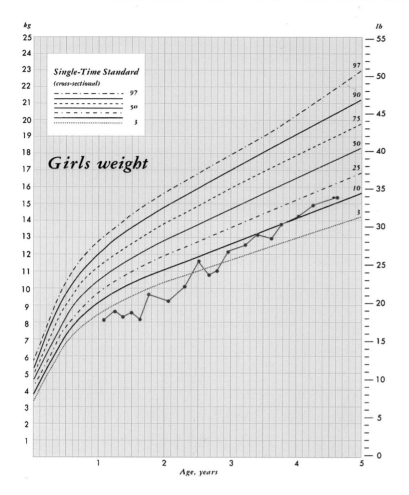

◀ **17.67**

This growth chart shows a 'saw-tooth' pattern. In infancy this girl had gastro-oesophageal reflux, and repeated episodes of infection-induced wheezing, but the dips in weight related to periods of neglect when the marital relationship deteriorated. Her mother would leave home, the father took over the childcare and the child would begin to thrive.

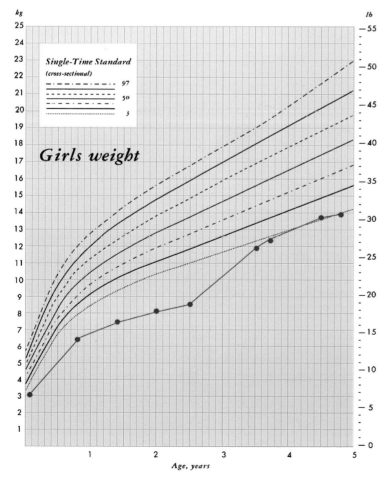

◀ **17.68**

This growth chart shows parallel poor centiles; this girl was physically neglected. Her mother described the huge meals she ate but the clinical diagnosis was that this child did not eat an adequate number of calories. Her height (not shown) grew along the 3rd centile and her weight gradually increased to a position just below the 3rd centile.

Chapter 18

Emotional Abuse

General characteristics of emotional abuse (after Skuse 1989)

Emotional abuse and deprivation cause unhappiness and damage to the child's developing personality which may be irreversible.

Emotional abuse, which is the commonest form of abuse and occurs in all social groups, may be missed, especially when the physical care is good and the child is stunted but appears as short and well nourished.

◆ Other forms of abuse (usually chronic abuse) are commonly associated with emotional abuse.

Emotional abuse may be recognized:
◆ during infancy:
  – failure to thrive;
  – recurrent infections;
  – chronic nappy rash;
  – global developmental delay;
  – unresponsive socially or 'frozen'.
◆ pre-schoolers:
  – short ± underweight;
  – unkempt, dirty, thin hair (NB there may be good physical care);
  – language and social skills poor, attention span short;
  – seeks out physical comfort from all.
◆ school child:
  – short ± underweight;
  – unkempt, dirty with poor, thin hair;
  – immature and lacking in confidence, poor concentration, learning problems;
  – over-active, aggressive, poor adult and peer relationships, withdrawn;
  – wetting ± soiling.
◆ teenagers:
  – unkempt, thin hair, dirty, badly dressed (NB physical care may be good);
  – short ± thin ± obese;
  – general health poor;
  – delayed puberty;
  – school failure with truanting and running away leading to stealing, sexual exploitation, alcohol and substance abuse;
  – self-harm.

▶ **18.1–18.5 Female aged 15 years**
She had been repeatedly abused by several family members. The burn at the base of the thumb was allegedly caused by the mother using a cigarette. The cross on the outer aspect of the shoulder raises the possibility of satanic abuse. This girl had a long history of self-harm including eating glass and she caused cuts to all four limbs.

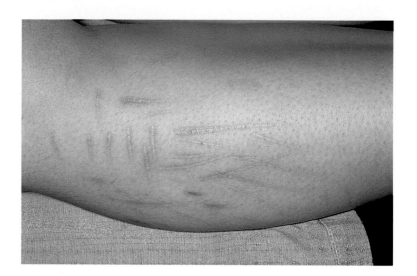

▶ **18.2**

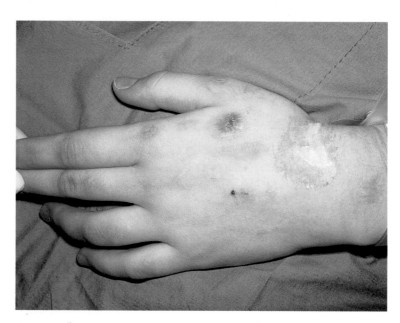

▶ **18.3**

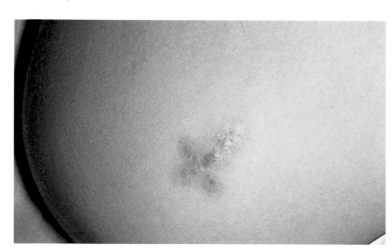

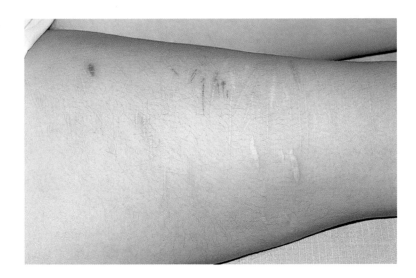

◀ **18.4**

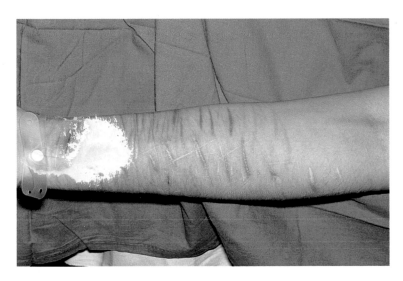

◀ **18.5**

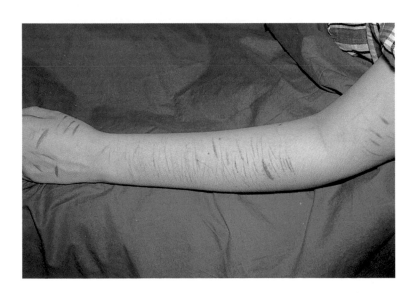

◀ **18.6 Female aged 14 years**
Girl with severe self-harm.

▶ **18.7 Female aged 10 years**
Girl with history of self-harm. Note irregular laceration on anterior aspect of shin. Self-harm in children should always be taken particularly seriously.

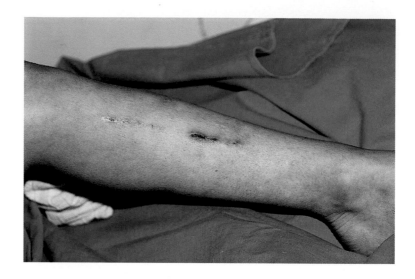

▶ **18.8 Male aged 10 years**
Boy with an ongoing history of sexual abuse. This lovebite was caused by himself.

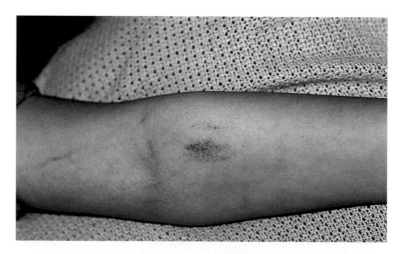

▶ **18.9–18.12 Male aged 10 years**
He was cared for in a children's home following sexual abuse at home. He has multiple self-inflicted lesions, which he chronically picked. Several of the lesions were also infected. There were concerns of possible further sexual abuse.

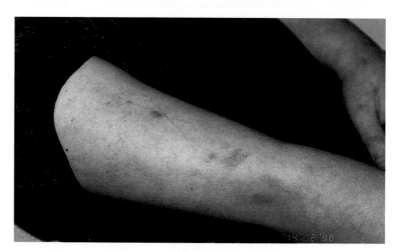

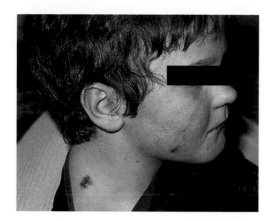

▲ 18.10

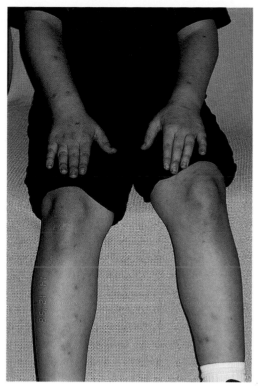

▲ 18.11

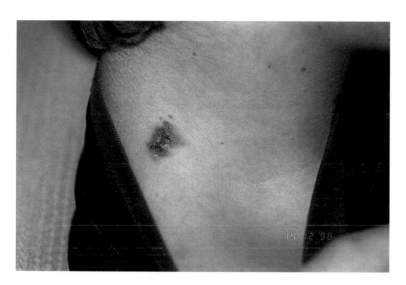

▲ 18.12

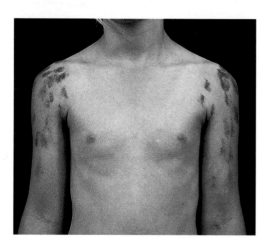

▲ 18.13 Female aged 10 years
She was taken by her mother for medical advice after finding these unusual marks: several classical paired bruises–pinch marks of self-harm. (Courtesy of Dr Kamalanathan.) The cause of this child's distress was not known.

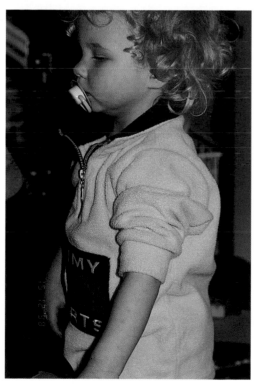

▲ 18.14 Female aged 3 years
Girl who bit her own arm. She has a history of sexual abuse.

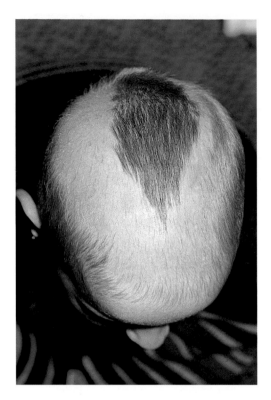

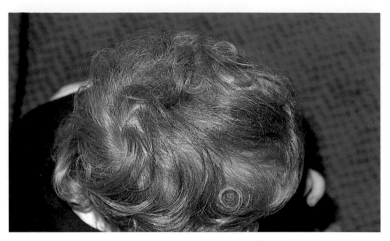

◄ 18.15, ▲ 18.16, ◄ 18.17 Female aged 4 years

Traumatic hair loss in a 4-year-old girl which was self-inflicted. It became clear during investigation that she was being sexually abused by her parents and her grandparents. Only when she was taken into foster care did her hair grow, as shown in Fig. 18.16. Figure. 18.17 of the genitalia shows an unusual shaped hymen with a tear at 6 o'clock.

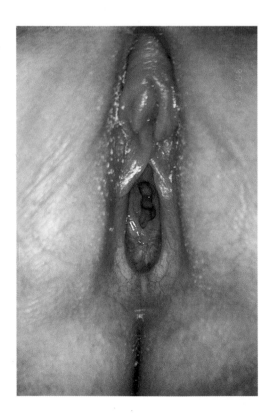

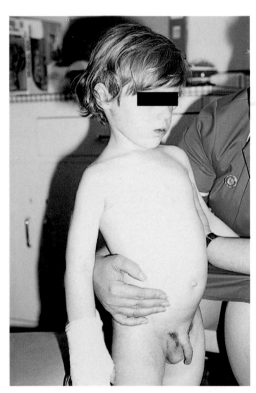

◄ 18.18 Male aged 5 years

Sad boy admitted to hospital because of diarrhoea. He had a healing scald in the perineum, a bruised penis and grossly abnormal anus. He was very anxious and fearful whilst in the hospital. His stepfather was heard to offer to buy him a bike if he kept their secret.

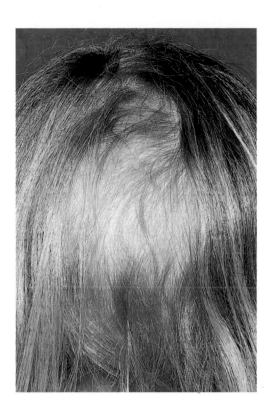

◀ **18.19 Female aged 7 years**
Child with history of emotional abuse involving her stepmother. Her stepmother repeatedly pulled out her hair when she didn't stand still to have it brushed. She was also physically abused with severe bruising of the face.

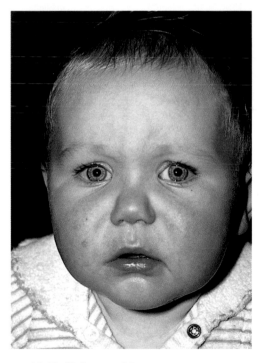

▲ **18.20 Male aged ?**
Anxious face of a toddler who was exposed to his mother's violent, aggressive verbal abuse.

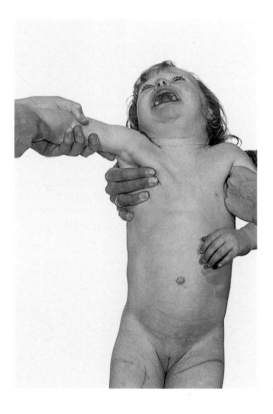

◀ **18.21 Female 2 years**
In pre-schoolers prolonged temper tantrums, including back arching are which is shown in this frightened little girl, occur in abused children.

▶ **18.22,** ▶ **18.23 Female aged 2 years**
Pathetic face of a rejected child. Her mother
decided that she was greedy and should not
be given any more to eat. She had dramatic
weight loss, which was reversed in hospital.
Her mother also complained that she couldn't
walk but within 24 hours she was running.
She also had hair loss.

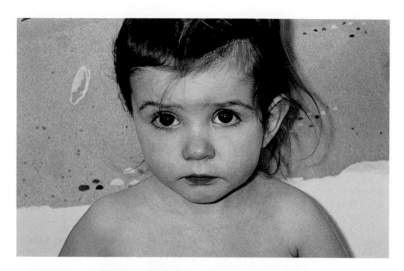

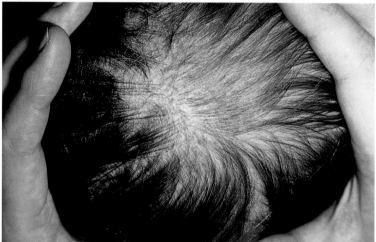

▶ **18.24–18.26 Male aged 10 months**
Infant boy who presented to the GP with
unexplained lesions on the forehead and knee.
Observation showed that the child's mother
also had picked lesions of the cheek and ear.
This mother was emotionally disturbed. The
lesions quickly healed when the cause was
pointed out to the mother. Follow-up
subsequently failed.

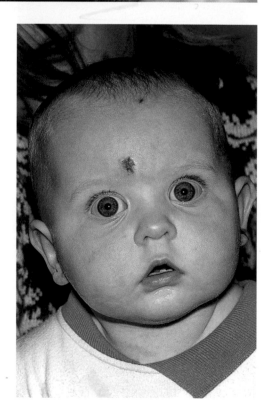

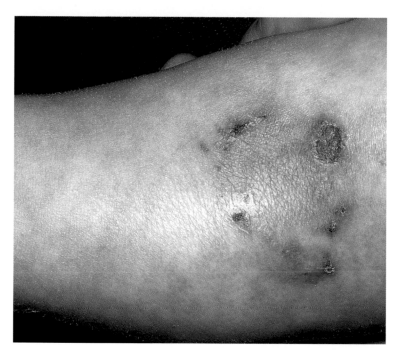

▲ 18.25

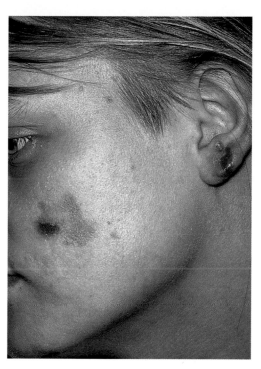

▲ 18.26

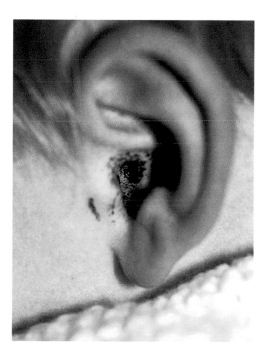

▲ 18.27 Male aged 18 months

Boy referred because of bleeding from the ear. The mother said that every time the temperature dropped in the house or outside her son's ears bled. The boy was also failing to thrive and had delayed development. He and his mother were admitted to a mother and baby home when the bleeding recurred several days after admission. The local general practitioner extracted a small tube of aluminium foil from the ear. The mother probably had been sexually abused but had also been physically and emotionally abused as a child by a member of her family. The diagnosis is Munchausen's syndrome by proxy (fictitious illness).

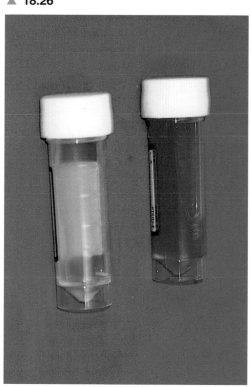

▲ 18.28 Female aged 6 years

She presented repeatedly with 'haematuria'. The urine smelt of vinegar and tomato seeds were seen on microscopy. She had previously been seen with glycosuria. The diagnosis was Munchausen's syndrome by proxy (fictitious illness).

SECTION 4

SEXUAL ABUSE

Chapter 19

Associated Non-sexual Injuries

Physical abuse and child sexual abuse (CSA) are closely related as part of the abuse, to ensure compliance, terrorize and maintain secrecy. Partner violence usually involves the children in one or more ways − the abuse may be emotional, physical, sexual and neglect − and the child may be abused by both carers. Research shows that physically abused mothers are more likely to hit their children.

Approximately 1 in 7 physically abused children are also sexually abused and 1 in 6 sexually abused children physically abused in the Leeds study. In a report of domestic violence 55% of the children were physically abused and 21% sexually abused.

Figure 19.2. shows the distribution of injuries in physically and sexually abused children, compared with physically abused children. The injuries sustained by the child may be very serious and may include murder.

The particular patterns associated with CSA include:

◆ grip marks round the upper arms, inner thighs and knees;
◆ signs of partial strangulation with petechiae of the upper eyelids, linear marks round the neck;
◆ bruises over the lower abdomen, especially the symphysis pubis;
◆ 'love bites' − usually on the neck, breast;
◆ sadistic injuries such as lacerations to the penis, perineum, anus, labia;
◆ burns, for example cigarettes burns to the genitalia, breasts, 'branding' with a heated implement;
◆ the injuries may be in 'abusive' sites such as genitalia but also on the back of the hand, neck, etc.;
◆ self-mutilation is relatively common in CSA − see Chapter 18.

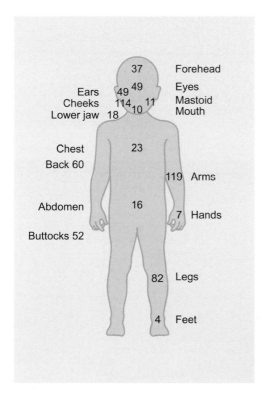

Fig. 19 1 Sites for superficial injury in 251 non-accidental injury cases. Sites, not number of children, are totalled. (Reproduced by courtesy of Dr M F G Buchanan).

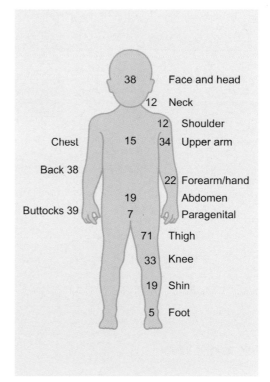

Fig. 19.2 Distribution of bruises by site in 110 physically and sexually abused children. Figures refer to the number of children. (Reproduced with permission from Hobbs C J, Wynne J M 1990 The sexually abused battered child. Archives of Disease in Childhood 65: 423–427.)

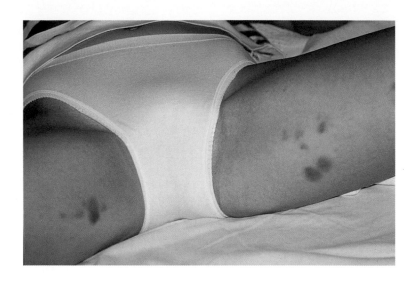

▶ **19.1,** ▶ **19.2 Female aged 9 years**
Girl who was sexually assaulted by her
19-year-old brother. Note the fingertip
bruising on the inner aspect of both thighs
(Fig. 19.1). Fingertip bruises on the inner
aspect of the left upper arm with superficial
scratching (Fig. 19.2).

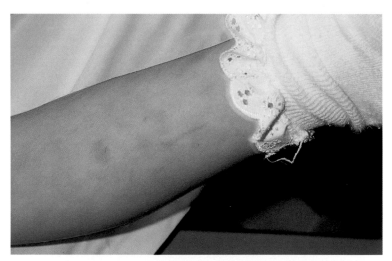

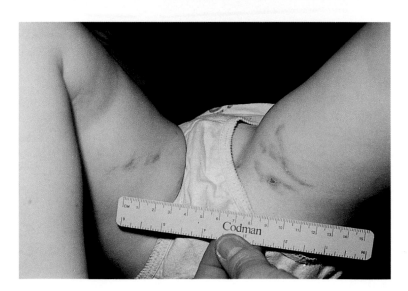

▶ **19.3 Female aged 4 years**
Girl who was sexually assaulted by a family
member. Note extensive scratching on inner
aspect of both thighs where she was
restrained.

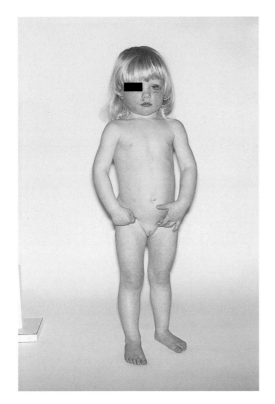

▲ 19.4

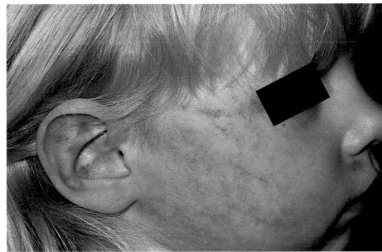

▲ 19.5

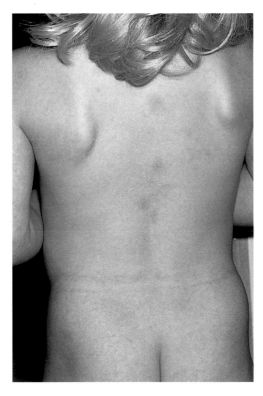

▲ 19.6

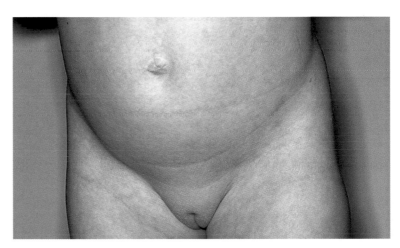

▲ 19.4, ▲ 19.5, ◄ 19.6, ▲ 19.7 **Female aged 3 years**
The mother returned after an evening out to find the child with a badly bruised face. Her partner admitted to hitting the child. There is a recent hand slap across the right side of the face with bruising in one ear (Fig. 19.5). There is also bruising on the mid and lower back (Fig. 19.6), the left groin, and a faint bruise is also visible on the right lower abdomen (Fig. 19.7). The other bruises were inflicted by gripping the child. The child disclosed sexual assault but there was no abnormality of genitalia or anus.

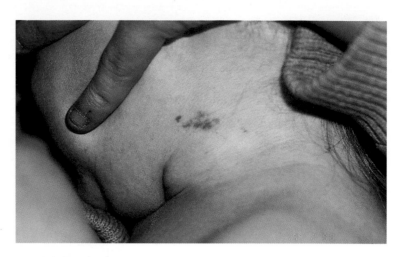

▲ **19.8 Female aged 3 years**
The bruise on her neck was noticed in the day nursery. The photograph shows a bruise on the left side of the neck, with the appearance of a 'love bite'. (Note: bruises such as these are highly correlated with sexual abuse.)

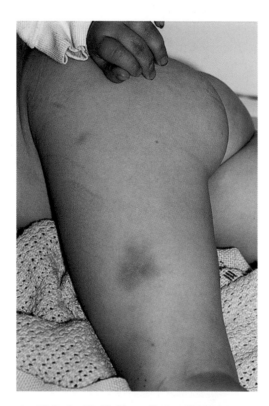 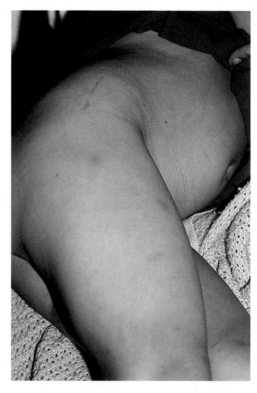

▲ **19.9, ▲ 19.10 Female aged 4 years**
She was seen in the clinic because her older sister had disclosed sexual abuse. A large, roughly triangular bruise is seen on the posterior aspect of the left upper thigh, with a smaller bruise on the buttock (Fig. 19.9). There were also scratches just above the knee and several further bruises on the outer aspect of the right thigh laterally (Fig. 19.10). Examination of the genitalia and anus showed signs consistent with vaginal and anal penetration. (Note: if one child in the family has disclosed sexual abuse, it is usual practice to examine all the other siblings. Whilst these injuries are non-specific they are worrying in their distribution, i.e. thigh, and the smaller round bruises may be fingertip bruising.)

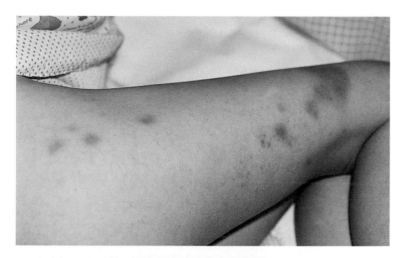

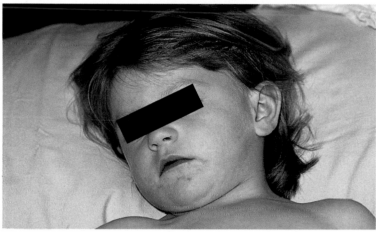

◀ **19.11 Female aged 7 years**
She was referred by a school nurse who noticed bruising on her thigh. There are multiple round bruises on the outer aspect of the right upper thigh and a larger triangular-shaped bruise on the lower thigh. The father admitted to sexually abusing this child, and also hitting her with a belt.

◀ **19.12,** ◀ **19.13,** ◀ **19.14,** ▼ **19.15**
Female aged 2 years
A miserable child who was being chronically sexually abused. She was brought to the A&E Department with a history that for several days she had had a band of bruising across the abdomen. She had extensive labial fusion and markedly dilated anus with prolapsing mucosa and reddening perianally. There was some swelling of the anal margin. Despite clear medical evidence from both experts the court sent this child home.

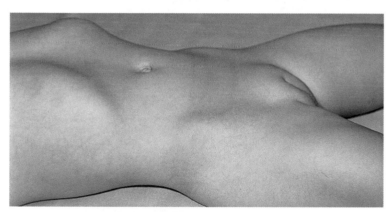

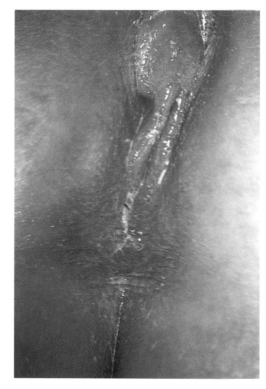

▲ **19.15**

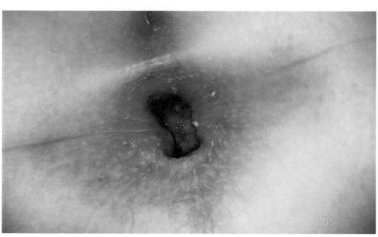

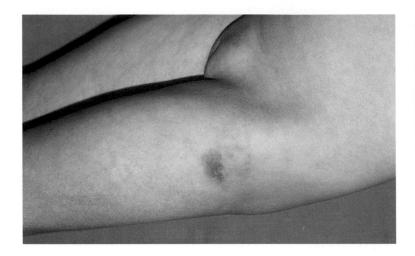

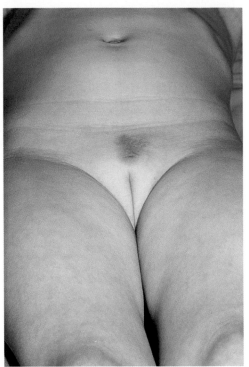

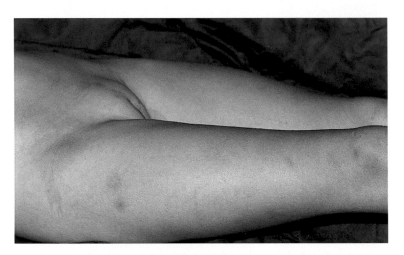

◄ **19.16,** ▲ **19.17,** ◄ **19.18,** ◄ **19.19**
Female aged 5 years

Initially the child was taken to the hospital
emergency department by her parents who
alleged that the girl's older cousin had sexually
assaulted her. Investigations revealed a recent
bruise on the symphysis pubis. Approximately
a year later the child was brought back to the
emergency department by her parents
because of serious vaginal bleeding. Again
bruising was seen on the symphysis pubis and
both outer thighs. Further investigation revealed
profuse bleeding from the genitalia with a large
clot at introitus, and a tear was seen to extend
from the posterior vaginal wall onto the
perineum. The genital signs were of vaginal
rape and the bruising associated with this.

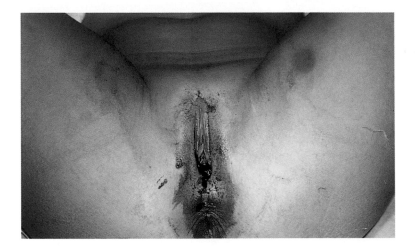

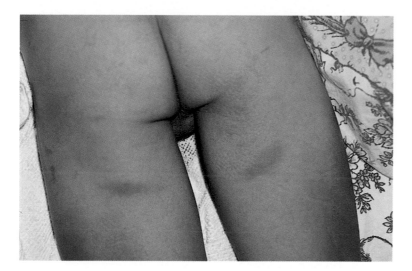

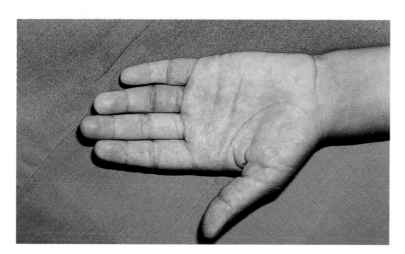

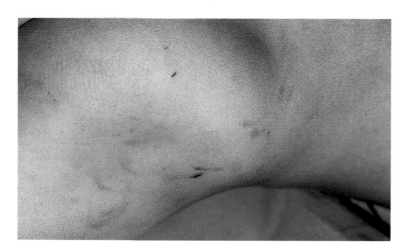

◄ ◄ ◄ **19.20–19.22 Male aged 4 years**
Social services referred the child after sexually
explicit play was seen at nursery school. The
photographs show linear bruises on the
posterior aspect of both upper thighs proximally,
bruising of the proximal phalanx of the fourth
and fifth fingers of the left hand and old healed
scratches on the outer aspect of the thigh and
buttock. Abnormal anal findings consistent with
penetration were also seen. These are unusual
injuries, all unexplained, combined with
abnormal anal findings, and later the child
disclosed abuse by his father and grandfather.

▶ **19.23 Female aged 2 years**

The mother moved into a friend's house, and shortly afterwards the child complained of a sore bottom. The doctor examined her and found an acute anal fissure and referred her to the paediatrician. The photograph shows an irregular recent bruise on the outer aspect of the right upper thigh. Examination of the anus showed an acute fissure, dilated veins, and perianal oedema. (Note: a diagnosis of anal abuse was made in this child and the older children in the household were subsequently taken into care because of multiple abuse, including physical abuse due to Munchausen's syndrome by proxy.)

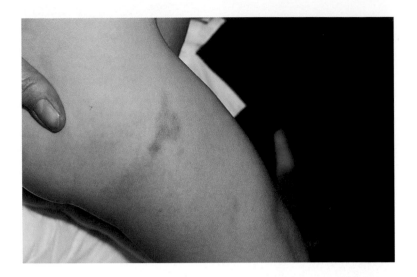

▶ **19.24 Male aged 4 years**

A child with unexplained bruising of the abdomen. He was presented at the A&E Department with an unexplained laceration to his penis.

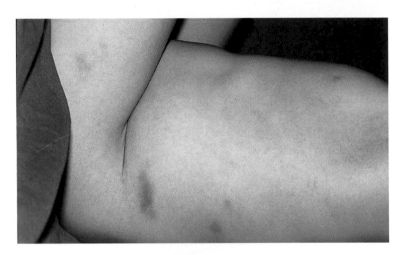

▶ **19.25 Male aged 2 years**

The child's father took him to the hospital emergency department saying that 24 hours earlier the child had fallen and hurt his arm. X-ray showed a metaphyseal humeral fracture and the child was also noted to have multiple facial bruising and an abnormal anus. The child was returned to the care of the father and stepmother and re-referred by his nursery with new injuries. Linear scratches are seen on the anterior and medial aspect of the right thigh. A small bruise on the dorsal aspect of the penis is also seen. The scratches are consistent with nail marks and the bruise with a nip to the penis.

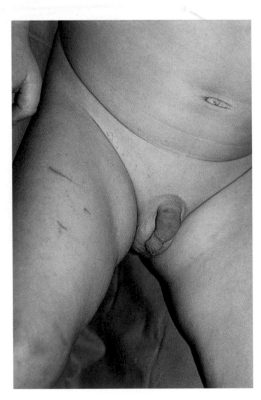

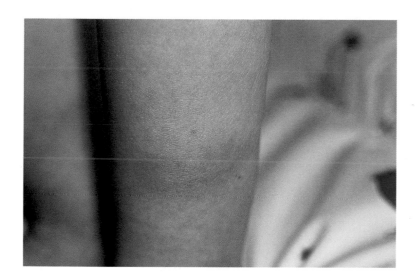

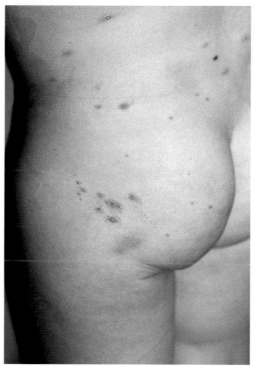

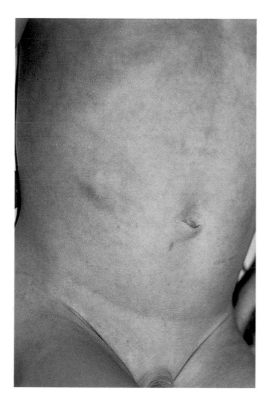

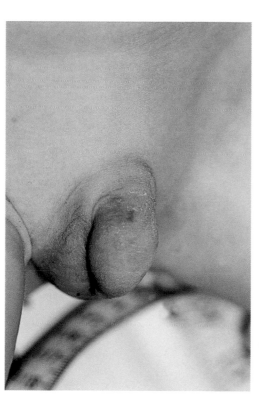

▲ ▲ ▲ ▲ **19.26–19.29 Male aged 18 months**
Presented at A&E with a penile injury and also unexplained bands of bruising on the posterior aspect of his lower thighs. He also had an old, untreated scald on his face and healing rib fractures. His general care was poor with scattered infected spots (Fig. 19.27). He was also underweight. He also had a linear bruise lateral to the umbilicus (Fig. 19.28). He had proximal bruising of the penis and a small healed laceration (Fig. 19.29).

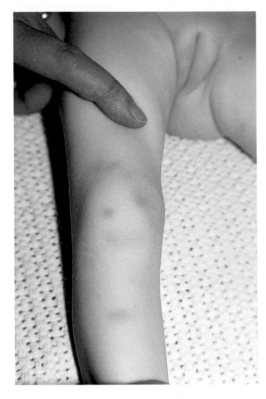

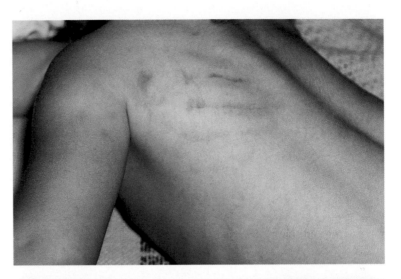

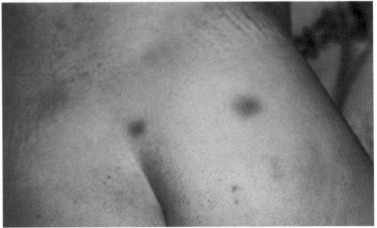

▲ **19.30 Female aged 15 months**
She was admitted to hospital following an emergency call claiming she had 'drowned in the bath'. Multiple circular bruises are seen on the right knee. Signs of sexual abuse, physical abuse and failure to thrive were all identified.

▲ **19.31, ▲ 19.32 Female aged 3 years**
The family was under supervision of the social services because of concern about Munchausen's syndrome by proxy. The mother told a social worker that the child had injured her back when she slipped in the bath. There is a clear adult hand print across the right upper back and three round bruises on the right buttock. The child made a very clear disclosure of sexual abuse following physical examination.

▶ **19.33 Female aged 2 years**
Child with extensive bruising on the left lower aspect of the abdomen. Bruising when seen on the lower abdomen, i.e. not over bony promontories, is highly correlated with sexual abuse.

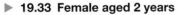

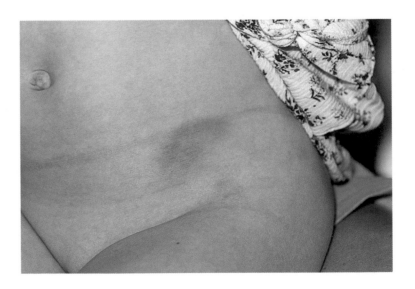

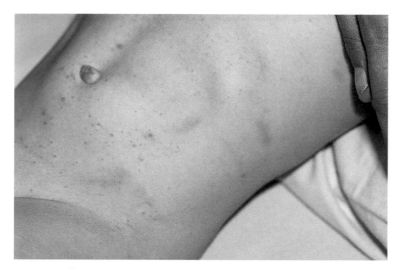

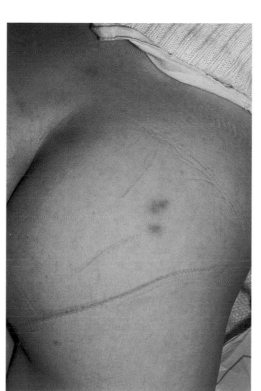

◀ **19.34 Female aged 14 months**
The mother took the child to the doctor because of 'soreness'. Social services were involved because of contact with a known child abuser. There is multiple bruising of different ages over the abdomen and left groin. There was also associated nappy rash and the genitalia were abnormal. This is very unusual bruising; abdominal bruising is frequently associated with sexual abuse.

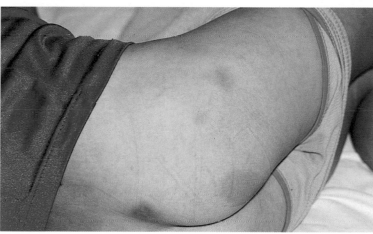

▲ **19.35 Male aged 7 years**
He told his parents that a man had tried to touch his bottom in the street. A large bruise is seen on the superior aspect of the natal cleft, purple in colour with brown edges, and two more bruises are seen on the lateral aspect of the right buttock. The bruise in the natal cleft is particularly unusual, but the bruises on the buttock are also relevant given the history. Abnormal anal signs were present too.

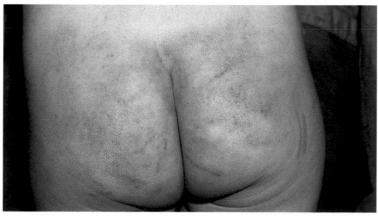

▲ **19.36 Female aged 5 years**
She was examined because her older sibling had been sexually abused. A pinch mark is seen on the right buttock. Pinch marks on the buttocks are always of great concern, and particularly in view of the family history in this case.

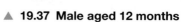

▲ **19.37 Male aged 12 months**
The mother complained to the social services that following an access visit to his father the child had a badly bruised bottom. There is extensive bruising over both buttocks, and finger marks are visible within the mass of bruising. This is a severe beating in a very young child. There was evidence of sexual abuse in an older sibling. 'Spanking' may have sexual connotations.

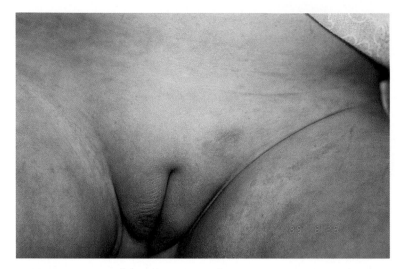

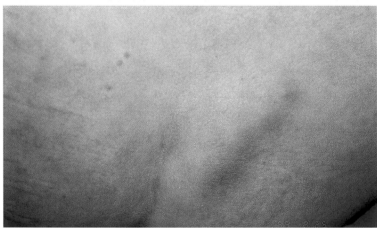

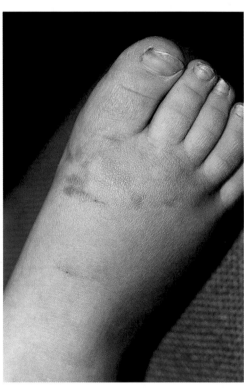

▲ 19.38, ▲ 19.39, ▶ 19.40 **Female aged 2 years**
Social services referred her when bruises had been seen at day nursery.
Bruising is seen in the left pubic area; there was also bruising on the
buttocks and dorsum of the right foot. Further examination showed anal
findings consistent with sexual abuse. Bruising in the pubic area is always
very worrying, and is unusual in accidental injury.

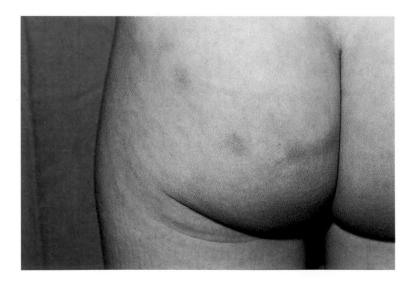

◀ 19.41 **Female aged 4 years**
She attended a routine paediatric follow-up
appointment, having been previously physically
abused, and also possibly emotionally abused
with an over-involved father and very anxious
stepmother. There is fingertip bruising of the left
buttock. Bruising of this nature is always of
great concern and raises a strong possibility of
sexual abuse.

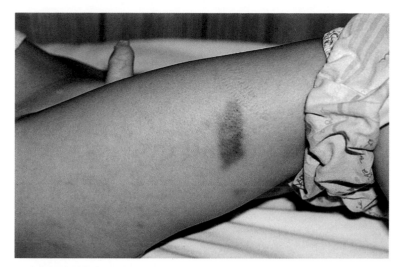

◀ 19.42 Male aged 6 years
He was referred by the family service unit after it had been discovered that his older sister had been sexually abused by their father. A large bruise is seen on the outer aspect of the right upper thigh, but also note several small fingertip bruises too. The bruise on the outer thigh is non-specific but may have been caused by a kick; the small fingertip bruising in this location is worrying. (Note the sustained erection, this is a very worrying sign in small boys.) Several other children in this family had evidence of sexual abuse.

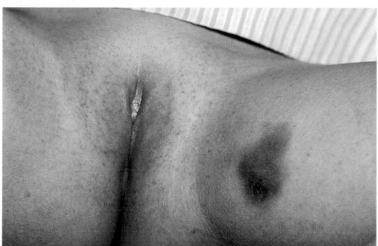

◀ 19.43 Female aged 5 years
During a games lesson when the child was sitting cross-legged the teacher noticed a bruise on the inner thigh, and also a similar bruise on the outer thigh. She remembered that some 2 weeks earlier the child had complained of having a sore bottom. There is a large irregular bruise on the inner aspect of the left thigh. The findings were consistent with anal and genital abuse. The child subsequently gave a very clear disclosure of genital and anal abuse by her father.

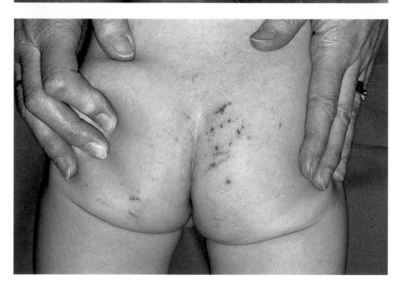

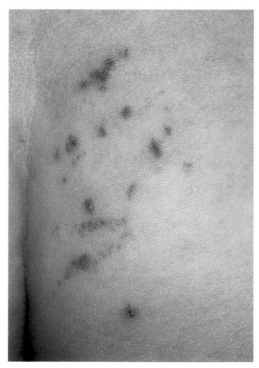

◀ 19.44, ▶ 19.45 Female aged 2 years
Child was previously known to the paediatric department because of extreme clinging, sore vulva, and a very anxious mother. She had been admitted to the local fever hospital when this 'unexplained' rash was seen. Scratch marks can be seen on both buttocks with linear scratch marks and small areas of skin loss. The child also had multiple anal fissures. These scratches are fingernail marks in a child who had also been sexually abused.

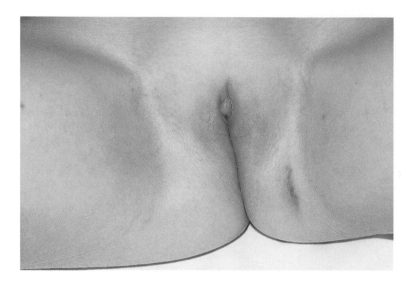

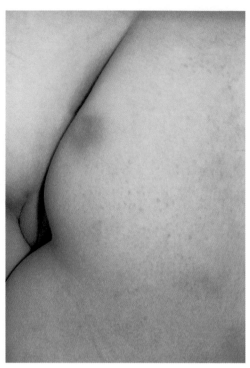

▲ **19.46,** ▶ **19.47 Female aged 6 years**

Over the previous months she had returned from access to her father with bruising about the face, but her grandmother was very anxious when she found bruising on the buttocks and in the groin and informed social services. The photographs show a linear bruise on the left groin and a bruise on the right buttock at the natal cleft. Examination showed signs consistent with anal abuse. The girl gave a very clear disclosure of physical and sexual abuse by her father occurring on access visits.

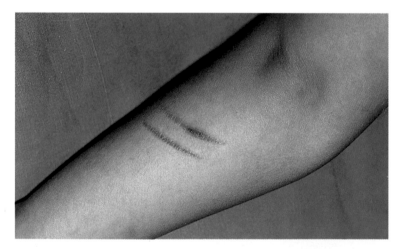

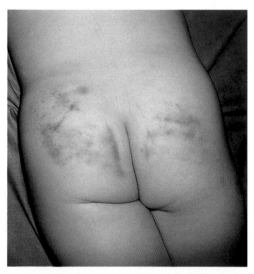

▲ **19.48 Female aged 7 years**

She told a neighbour that her father had been hurting her. Social services were contacted. There is an unexplained burn on the outer aspect of the left forearm; also note the small brown bruise just above the wrist. Examination of the genital area showed marked reddening. Both the burn and the reddening were unexplained, and it was some months before this child could be protected when care from her mother deteriorated to even more unacceptable levels.

▲ **19.49 Male aged 4 years**

He had been recently seen in the hospital emergency department with a fractured clavicle which had been accepted as being due to an accident. A second medical was requested by social services after it was realized that his father was a convicted child abuser. The photograph shows severely beaten buttocks. No abnormality was seen of the genitalia or anus. There is clearly serious non-accidental injury, and the possibility of sexual abuse remains.

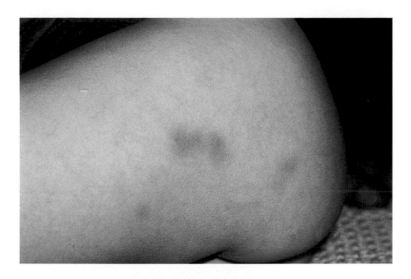

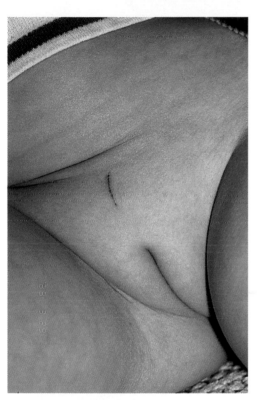

▲ 19.50, ◄ 19.51 Female aged 24 months

She was examined because her younger half-brother had severely beaten buttocks (Fig. 19.37). Grip marks are seen on the outer aspect of the left upper thigh/buttocks, and there is a scratch on the pubis. These are genital signs consistent with sexual abuse.

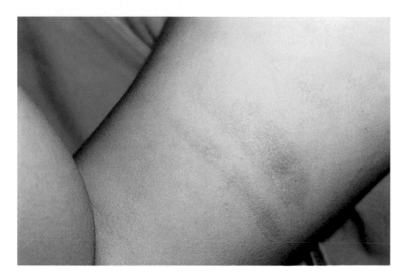

◄ 19.52 Female aged 3 years

She was seen in the paediatric clinic because her older brother had disclosed that his parents had sexually abused him, after he had been received into foster care. This girl was mute. There are healing linear burns on the posterior aspect of the right upper thigh. There was also a severe degree of labial fusion and abnormal anus. Unexplained burns are always of great concern. Burns are related to sadistic abuse and in particular sexual abuse. There is also an association between mutism and sexual abuse.

▶ **19.53,** ▶ **19.54 Female aged 16 years**
Child told her social worker that she had been
sexually abused (again). She lived between the
Safe House and a violent family. The
photographs show a cigarette burn on the
right breast and inner aspect of the left thigh.
On further examination she had a total of
16 burns. These were caused by an
unidentified assailant, and not thought to be
self-inflicted. This was a severely damaged
girl caught up in a violent relationship.

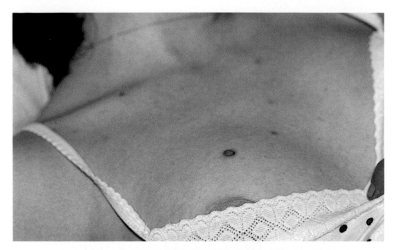

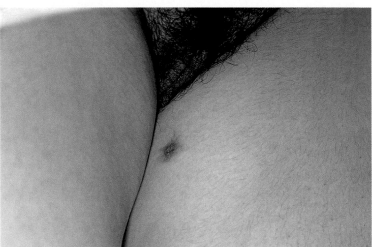

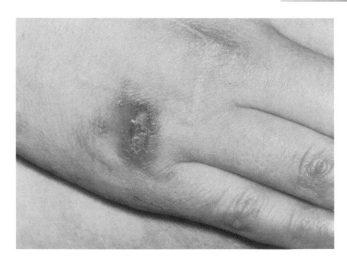

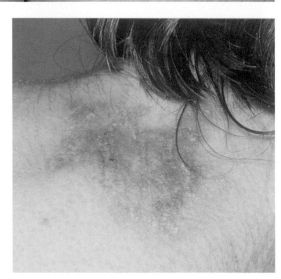

▲ **19.55,** ▶ **19.56,** ▶ **19.57,** ▶ **19.58**
Female aged 11 years
She was referred by her special school when bruising about the face was noted. The photographs
show a healing burn on the back of the neck (Fig. 19.56), an almost healed burn on the dorsum of the
right hand across the knuckles (Fig. 19.55), bruises on the dorsum of both feet (Fig. 19.57) and a
large bruise on the inner aspect of the right thigh (Fig. 19.58). There were signs consistent with genital
and anal abuse. These were inflicted burns on the back of the neck and on the back of the hand. The
injury to the feet is consistent with stamping, and of the inner thigh with a kick (see Chapter 12). The
child subsequently disclosed sexual abuse by the stepmother. The younger stepbrother had been
encouraged to stamp on the girl's feet. These injuries were seen in the context of sadistic abuse,
which also included the child having a polythene bag put over her head.

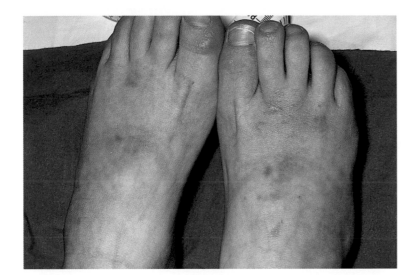

◄ **19.57**

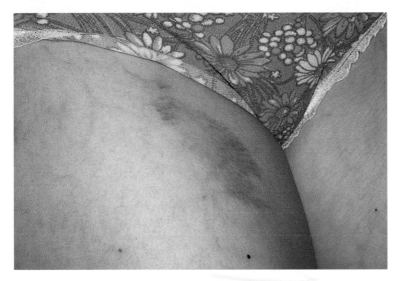

◄ **19.58**

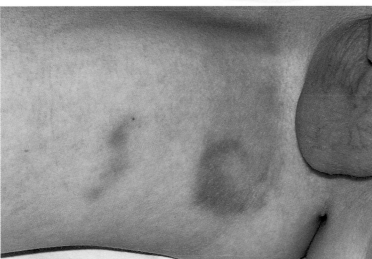

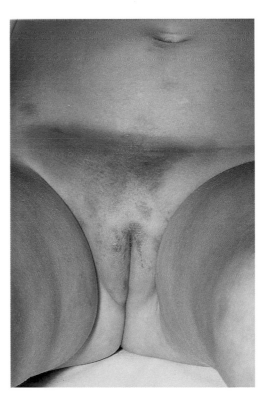

▲ **19.59 Male aged 11 years**

The social services requested that the child be seen in the paediatric clinic after he had been seen visiting a known child abuser. There is an unexplained circular bruise on the inner aspect of the right upper thigh, and a probable pinch mark. Further examination showed a markedly abnormal anus. The circular bruise is unexplained, but is in a worrying site as are the pinch marks. The boy later disclosed sexual abuse by the known child abuser.

▲ **19.60 Female aged 10 months**

The mother took the child to the hospital emergency department because of concern about bruising on her abdomen. There is extensive bruising in the pubic area and lower abdomen. This is an old photograph from the early 1970s; sexual assault was questioned but not confirmed.

▶ 19.61 Male aged 4 years

The mother sought help from social services after separation from her husband. The oldest daughter had nightmares, and profuse vaginal discharge. Examination of her sister revealed signs consistent with abuse. All the children were examined. The boy showed a circular bruise on the right pubic area. He also had an abnormal anus. The child initially said the injury was due to handle bars on his bicycle. He later went on to disclose sexual abuse by his father. This is an unexplained bruise in an unusual site, and may be a suction bruise.

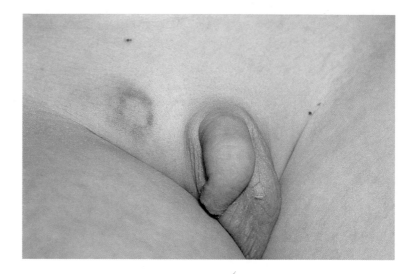

▶ 19.62 Male aged 5 years

He was seen in the clinic after it had been found that his younger sister, who had been admitted to hospital because of severe physical abuse, had been sexually abused. The father asked the boy to say that he had bruised his buttocks after having fallen off a gate. Investigation revealed an incomplete circular bruise consistent with a bite; there were also abnormal anal signs. It was felt that this was an adult bite, but the opinion of the forensic orthodontologist was not sought.

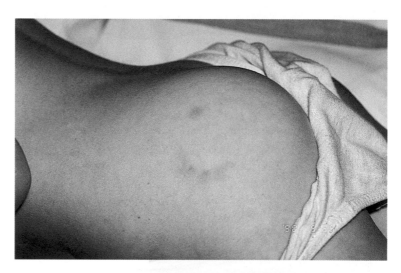

▶ 19.63 Female aged 3 years

Child told her mother that her mother's partner had rubbed her tuppence. There is a linear bruise on the right buttock, and linear and circular bruises on the lateral aspect and posteriorly on the right thigh. The genitalia were reddened. The bruises are suggestive of fingertip bruising, and the reddening is consistent with rubbing.

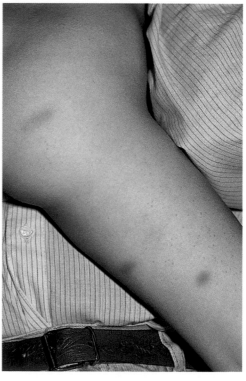

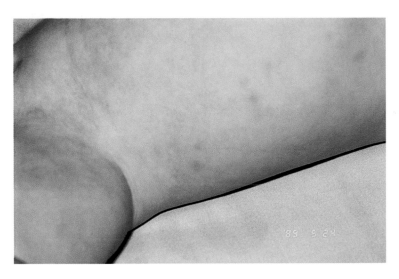

▲ **19.64**

◀ **19.64,** ◀ **19.65,** ▼ **19.66,** ◀ **19.67,**
▶ **19.68,** ▶ **19.69,** ▶ **19.70,** ▶ **19.71**
Female aged 18 months
She was seen for routine follow-up in the failure to thrive clinic when bruising was noticed. The photographs show multiple pinches and fingertip bruising on the abdomen, a probable bite on the left lower leg, a linear bruise on the left calf posteriolaterally, scratches about the right knee with a bruise on the front of the knee, a bruise on the outer aspect of the right upper arm and right chest, a bruise on the outer aspect of the right lower arm, a laceration on the lateral border of the left foot and recent and healed scratches on the face. Further examination showed genital and anal abnormality. These are multiple bruises and fingernail scratches in a child already known because of failure to thrive. These injuries are consistent with repeated physical abuse in association with sexual abuse.

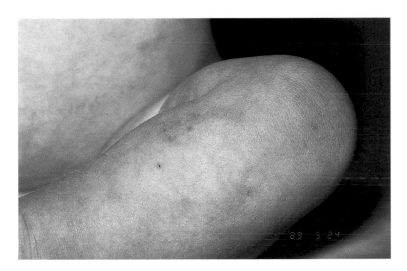

▲ **19.65**

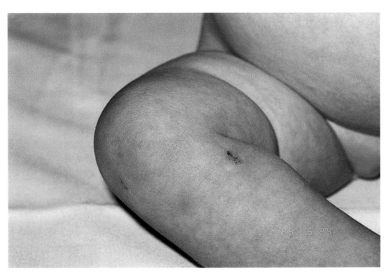

▲ **19.67**

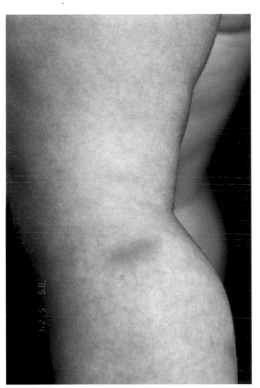

▲ **19.66**

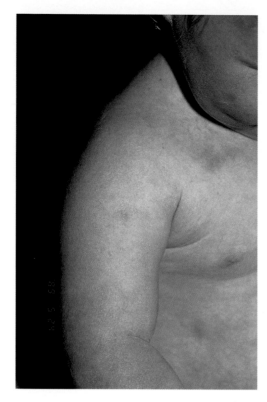

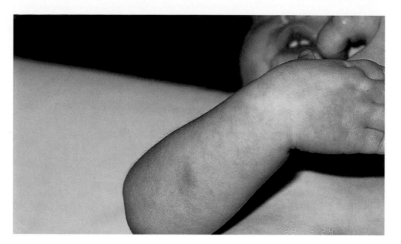

▲ 19.69

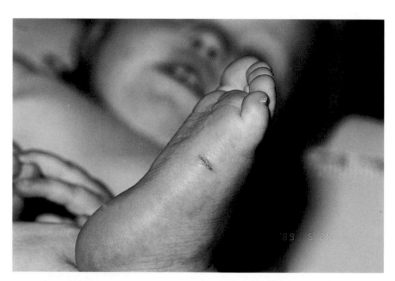

▲ 19.70

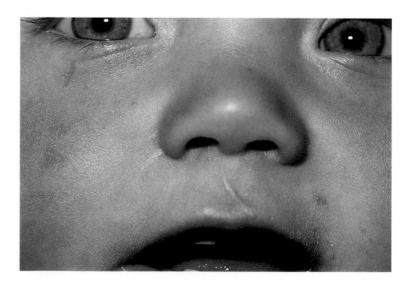

▲ 19.71

▲ **19.68–19.71**
Female aged 18 months (continued)

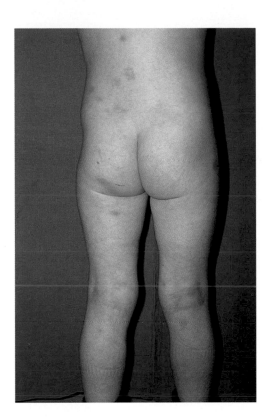

◀ 19.72 Female aged 3 years

She was seen for examination after it was disclosed to the girl's mother that her 12-year-old sister was abusing her. Multiple, fingertip bruising of the left lower back, the left buttock, the posterior aspect of the left thigh and the right outer thigh can be seen. Her genitalia were normal. This child had far too many bruises suggestive of fingertip bruising. She was seen again 3 months later with grossly abnormal genitalia and anus where she had been sexually abused by an adult.

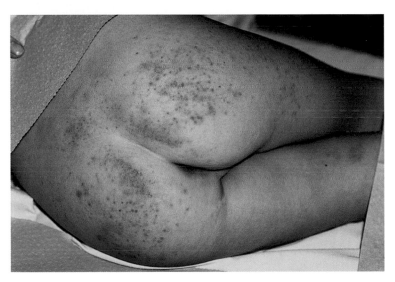

◀ 19.73 Female aged 5 years

The child returned home with a rash on her buttocks after a contact visit with her father. Her mother took her to the doctor who referred her to hospital. Extensive bruising and petechial haemorrhages can be seen over both buttocks. The anus was abnormal. The signs are consistent with a beating of the buttocks and sexual abuse.

Chapter 20

Normal Ano-genital Findings

The normal genitalia:
(a) female
- prepubertal;
- postpubertal.

(b) male.

Prepubertal

Girls in the UK currently reach the menarche at 12.8 years but the first effects of oestrogen are seen in the neonatal period and early infancy due to transplacental transfer of maternal hormones.

In early infancy there are signs caused by maternal hormones and subsequent 'withdrawal' and include:

- breast swelling in both boys and girls;
- thick, abundant, pale hymen;
- white vaginal discharge;
- vaginal bleeding (withdrawal of maternal oestrogen).

Congenital anomalies

- imperforate hymen;
- 'congenital absence' of the hymen has not been reported in a large series of examinations of normal newborn infants but 3–4% girls may have anatomical variants such as hymenal tags, septate hymen.

In practice, an 'absent' hymen is seen only as part of a more widespread congenital anomaly or abuse.

As the infant grows the effects of maternal oestrogen diminish and the configuration of the hymen changes.

- The hymen becomes thinner and has a sharp free edge.
- The vasculature of the hymen is clearly visible and gives the appearance of reddening (which is normal and not, for example, inflammation).
- The configuration changes with age from infancy, where annular, sleeve or fimbriated hymen are the usual forms, until 2 to 3 years, when a crescentic shape becomes more common.
- In a crescentic hymen there is a relative lack of tissue anteriorly and symmetrical shallow notches at 10 and 2 o'clock.
- The horizontal hymenal measurement is usually less than 0.4 cm prepubertally and by puberty 1.0 cm. Note the method of examination, which affects the appearance of the hymen:
  − supine (separation, traction)
  − knee−chest

- Congenital notches are not seen in the posterior hymen; thus posterior notches are highly correlated with penetrative trauma.
- A few mm of a superficial labial fusion is commonly seen when the infant is in nappies.
- Reddening is commonly seen.

Postpubertal girl

Sexual maturation is suppressed during childhood but by the age of 11.5 years the average girl in the UK has breast development stage 2 with the presence of glandular tissue in the subareolar region and the nipple and breast tissue project as a single mound from the chest wall (Marshall & Tanner, 1969). The average age of menarche is 12.8 years by when the breast development is Tanner 4−5 (fully developed). The development of external genitalia, bar pubic hair (adrenal androgens), is oestrogen dependant. The labia majora and minora grow in size and thickness under the influence of oestrogen. At the same time, again under the influence of oestrogen the hymen thickens and the hymenal opening grows to the adult size of 1 cm. (Garden 1998). The vagina lengthens and the lining thickens and begins to secrete mucus. The final length is around 10 cm.

- Precocious puberty in girls is usually familial and in girls benign apart from social adjustment, adrenarche is the isolated development of pubic and axillary hair and thelarche is the development of breasts.

Reference

Marshall WA, Tanner JM (1969) Variations in the pattern of pubertal changes in Girls. *Arch Dis Child* **44:291-303**

Further Reading

Garden AS (1998) Gynaecological development p.3−14 in: *Paediatric and Gynaecological Gynaecology.* ed: AS Garden, Arnold: London

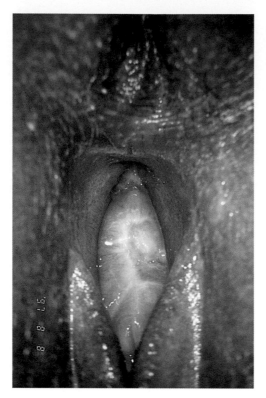

▲ **20.1 Female aged 12 years**
Teenage girl in early puberty with fleshy pale hymen. Slight irregularity at the posterior fourchette. Examination of teenage girls is not adequate by inspection alone. Some form of digital examination is necessary.

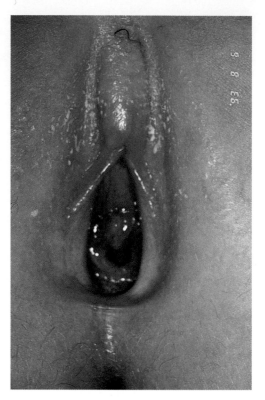

▲ **20.2 Female aged 2 years**
A crescentic opening in a fleshy hymen.

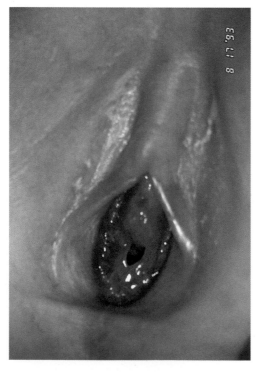

▲ **20.3 Female aged 3 years**
A crescentic hymen and semi-transparent smooth margin with no disruption of blood vessels.

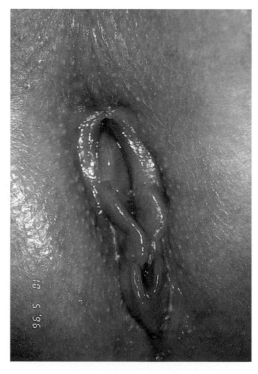

▲ **20.4 Female aged 6 months**
Infant with normal fleshy hymen.

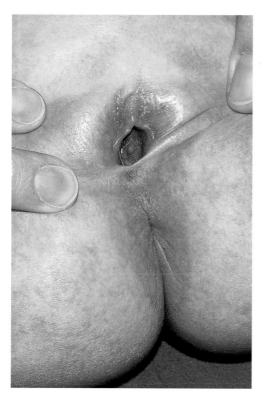

▲ **20.5 Female aged 2 years**
A fleshy hymen with a redundant free edge and normal anus.

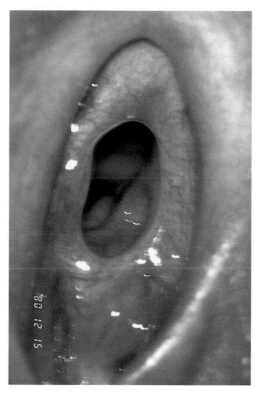

▲ **20.6 Female aged 4 years**
High magnification view demonstrating an annular hymen with a sharp edge and clear vascular pattern.

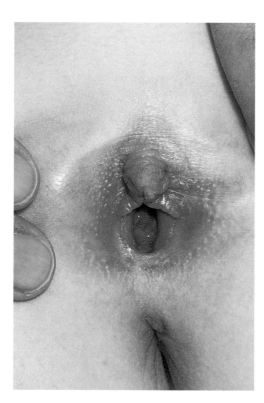

▲ **20.7 Female aged 2 years**
A closed fleshy hymen.

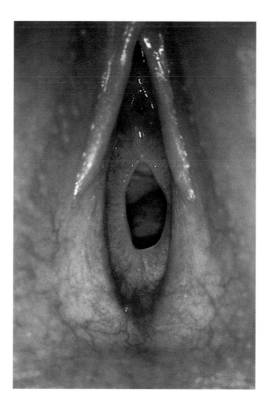

◀ **20.8 Female aged 6 years**
A high magnification view which gives the appearance of a gaping but smooth semi-translucent free edge and an undisturbed vascular pattern. Annular hymen.

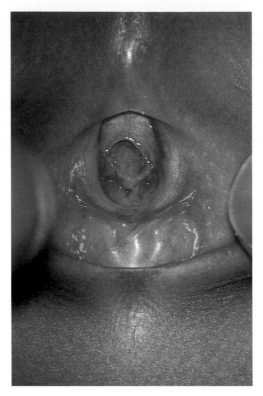

▲ **20.9 Female infant**
Genitalia of infant demonstrating annular hymen with clear blood vessel pattern running to sharp margin. Labial traction initially makes this look a rather wide hymenal opening but note magnification.

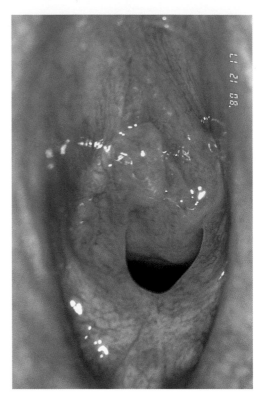

▲ **20.10 Female aged 5 years**
A high magnification view of a crescentic hymen.

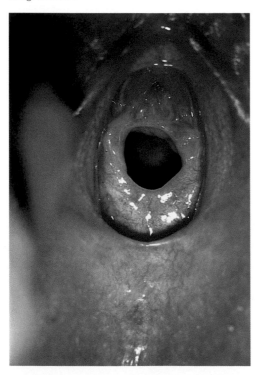

▲ **20.11 Female infant**
A high magnification view of an annular hymen.

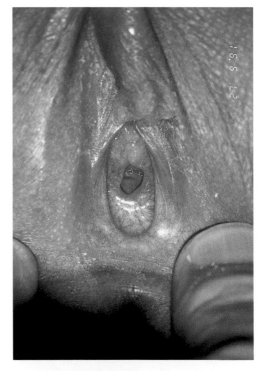

▲ **20.12 Female aged 3 years**
Annular hymen in a 3 year old. The hymen is abundant. Note again the clear vascular pattern. High magnification.

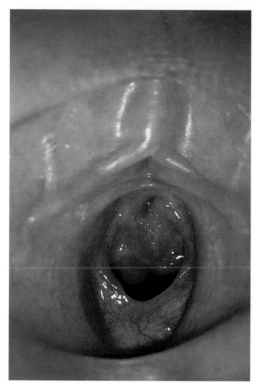

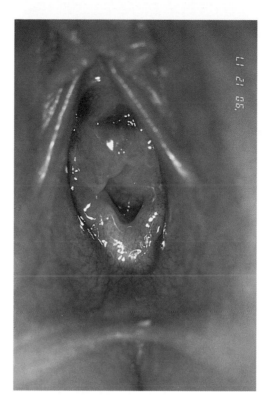

▲ **20.13 Female aged 6 years**
A high magnification view of a crescentic hymen. Note the thin posterior rim which is almost translucent with clearly visible blood vessels. There is little hymenal tissue anteriorly.

▲ **20.14 Female aged 1 year**
A high magnification view of the fleshy redundant hymen of infancy leading to a distorted view of the hymenal opening.

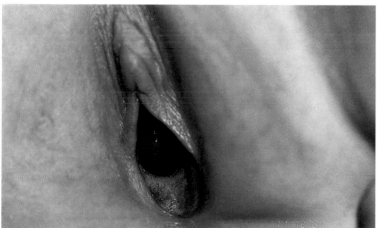

◀ **20.15 Female aged 6 years**
A normal crescentic hymen in a child with vulvitis.

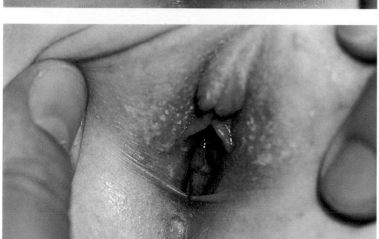

◀ **20.16 Female aged 1 year**
Mild vulvovaginitis but fleshy hymen of infancy.

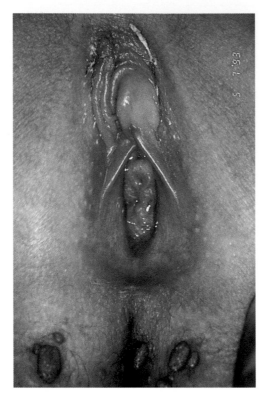

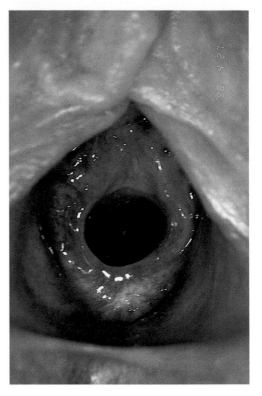

▲ **20.17 Female aged 1 year**
Fleshy redundant hymen of infancy. The perianal warts need to be investigated as a possibly sexually transmitted disease.

▲ **20.18 Female aged 5 years**
Girl with annular hymen and small notch at 12 o'clock. Notches like this in the midline are usually thought to be normal.

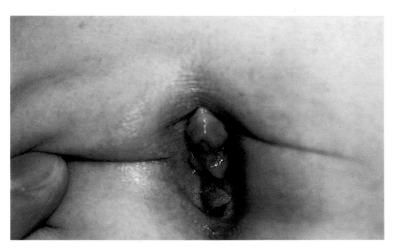

▲ **20.19 Female aged 12 months**
Infantile hymen with fleshy tag.

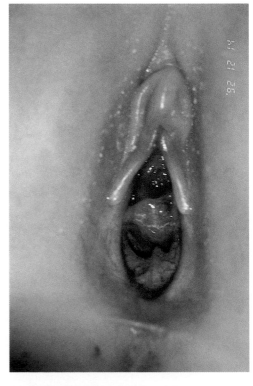

▲ **20.20 Female aged 7 years**
Septal remnant at 6 o'clock seen in a normal crescentic hymen.

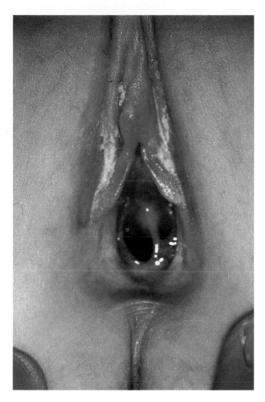

▲ **20.21 Female aged 5 years**
Septate hymen.

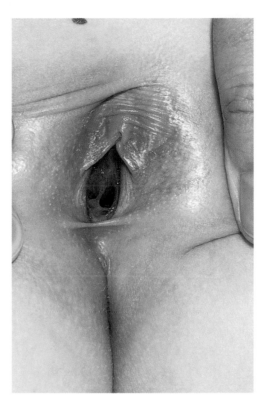

▲ **20.22 Female aged 4 years**
Multiperforate hymen.

◄ **20.23 Female aged 7 years**
High magnification of a septate hymen.

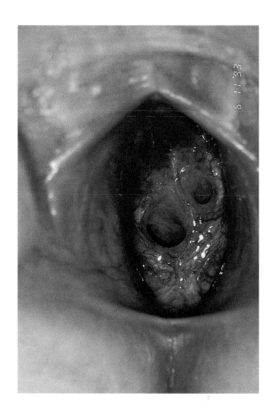

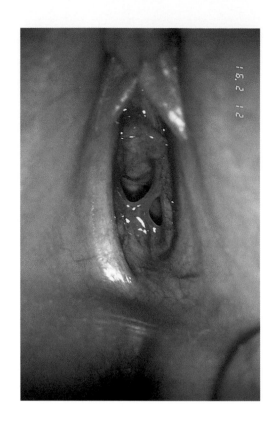

▶ **20.24 Female aged 5 years**
Septate hymen.

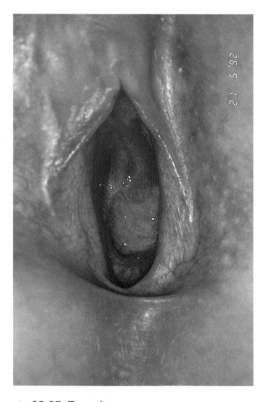

▲ **20.25 Female**
Unusual appearance with a 'flap of hymen' forming across the hymenal opening. This may be a normal variant.

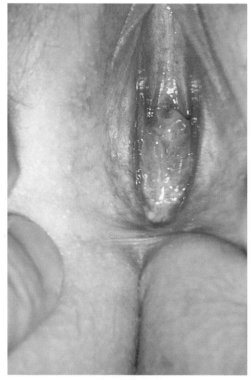

▲ **20.26 Female aged 10 years**
The effect of oestrogen on the hymen at puberty – note thickened, pale tissue, and vasculature less evident.

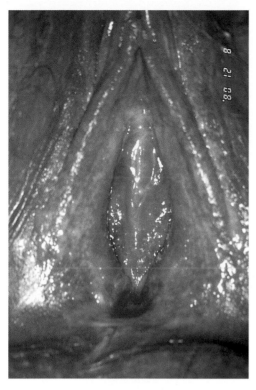
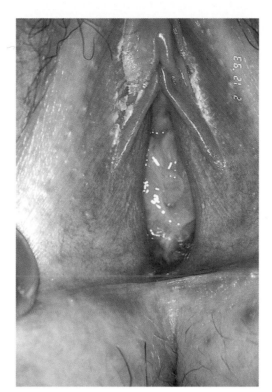

▲ **20.27,** ▲ **20.28 Female aged 12 years**
Normal oestrogenized hymen.

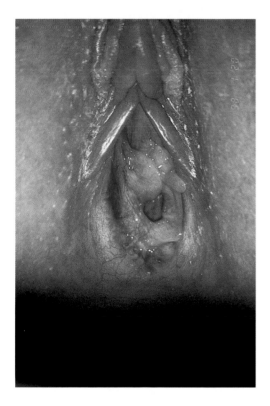

◀ **20.29 Female aged 8 years**
Girl with unusual but probably normal genital
findings including the 2 flaps of tissue anteriorly.
The abundance and pallor of the hymen
suggests there may be an early oestrogen
effect here.

The perineum, anus and perianal region

◆ The perineum should be free from scarring.

◆ The perianal skin is dry and smooth.

◆ The anus: there are radiating skin folds which are largely symmetrical;

    ◆ skin tags at 6 and 12 o'clock may be 'congenital';

    ◆ anal fissures are not seen (i.e. asymptomatic);

    ◆ depressed, shiny areas at 6 and 12 o'clock are normal – they may be mistaken for scars;

    ◆ the anus is examined in the left lateral position, the buttocks are parted and the anus is inspected over 30 seconds – young children initially have a closed, external anal sphincter but after 10–15 seconds the sphincter relaxes but as the internal sphincter remains shut the phenomenon of 'reflex' anal dilatation is not observed;

◆ dilated veins may become visible if the buttock separation is prolonged;

Note: some practitioners prefer to examine children in the knee–chest position, and the period of inspection should not be prolonged;

◆ the anal tone is such that the anus remains closed on buttock separation – digital examination is not recommended.

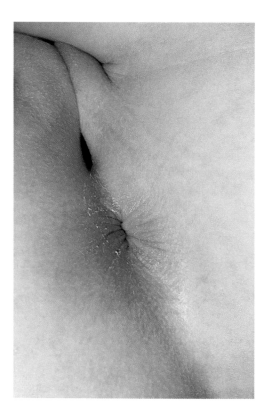

▲ **20.30 Female infant**
A normal anal sphincter.

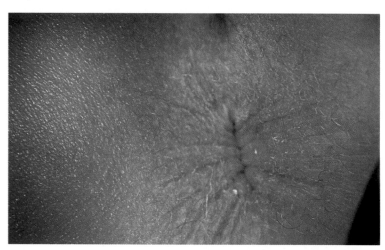

▲ **20.31 Male aged 5 years**
A normal anal sphincter in pigmented skin.

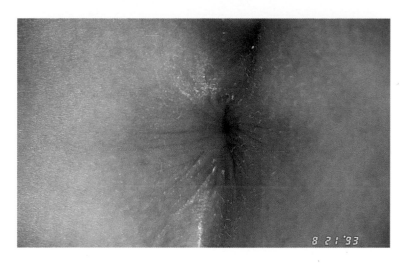

◀ **20.32 Female aged 7 years**
A normal anal sphincter, but note there are often rather shiny areas at 6 and 12 o'clock which superficially look like scars.

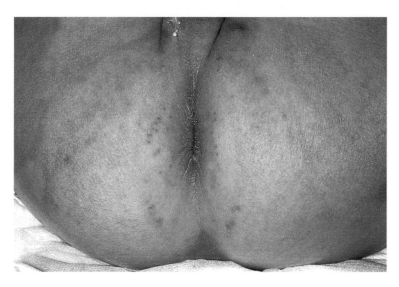

◀ **20.33 Male aged 10 months**
Slight perianal reddening and mild nappy rash. Some perianal reddening is common in babies still in nappies.

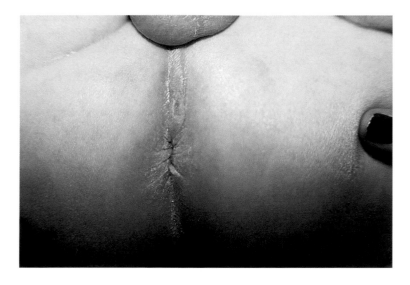

◀ **20.34 Male aged 4 years**
Prominent raphe.

Chapter 21

Genital Injuries in Boys

Injuries to the genitalia in boys were thought be rare, in the order of 3% of sexually abused boys. With increasing knowledge it is evident that toilet seats have been much maligned.

The injuries seen more commonly include:

- bruising to the penis and scrotum, petechiae and swelling are associated with sucking injury;
- a torn frenulum (of the penis) caused by forced retraction of the foreskin;
- an incised wound to the penis, usually proximal and on the dorsal surface but may be circumferential;
- a red circumferential mark due to a ligature;
- contact burn, scald;
- bites;
- damage to the urethral meatus due to insertion of a foreign body;
- urethral discharge, warts, vesicles due to a sexually transmitted disease.

The differential diagnosis of genital abnormality:

- accidental injury such as dog or horse bite, straddle injury (but check the history carefully), zip injury;
- complications of ritual circumcision;
- excessive washing, handling of the penis and forced retraction of the foreskin;
- forceful masturbation – but ensure this is not inflicted in young boys but also adolescence;
- paraphimosis with swelling, inflamed glans penis due to a tight foreskin which has been retracted and stuck at the coronal sulcus;
- as for bruising – bleeding and clotting disorder.

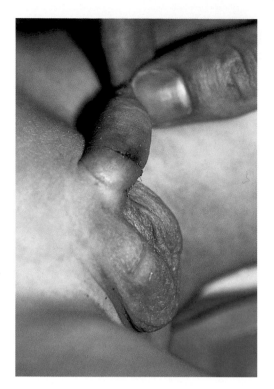

◀ 21.1 Male
Pre-school child with laceration of the inferior aspect of the penis proximally. The lesion extended two-thirds of the circumference of the penis. The family suggested that the child had pulled his own penis, causing this laceration.

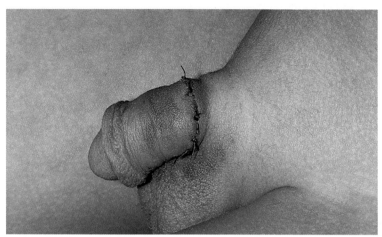

▲ 21.2 Male aged 4 years
He was brought to the hospital emergency department by his parents. History was later provided that he must have caught his penis on a tile sticking out from the wall. There is a circumferential skin-deep laceration of the base of the penis. The diagnosis is an unexplained severe injury. Note blood tracking down into the scrotum.

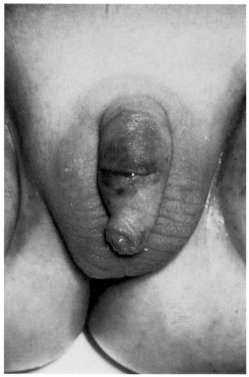

▲ 21.3 Male aged 5 years
He was brought to the hospital emergency department by his mother after a female babysitter aged 13 years had sawn the penis with a bread knife after warning the child to stop masturbating in front of the television. There is a deep incision of the penis. The babysitter was later found to have been repeatedly sexually abused for the previous 6 years.

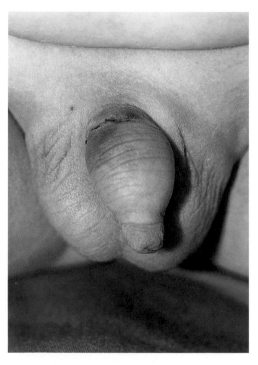

▲ 21.4 Male aged 2 years
Incised wound on the anterior aspect of the penis and local bruising. The history as given was that this child went into a 'portaloo' on his own and came out injured.

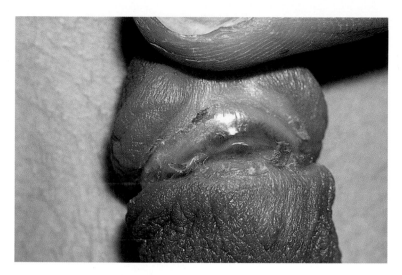

▲ **21.5 Male aged 5 years**
He was taken to the doctor by his parents who referred him on to the hospital. The photograph shows marked swelling at the distal end of the penis. Hairs were removed from around the coronal sulcus. There are signs of an early infection. No satisfactory history was available.

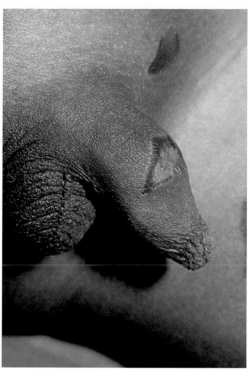

▲ **21.6 Male aged 2 years**
The child had developmental delay. He was noticed to have burns on his thigh and penis at day nursery. A healing triangular burn is seen on the dorsum of the penis. The mother admitted to burning the child.

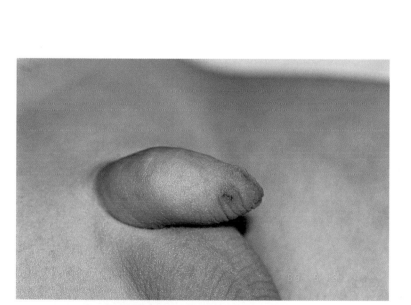

◀ **21.7 Male aged 3 years**
He was seen in the follow-up paediatric clinic because of previous sexual abuse. A small laceration is seen at the distal end of the penis. This is probably a fingernail scratch.

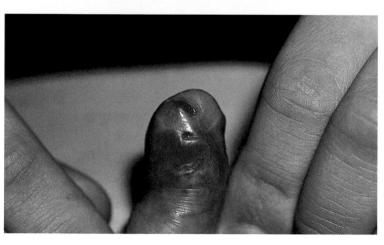

◀ **21.8 Male aged 8 years**
He gave a history of forceful painful masturbation by a stranger at the swimming baths.

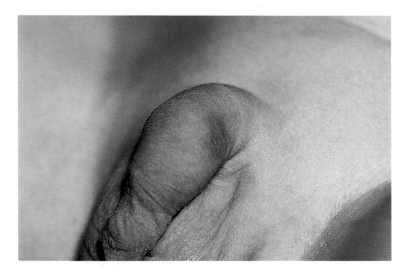

▲ **21.9 Male aged 3 years**
Day nursery referred the child because of scratches on his thigh and a bruised penis. There was a past history of repeated physical and sexual abuse. Clear bruising is evident at the base of the penis. This is probably due to pinching.

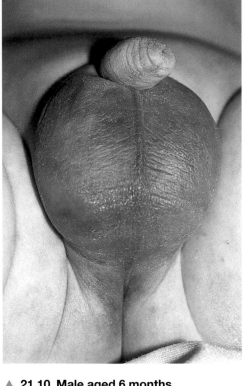

▲ **21.10 Male aged 6 months**
Infant who was kicked in the groin by his father. Extensive swelling and bruising of the scrotum.

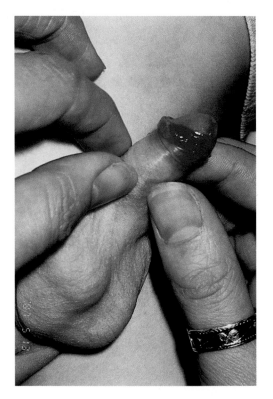

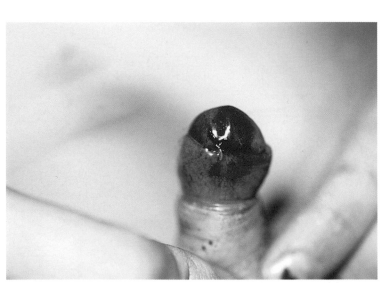

▲ **21.11, ▲ 21.12 Males aged 4 years**
Similar injuries in two boys who were playing out in the street and were assaulted by an elderly woman. There was trauma to the foreskin in both children.

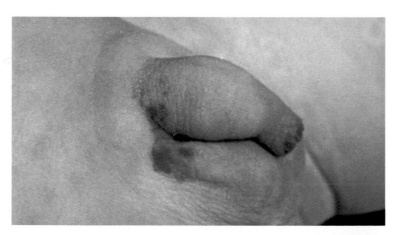

◀ 21.13 Male aged 2 years
Boy with bruising at the base of penis and scrotum. The boy was being toilet trained. His pre-adoptive mother murdered him.

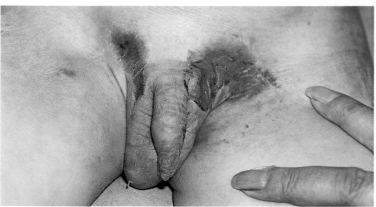

◀ 21.14 Male aged 6 years
He was sent to the local infectious diseases hospital by his doctor because of bloody diarrhoea. The child told a nurse that his father had poured a jug of hot water over him. There is a scald in the groin with signs of early healing. There were also marked anal signs. The diagnosis is inflicted scald in association with anal abuse.

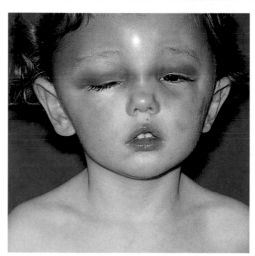

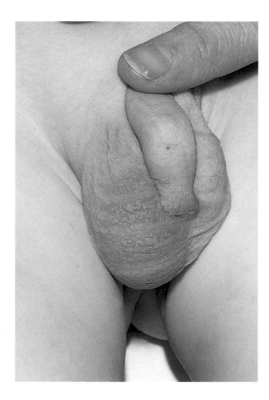

▲ 21.15, ▶ 21.16, ▶ 21.17, ▶ 21.18, ▶ 21.19 Male aged 3 years
He returned home from access with his father with severe facial bruising. The photographs show a tense, swollen forehead with bruising to the orbit and nose. There is an additional bruise on the cheek, fingertip bruising in the right loin, paired contact burns on the thigh, a swollen blistered scrotum and petechiae on the penis. A photograph of the scrotum 24 hours later shows swelling settling but a blister is evident as well as bruising of the foreskin. This was a severe physical and sexual assault. Note the complex contact burns; he had several pairs of burns on his abdomen and legs as well as on the genitalia.

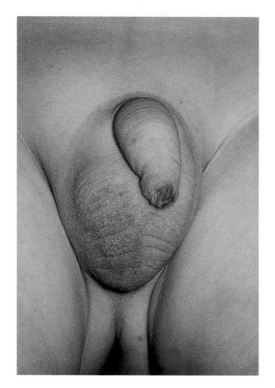

▲ 21.17

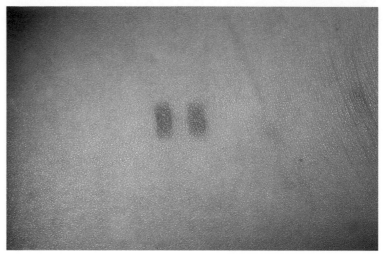

▲ 21.18

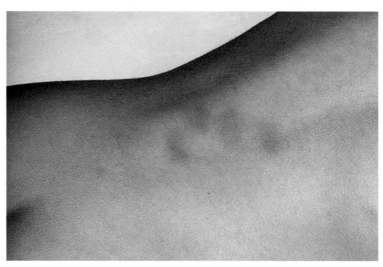

▲ 21.19

▶ **21.20 Male aged 3 years**
He was referred by his day nursery to social services after he complained about a 'sore willy' and drew what looked like sexualized pictures. The photograph shows a swollen smooth distal end of the penis. It was not possible to retract the foreskin. The diagnosis is xeroderma obliterans, the male equivalent of lichen sclerosus.

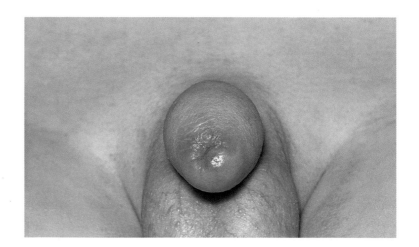

Chapter 22

Genital Findings in Sexually Abused Girls

The diagnosis of child sexual abuse (CSA) may be straightforward but on other occasions is extremely difficult and in these circumstances the 'jigsaw' may be very useful in linking the pieces of information which are available (see Chapter 1).

Building up a diagnosis in this way will make the opinion more robust and diminish the likelihood of mistakes.

General features

- Disclosure of CSA remains the mode of presentation in over 50% of referred girls: sexualized play or sexual precocity may occur.
- Girls disclose when they are ready; this in practice means safe.
- False allegations are rare, possibly 1–2%, and children are likely to diminish rather than exaggerate their abuse. When a child discloses re-abuse there may be a slightly increased chance of falsehood and it is also alleged that teenagers are more likely to lie about abuse. Mothers in difficult custody cases may be put in a difficult position if their child discloses on separation (when they feel safe) and she may be accused of malevolent manipulation.
- The vast majority of abuse is within the home by someone the child knows and the prognosis is improved if the mother believes the child.
- Children's stories should always be carefully evaluated, taking into account the child's developmental level, their language and note taken of anxiety, fear, sensory or other disability. Ideally a developmental psychologist would assess the child, rather than the police and social worker.
- 15% of children are physically abused in addition to the CSA, bruises, laceration and burns (i.e. sadistic, inflicted injury).
- Symptoms such as vaginal bleeding are good markers of CSA and CSA should be also on the differential diagnosis of dysuria, recurrent vaginal discharge and rectal bleeding.
- Sexually transmitted diseases (STD) – see Chapter 25.
- Forensic tests are described later.
- A positive pregnancy test/pregnancy is proof of CSA.
- Psychosomatic disease, alcohol and substance abuse, self-harm and conduct disorder are associated with CSA.

The examination is a 'whole child exam' and involves an assessment of the child's growth, development and emotional well being, as well as signs associated with any abuse.

Investigations include tests for the differential diagnosis of bruising, STD, and if the assault was recent (within 72 hours for prepubertal and up to 5 days for postpubertal girls), forensic tests (for saliva, semen, blood, lubricant, etc.)

Recording findings is important (as in all clinical findings)

- Contemporaneous handwritten notes and diagrams, dated and signed.
- Photography, preferably whilst using a colposcope, use a camera with a data bank.

Points to note during the examination

- Was the child angry, sad, appropriately shy?
- Was the child's behaviour sexualized? Did the child 'flirt' with the doctor, begin to masturbate, have a sustained erection (boys)?

Physical signs associated with CSA

1. A recent tear(s) in the hymen.
2. Attenuation of the hymen – this refers to thinning and destruction of the hymen; the result may be that only a thin rim of hymen remains.
3. An enlarged hymenal opening which may gape on inspection; labial traction gives the largest dimensions.

   - at 5 years an opening of 5 mm is unusual but not proof of abuse;
   - by puberty 10 mm is average;
   - the effect of puberty is to thicken and enlarge the hymen, which also becomes more elastic; hence although inspection is adequate, prepubertally digital examination is mandatory once the effects of oestrogen are seen:
     - at puberty 10 mm is average;
     - 15–20 mm is compatible with digital penetration;
     - 35 mm is compatible with penile penetration;
     - tears or notches of the hymen are demonstrated on digital examination, glass-rod or a cotton wool bud at puberty – tears caused in the hymen prepubertally may be visible postpubertally.
       The hymen may be 'rubbed' away by repeated penetration but this is very variable and considerable amounts of hymen may remain.

4. Notches in the posterior hymen are not seen as a congenital variant and are highly correlated with abuse.
5. Anterior notches may be part of a crescentic hymen but should be shallow, symmetrical and at 10 and 2 o'clock but the hymen may be traumatized anteriorly too.
6. Prepubertally the hymen has a smooth, thinned margin – rubbing or penetration may result in tears, notches, concavities, local thickening and irregularities, dilatation and secondary obliteration.
7. Bleeding, an area of friable tissue or scarring at the posterior fourchette may be associated with CSA.
8. Labial fusion which is posterior, superficial and short in length in infants is common, but thick, long irregular posterior fusion may be traumatic in older children.
9. Reddening, non-specific vaginal discharge is associated with CSA but not proof.
10. A dilated urethral opening is compatible with penetration.
11. Other forms of abuse – see Chapter 19.
12. Vaginal foreign objects are found rarely but may present with a purulent vaginal discharge.
13. An STD, pregnancy.
14. Forensic tests – blood, saliva, semen.

▶ **22.1 Female aged 1 year**
Markedly wrinkled, flattened labia majora. Note the gaping hymenal opening. The midline raphe is probably normal. Signs: flattened labia, gaping hymenal opening.

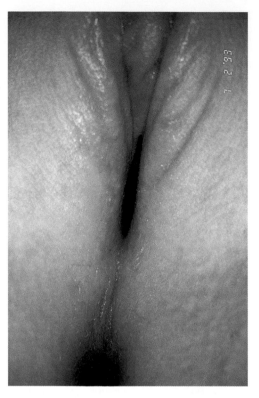

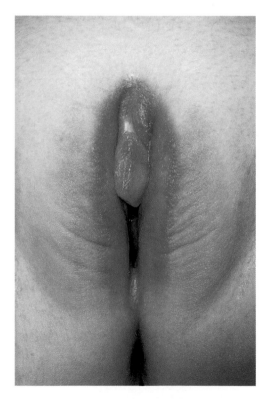

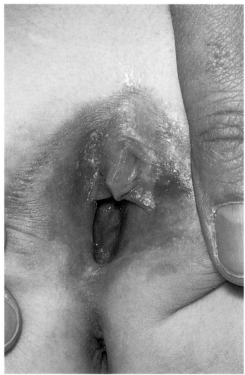

▲ **22.2, ▲ 22.3 Female aged 3 years**
Flattened, wrinkled labia majora with tramline reddening. A smooth posterior fourchette is seen. There is marked oedema with vulvitis and discharge. Signs: reddening, swelling.

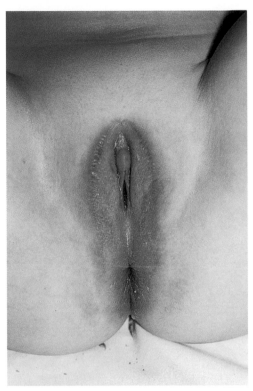

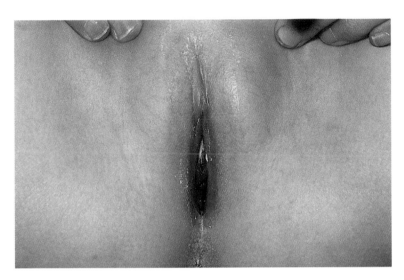

◄ 22.4 Female aged 5 years

Flattened labia, with marked reddening extending from the genitalia across the perineum and perianally. Signs: flattened labia, symmetrical reddening.

▲ 22.5 Female aged 5 years

Marked reddening and oedema of the labia minora and hymen. Signs: reddening, swelling.

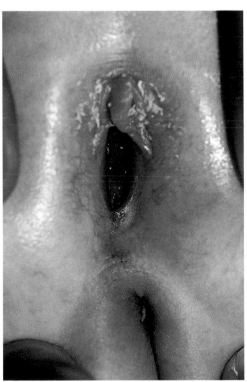

◄ 22.6 Female aged 4 years

Marked reddening and swelling of the hymen and perihymenal tissues. Signs: reddening, swelling.

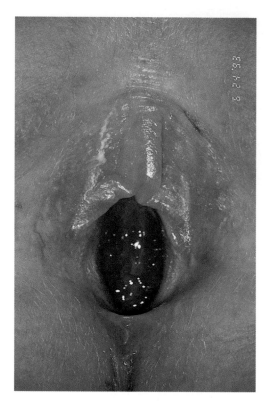 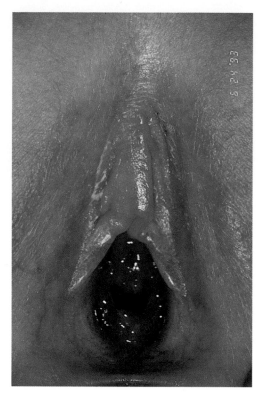

▲ **22.7, ▲ 22.8 Female aged 11 years**
Marked swelling and reddening of the hymen and perihymenal tissues. An asymmetrical hymenal opening is also seen. Signs: reddening, swelling, asymmetrical hymenal opening.

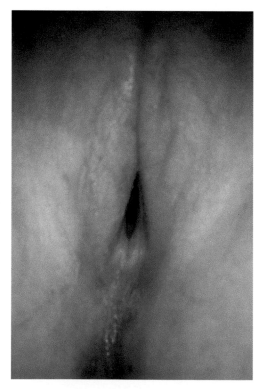

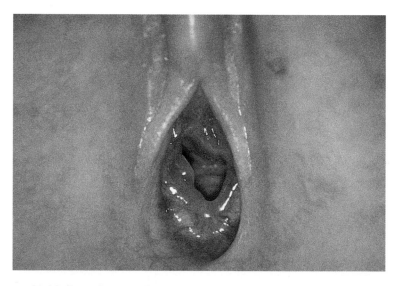

▲ **22.10 Female aged 8 years**
Reddened, swollen and markedly asymmetrical hymenal opening with notch at 2 o'clock and a bump at 3 o'clock. Signs: reddening, swelling, notch in hymen at 2 o'clock.

▲ **22.9 Female aged 5 years**
Flattened labia majora with a scooped out appearance posteriorly. Labial fusion is also seen. Note the gaping hymenal opening. Signs: flattened labia, labial fusion.

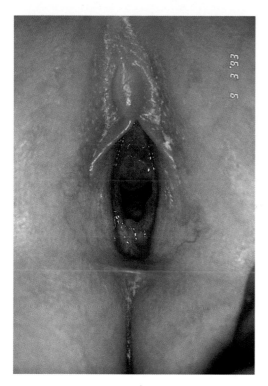

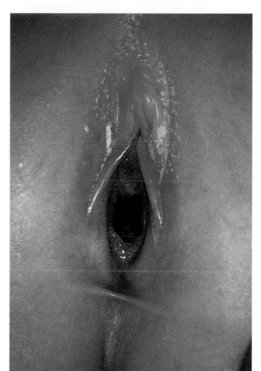

▲ 22.11 Female aged 5 years
Reddening with swelling and an irregular hymenal opening. Signs: reddening, swelling, gaping, irregular hymenal opening.

◀ 22.12 Female aged 6 years
The photograph shows reddening with a gaping dilated hymenal opening, attenuated hymen, and some rolling of hymenal edge. Note the vaginal ridge adjacent to the hymen at 5 o'clock. Signs: reddening, gaping and dilated hymenal opening, attenuated hymen.

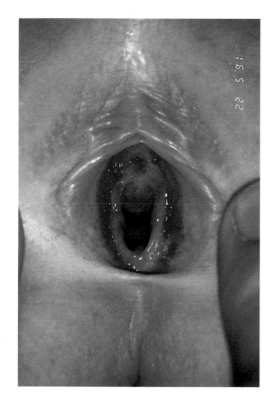

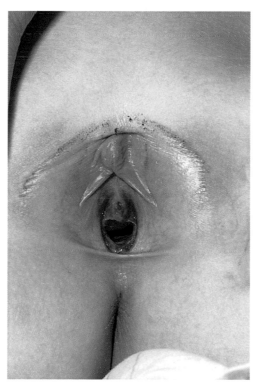

▲ 22.13 Female aged 5 years
There is uniform perihymenal reddening with a gaping, dilated hymenal opening, with little hymen persisting posteriorly. Note vaginal ridges at 3, 6 and 9 o'clock. Signs: reddening, gaping, dilated hymenal opening, attenuation.

▲ 22.14 Female aged 7 years
A gaping hymenal opening is seen with attenuation of the hymen and a recent tear at 5 o'clock. Signs: gaping hymenal opening, attenuation, tear at 5 o'clock in hymen.

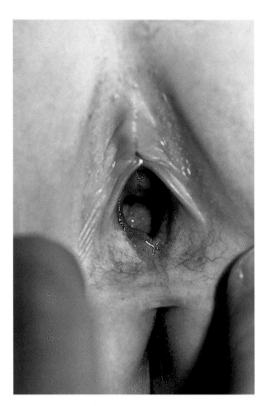

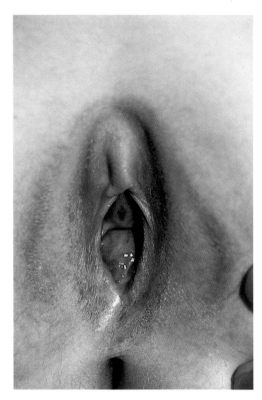

◀ **22.15 Female aged 6 years**
There is a gaping hymenal opening with a notch at 6 o'clock and a bump at 7 o'clock, and a rolled edge to the hymen. Signs: gaping hymenal opening, notch in hymen, bump, rolled edge to hymen.

▶ **22.16**

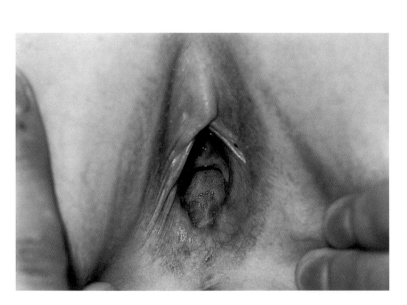

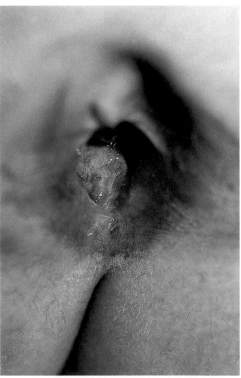

▲ **22.16**, ▲ **22.17**, ▲ **22.18**
The photographs show dry reddened skin and a gaping vagina with only remnants of hymen left posteriorly. An old scar is visible on the posterior vaginal wall between remnants of the hymen. Note the smooth posterior vagina walls. The angled view (Fig. 22.18) shows friability at the posterior fourchette with localized disruption and scarring. Signs: reddening, gaping vagina, scar, friability at fourchette, remnants of hymen.

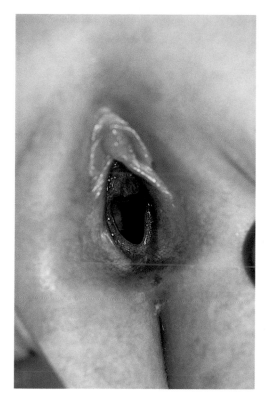

▲ **22.19 Female aged 5 years**
There is a dilated, gaping hymenal opening with reddish/purple adjacent tissues. The hymen is attenuated, persisting as a thin rim. The fourchette skin is friable with surface bleeding. Signs: reddening/purple, dilated, gaping hymenal opening, attenuated, friable posterior fourchette.

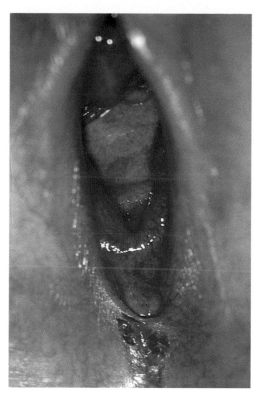

▲ **22.20 Female aged 4 years**
The posterior fourchette is friable and bleeds when the labia are separated. There is a deep notch in the hymen at 6 o'clock. Signs: friable posterior fourchette, notch in hymen.

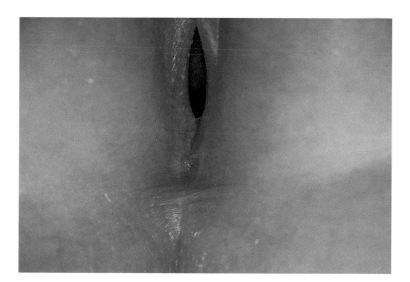

▲ **22.21 Female aged 8 years**
There is marked reddening of the labia and perineum with labial fusion traumatically separated. A gaping hymen is visible. Signs: reddening, labial fusion, gaping hymenal opening.

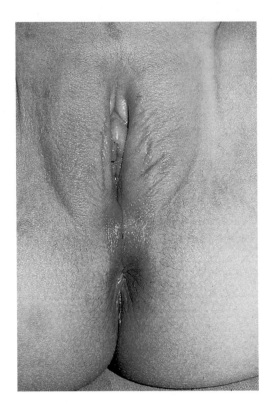
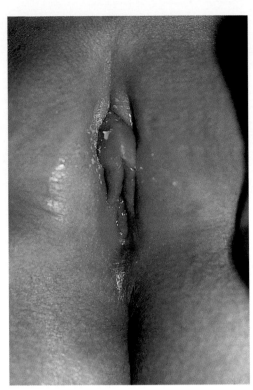

▲ **22.22**, ▲ **22.23 Female aged 1 year**
Figure 22.22 shows flattened, wrinkled labia. A midline tear can be seen extending posteriorly.
The resulting scar is seen in Fig. 22.23. Signs: flattened labia, tear, scar.

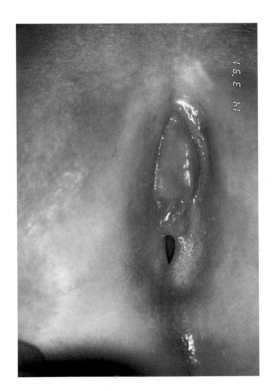
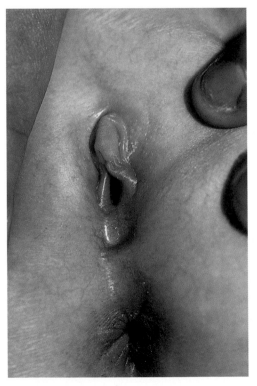

▲ **22.24 Female aged 9 years**
A very unusual appearance due to extensive
posterior labial fusion. Signs: labial fusion.

▲ **22.25 Female aged 2 years**
There is labial fusion with a visible line of fusion.
Signs: labial fusion.

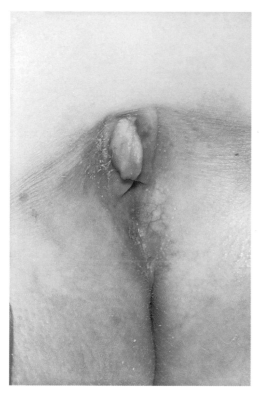

▲ **22.26 Female aged 9 years**
Very extensive, thick posterior labial fusion is
seen in an older child. Signs: labial fusion.

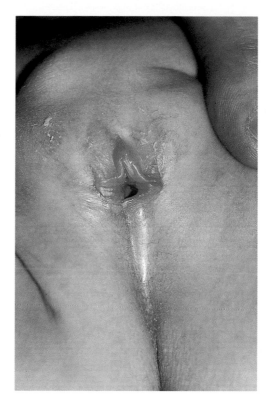

▲ **22.27 Female aged 2 years**
Extensive thick posterior labial fusion.
Signs: labial fusion.

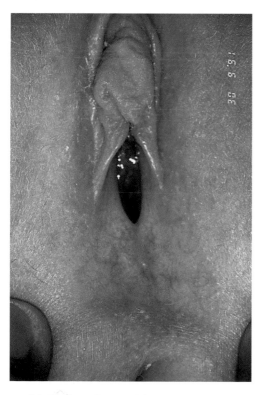

▲ **22.28 Female aged 3 years**
Posterior labial fusion, with a gaping, elongated
hymen. Signs: labial fusion, gaping hymen.

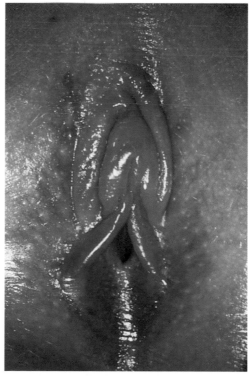

▲ **22.29 Female aged 3 years**
Posterior labial fusion. Signs: labial fusion.

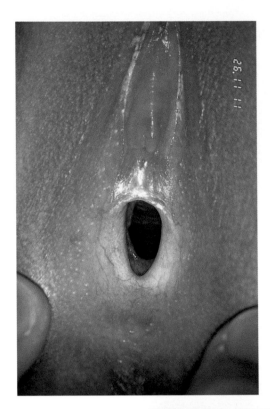

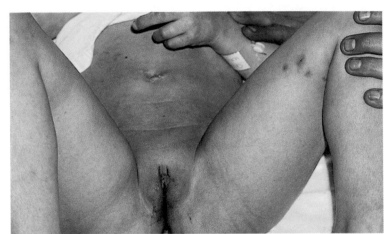

◀ **22.30 Female aged 6 years**
Anterior and posterior fusion of the labia. Note the gaping hymenal opening, with a notch at 9 o'clock. Signs: labial fusion, notch in hymen.

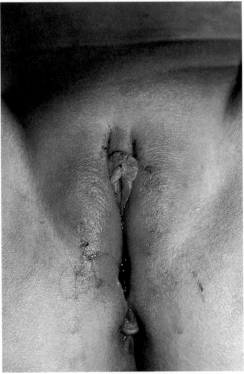

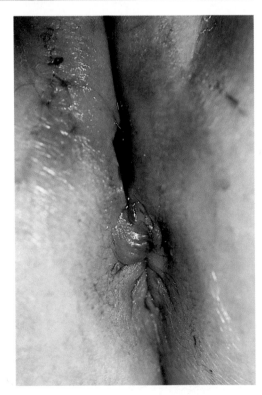

▲ **22.31,** ▲ **22.32,** ▲ **22.33 Female aged 4 years**
The photographs show scratch marks on the inner thigh, and reddening and bruising to the labia. The labia are seen to be swollen and bruised. There is a blood clot at the introitus with a midline tear. An anterior anal haematoma is seen at the posterior end of the tear. The tear extends through the posterior vaginal wall, posterior fourchette and across the perineum to the anterior margin of the anal sphincter. The anal sphincter is intact. Signs: scratching, swelling of labia, tear, haematoma, tag.

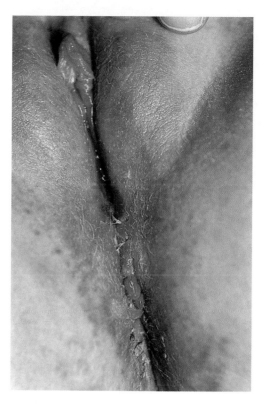

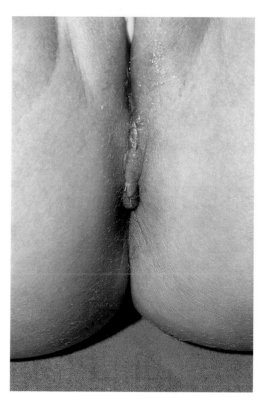

▲ 22.34, ▲ 22.35 Female aged 4 years
Same child as in Figs 22.31, 22.32 and 22.33. These photographs were taken
4 weeks later at a follow-up and show healing.

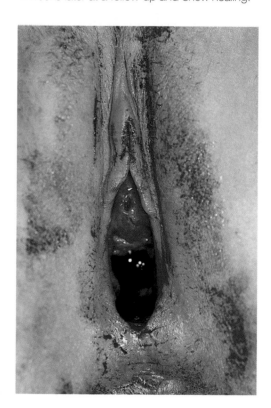

◄ 22.36 Female aged 5 years
An extensive blood clot is visible with a gaping,
but largely deficient, hymenal opening and a
tear through the posterior vaginal wall and
posterior fourchette onto the perineum.
Signs: gaping hymen.

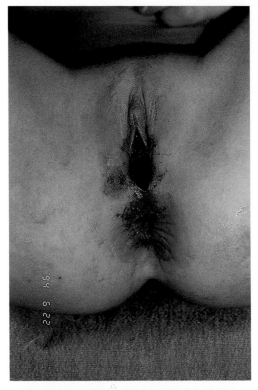 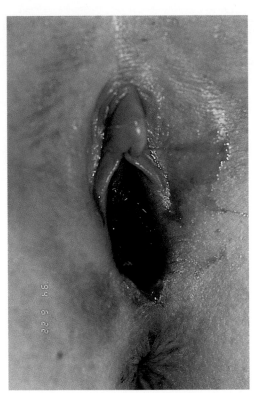

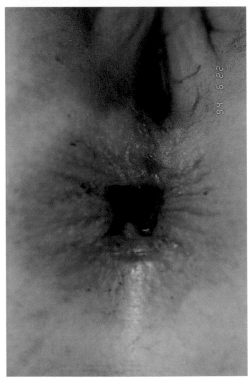 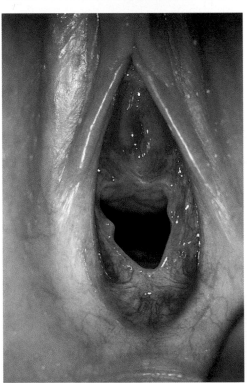

▲ **22.37, ▲ 22.38, ▲ 22.39 Female aged 5 years**

The photographs show a bruise to the right of the labia, dilated hymenal opening, disrupted hymen and a torn posterior fourchette. There is a gaping anus, with anterior abrasion, and red and swollen anal margin. Signs: bruise, reddening, disrupted dilated hymen, torn posterior fourchette, gaping anus, abrasion.

▲ **22.40 Female aged 8 years**

Dilated hymenal opening with bumps at 3 and 9 o'clock, and a deep rounded notch posteriorly. Signs: dilated hymenal opening, bumps, notch.

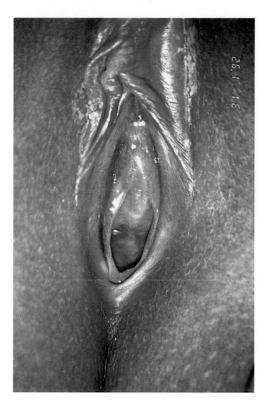 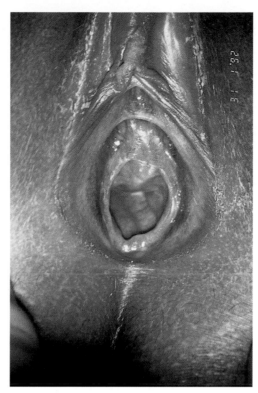

▲ **22.41**, ▲ **22.42 Female aged 9 years**
Figure 22.41 shows the shape of the hymenal opening with labial separation, and Fig. 22.42 with labial traction. A dilated hymenal opening is seen, and attenuation of the hymen, with a small notch at 7 o'clock. Signs: dilated hymenal opening, attenuated hymen, notch.

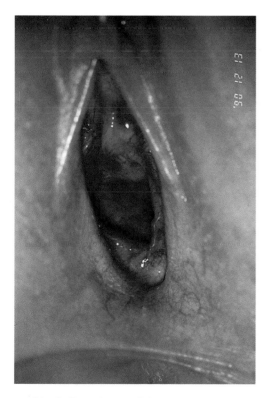 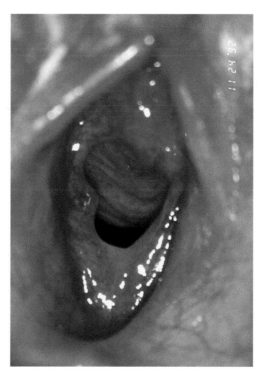

▲ **22.43 Female aged 6 years**
There is reddening of the hymen and vaginal wall with a dilated hymenal opening which is asymmetrical with notches at 3 and 5 o'clock. Signs: reddening, dilated hymenal opening, notch.

▲ **22.44 Female aged 6 years**
A reddened, dilated hymenal opening is seen with marked asymmetry giving a 'ballooned effect' (notch) at 10–11 o'clock. There is still hymen present circumferentially with a bump at 9 o'clock. Signs: reddening, dilated hymenal opening, notch.

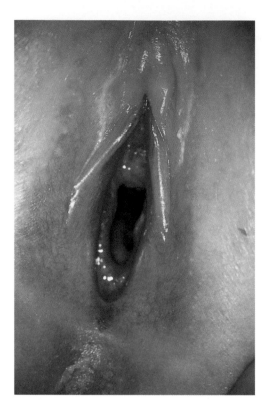 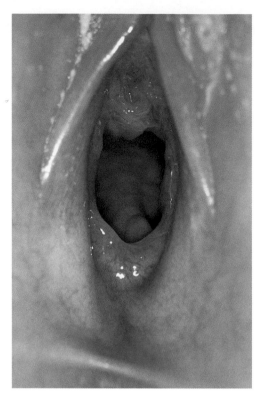

▲ **22.45, ▲ 22.46 Female aged 4 years**
Reddening with vertical elongation of the hymenal opening is seen in Fig. 22.45. There is a rolled edge to the hymen, a bump at 9 o'clock, and a friable fourchette. Figure 22.46 is a follow-up photograph taken 2 years later. This picture is taken with greater magnification but shows a markedly dilated hymenal opening, with attenuation, particularly laterally. There is little hymen anteriorly. A prominent vaginal ridge is seen. Signs: reddening, dilated hymenal opening, rolled edge to hymen, friable fourchette, vaginal ridge.

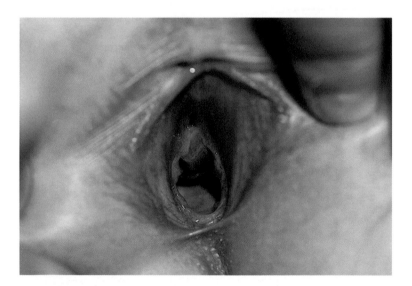

▲ **22.47 Female aged 10 years**
There is reddening with a dilated gaping hymenal opening. An asymmetrical shape is seen with little hymen remaining (attenuated). There are bumps at 3 and 9 o'clock and a notch at 12 o'clock. Signs: reddening, dilated hymenal opening, attenuated hymen, notch, bumps.

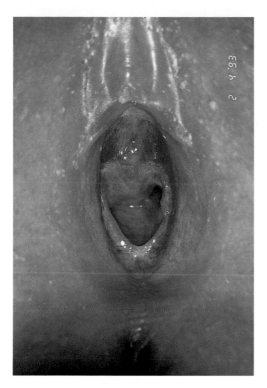

▲ **22.48 Female aged 8 years**
There is some reddening with a gaping, dilated hymenal opening. A vaginal ridge is shown clearly at 3 o'clock and there is a bump at 2 o'clock where the ridge joins the hymen. The hymenal edge is rolled and attenuated.
Signs: reddening, dilated hymenal opening, attenuation of hymen, vaginal ridge.

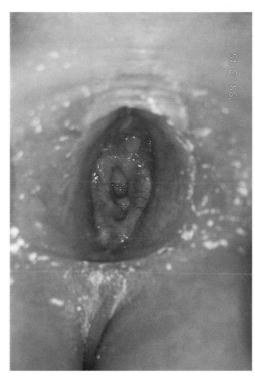

▲ **22.49 Female aged 6 years**
There is reddening with an unusual-shaped hymenal opening with a deep, wide notch at 6 o'clock and adjacent hymenal remnant.
Signs: reddening, notch, hymenal remnant.

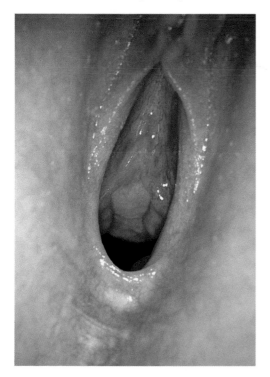

▲ **22.50 Female aged 6 years**
The hymenal opening looks to be dilated but a clear view is not obtainable because of the posterior labial fusion. Signs: gaping hymenal opening, labial fusion.

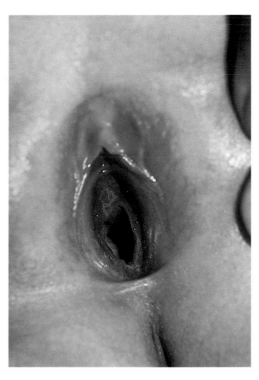

◀ **22.51 Female aged 7 years**
A markedly red introitus is seen. The surface are was very friable and bled on contact. The hymenal opening is gaping, dilated, irregular, and attenuated with a recent tear at 6 o'clock.
Signs: reddening, friable, dilated, attenuated hymenal opening, tear.

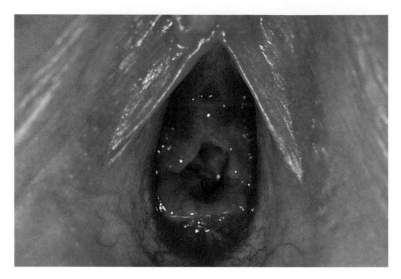

▲ **22.52 Female aged 4 years**
A reddening, fleshy hymen is seen with transection at 9 o'clock.
Signs: reddening, transection.

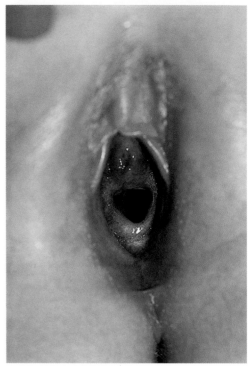

▲ **22.53 Female aged 8 years**
There is reddening, with a dilated, gaping
hymenal opening with fixed shape. The
hymenal edge has a rolled appearance. The
urethra is prominent. Signs: reddening, dilated
hymenal opening, rolled edge to hymen.

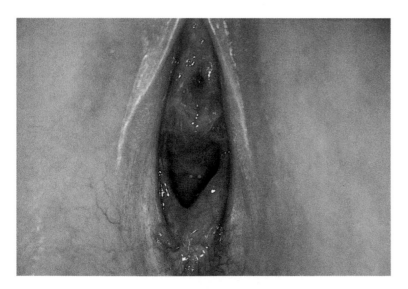

▲ **22.54 Female aged 6 years**
Reddening is seen, with a triangular-shaped dilated hymen with fixed
shape. There is a deep notch at 6 o'clock. Vascular hyperaemia is visible
at the posterior fourchette. Signs: reddening, dilated, fixed hymenal
opening, notch.

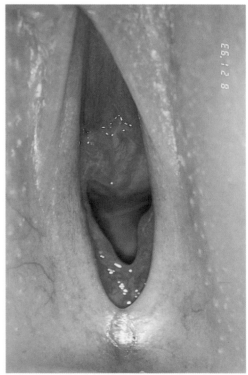

▲ **22.55 Female aged 10 years**
Asymmetrical hymenal opening with a deep
notch at 6 o'clock. Signs: asymmetry of
hymenal opening, notch.

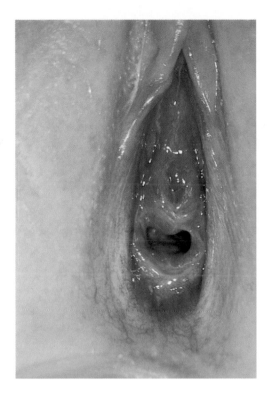

▲ **22.56 Female aged 5 years**
A thickened hymen is seen with constant shape, not dilated. Signs: thickened hymen.

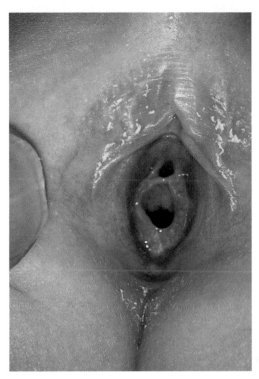

▲ **22.57 Female aged 4 years**
There is localized reddening with a markedly dilated urethral opening. The hymen is also gaping with little hymen persisting between 9 and 12 o'clock (attenuated). Signs: reddening, urethral dilation, gaping hymenal opening, attenuated hymen.

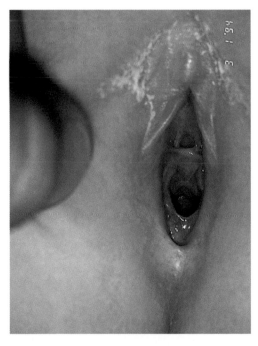

▲ **22.58 Female aged 3 years**
There is generalized reddening with marked dilatation of the urethral opening. A minimal amount of hymen is present anteriorly. The hymenal opening is dilated. Signs: reddening, dilated urethral opening, dilated hymenal opening.

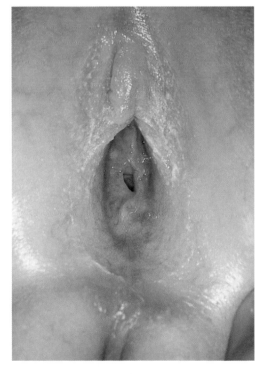

▲ **22.59 Female aged 3 years**
A distorted asymmetrical hymenal opening is seen with thickened scarred tissues posteriorly at 7 o'clock. Signs: distorted hymenal opening, scar.

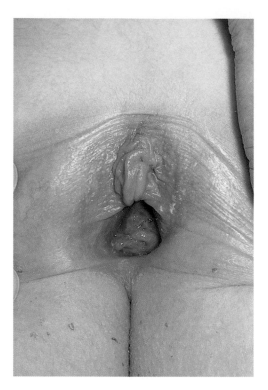

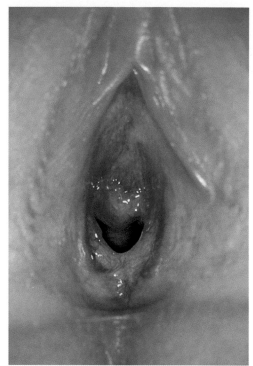

▲ **22.60 Female aged 9 years**
A disorganized fleshy hymen is seen.
Sign: obliterated hymen.

▲ **22.61 Female aged 11 years**
Reddening is seen with a gaping dilated
hymenal opening. There is marked asymmetry
anteriorly with a notch at 1 o'clock, and a bump
at 9 o'clock. Signs: reddening, gaping dilated
hymenal opening, bump.

▶ **22.62 Female
aged 8 years**
She was referred
after a foreign body
(a coil of cotton) had
been removed from
her vagina. A dilated
gaping hymenal
opening with an
irregular thickened
margin. Children
who insert foreign
bodies have almost
always been
sexually abused.
Signs: gaping
hymenal opening,
thickened margin.

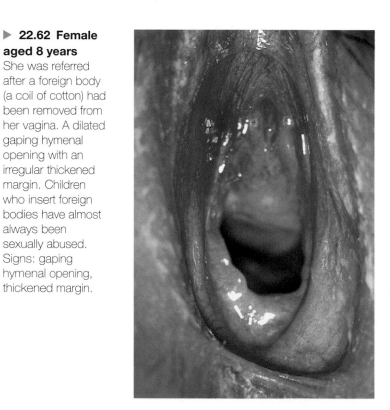

▲ **22.63 Female aged 3 years**
Hymenal opening is obliterated.
Sign: obliterated hymenal opening.

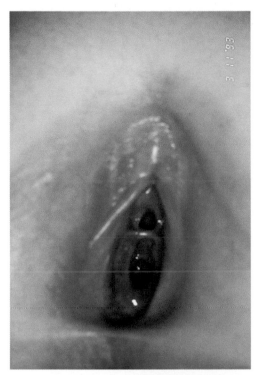

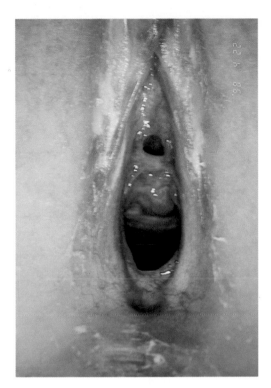

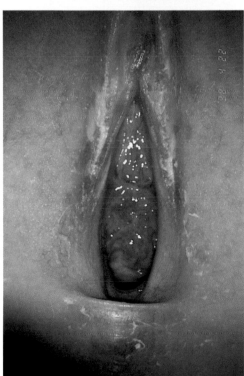

▲ **22.64,** ▲ **22.65,** ◀ **22.66,** ▶ **22.67,**
▶ **22.68 Female aged 3 to 8 years**
The evolution of the physical findings over a
5-year period from age 3 to 8 years.
Figure 22.64 shows the child when aged 3.
The initial findings were of generalized
reddening with marked dilatation of the urethral
opening. The hymen is an unusual shape with
a sharp V at 6 o'clock and a probable concavity
anteriorly. The degree of urethral dilatation is of
concern, as are the abnormalities of the hymen.
Four years later after it was thought the child
had been protected she presented with pelvic
inflammatory disease and unilateral salpingitis.
Figure 22.65 (green filter) shows marked
abnormality with a wide urethral opening,
attenuated hymen, and on the anterior vaginal
wall was a mass of granulation tissue. Further
views demonstrate the large area of granulation
tissue. The anus (Fig. 22.68) shows a posterior
anal fissure, irregular skin folds and dilated
veins. The clinical opinion was that this child
had been sexually abused for many years and
had not been protected. Long-term infertility
may be an outcome.

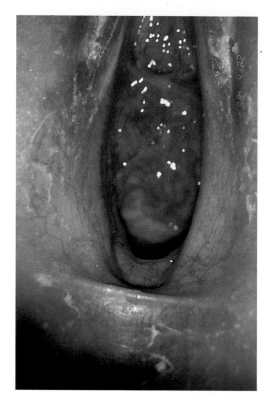

▲ **22.67**

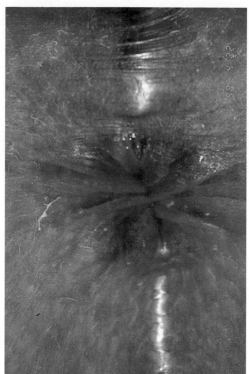

▲ **22.68**

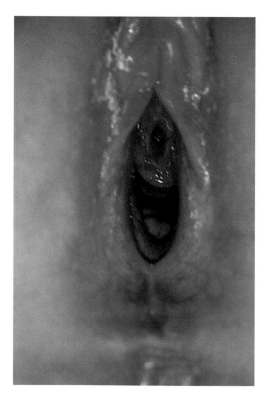

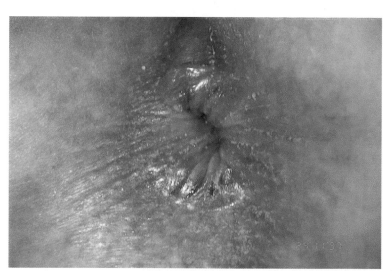

◀ **22.69, ▲ 22.70 Female aged 6 years**
There is very marked periurethral swelling, the hymen is gaping with a rolled edge and there is some labial fusion posteriorly. The anus showed an anterior skin tag with healing fissures and patchy dilated veins perianally.

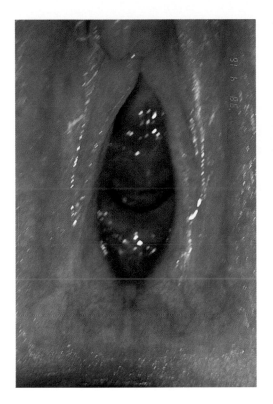

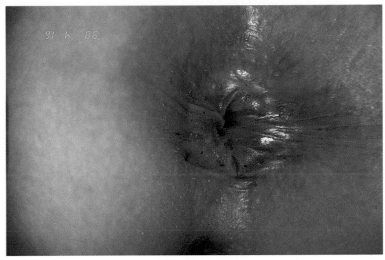

◀ 22.71, ▲ 22.72 Female aged 8 years

Prepubertal girl with periurethral and hymenal swelling. Crescentic hymen. There is a white streak running down the posterior fourchette which is a normal finding and not a scar. The anus shows a swollen anal margin, multiple fissures and dilated veins.

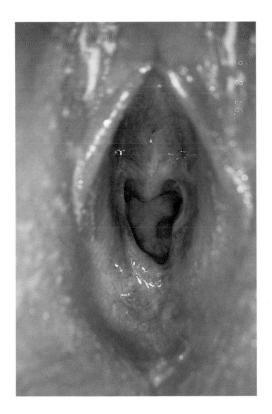

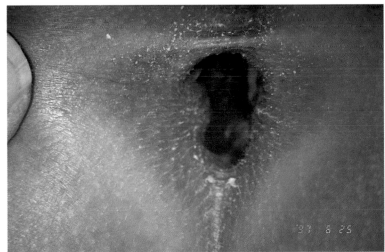

◀ 22.73, ▲ 22.74 Female aged 6 years

Prepubertal girl with unusual-shaped hymen with a large notch at 5 o'clock and a thickened narrowed hymen. There is possible scarring at the posterior fourchette and posterior hymen. The anus shows very marked reflex anal dilatation with rectal mucosa and a small amount of stool visible.

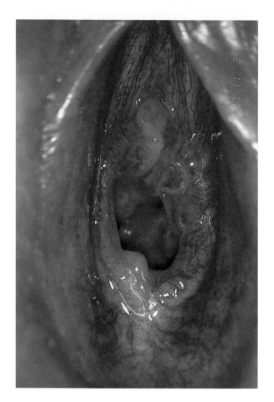

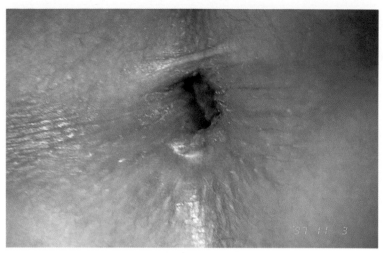

◀ 22.75, ▲ 22.76 Female aged 8 years

Prepubertal girl with swollen and hyperaemic tissue of the periurethra and hymen. There are two flaps of hymen anteriorly, partially obscuring the urethral opening. There is a wide healed notch at 5–6 o'clock and a bump on the hymen at 7 o'clock. Examination of this girl in the knee–chest position would probably have made the configuration of the posterior hymen clearer. The anus demonstrated reflex anal dilatation with dilated veins posteriorly and a probable healed fissure at 7 o'clock. Rectal mucosa is visible.

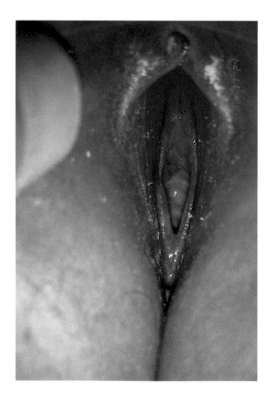

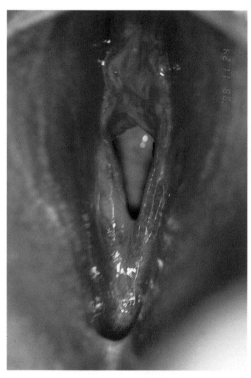

▲ 22.77, ▲ 22.78, ▶ 22.79 Female aged 9 years

An obese prepubertal girl. Intense erythema with an attenuated hymen and a sharp V at 6 o'clock. There is a large amount of hymenal tissue anteriorly with an asymmetrical appearance. There is also minimal labial fusion posteriorly. The anus is lax (Fig.22.79).

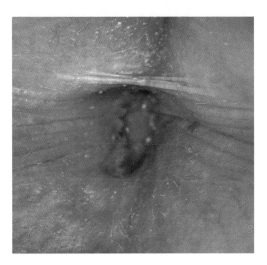

▲ 22.79

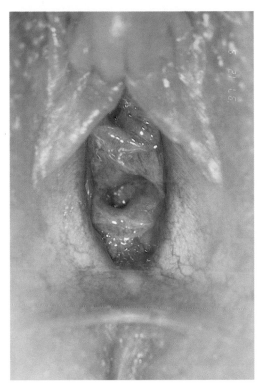

▲ 22.80 **Female aged 7 years**
Green filter image to demonstrate the unusual vessel pattern and thickened hymen posteriorly in this girl. There is redundant hymen anteriorly which also has a thickened appearance.

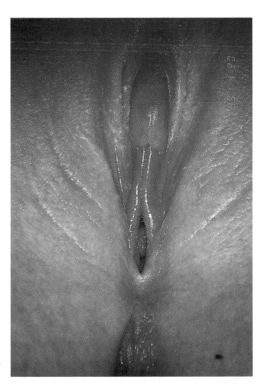

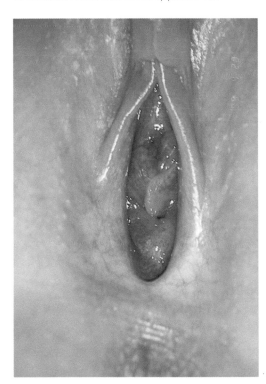

▲ 22.81, ▲ 22.82 **Female aged 6 years**
Prepubertal girl with flattened wrinkled labia and anterior labial fusion. Note the thickened skin tag across the perineum towards the anus. The photograph taken with a green filter (Fig. 22.82) shows the redundant hymen flaps anteriorly. The hymen is swollen posteriorly. At the age of 4 or 5 it would be expected that the hymen would have thinned out and have a clear margin. This redundant hymen is very unusual after this age.

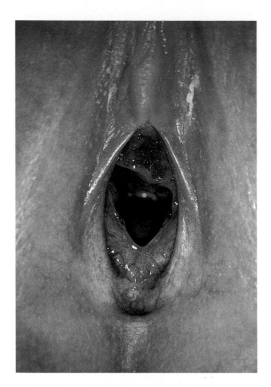 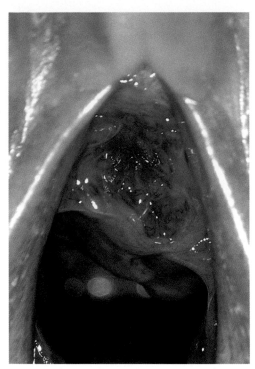

▲ **22.83,** ▲ **22.84 Female aged 8 years**
Prepubertal girl with a very abnormal appearance of the hymen and periurethral tissues. In the margin of the hymen there are dilated vessels and the shape of the hymen is unusual, with concavity at 10–11 o'clock and a sharp V at 6 o'clock. The high-powered view of the periurethral area (Fig. 22.84) shows distorted periurethral tissue. Note the dilated vessels on the anterior vaginal wall. The child also had perianal warts.

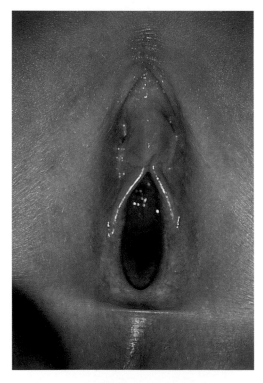 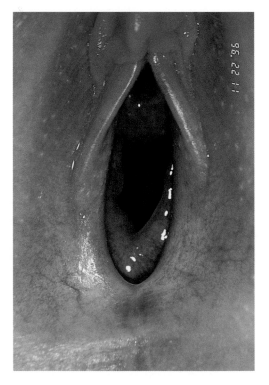

▲ **22.85,** ▲ **22.86 Female aged 5 years**
Prepubertal girl demonstrating erythema, deficient hymen anteriorly and a marked persisting notch at 8 o'clock. There is also a V-shaped notch at 6 o'clock. There is a small area of labial fusion. The high-powered view (Fig. 22.86) shows the persisting rounded notch at 8 o'clock and the V-shaped notch at 6 o'clock.

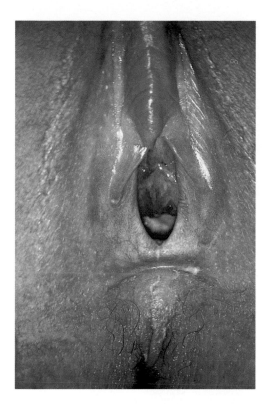

◄ 22.87 Female
Prepubertal girl with extensive labial fusion obscuring the view of the posterior hymen. The hymenal opening is gaping and the anterior vaginal wall has a swollen appearance.

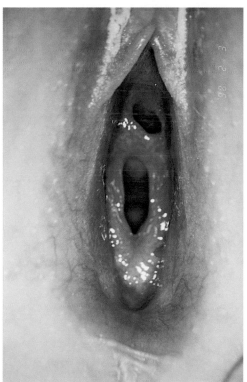

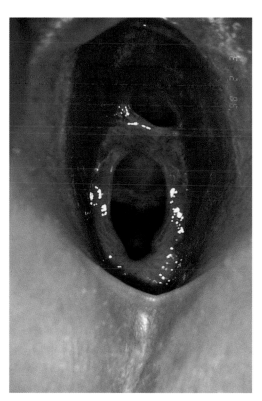

▲ 22.88, ▲ 22.89 Female aged 8 years
Prepubertal girl. The green filter view (Fig. 22.88) shows a markedly dilated urethral opening. The hymen is long with a notch at 6 o'clock (labial separation). The next view, (Figure 22.89) using labial traction method of examination shows marked erythema; it demonstrates the gaping urethral opening well and also the concavity at 6 o'clock. This is more clearly seen than in Figure 22.88 where labial separation was used.

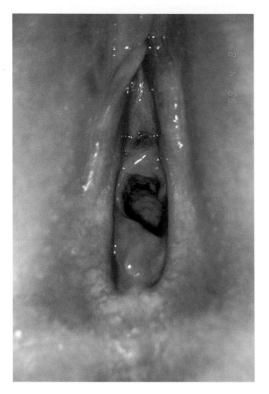

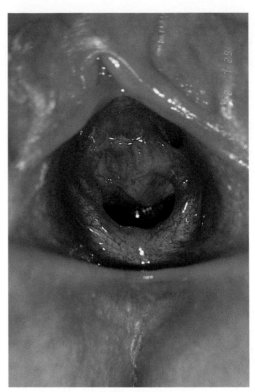

▲ **22.90 Female aged 2 years**
Prepubertal girl with gaping hymenal opening, an unusual appearance anteriorly with a notch at 5 o'clock and appearance of attenuation of the lateral hymen.

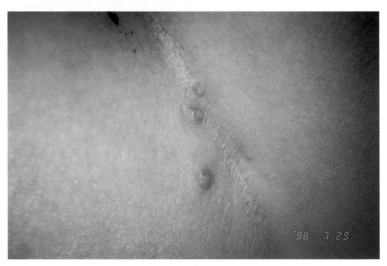

▲ **22.91,** ▲ **22.92 Female aged 4 years**
Prepubertal girl with gaping hymen which is swollen; at 10–12 o'clock there is a large notch. This is a high-powered picture and demonstrates the vasculature well. The child also had warts in the anal cleft.

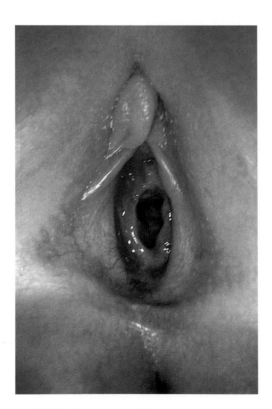

▲ **22.93 Female aged 3 years**
Prepubertal child with attenuated hymen laterally, notch at 6 o'clock and vaginal ridge at 9 o'clock.

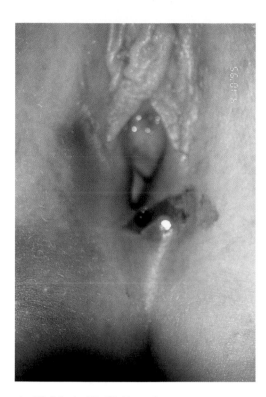
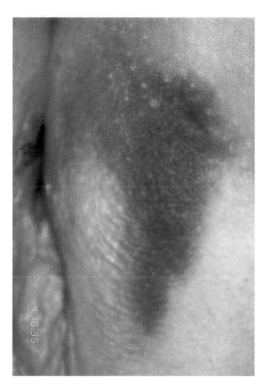

▲ **22.94,** ▲ **22.95 Female**
Deep laceration of the posterior fourchette with bruising of one labium majus. The hymen isn't well visualized but abnormal. History of fall on roller boots but considerable concern was expressed.

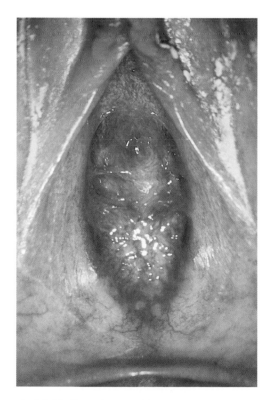
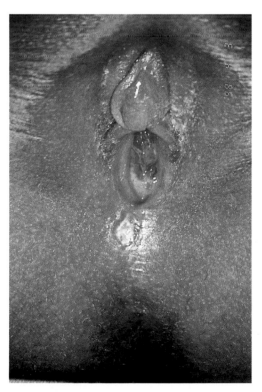

▲ **22.96 Female aged 7 years**
Secondarily obliterated hymen with scarring shown clearly by the green filter.

▲ **22.97 Female**
Recent midline tear in the posterior fourchette. Swollen traumatized hymen with contact bleeding.

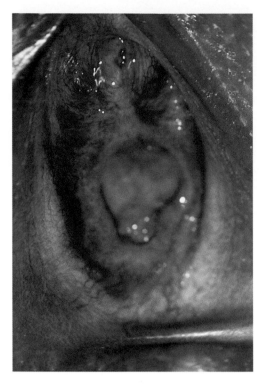

▲ **22.98 Female aged 18 months**
Annular hymen. There is a large concavity from
6–7 o'clock.

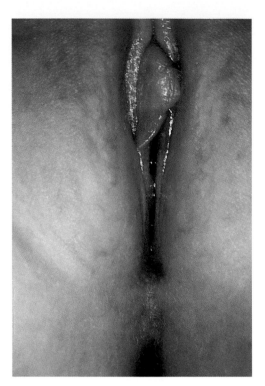

▲ **22.99 Female aged 3 years**
Recent trauma at the posterior fourchette which
is friable.

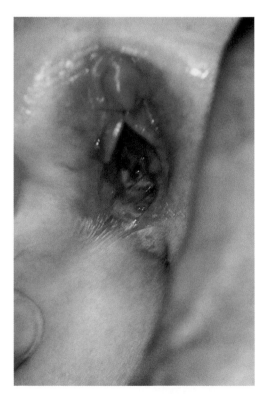

▲ **22.100 Female aged 3 years**
Severely disrupted hymen with multiple
haemorrhagic areas. Only remnants of hymen
are present.

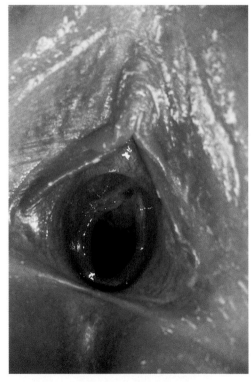

▲ **22.101 Female**
Attenuated hymenal rim with smooth edge,
widely dilated. Notch at 12 o'clock.

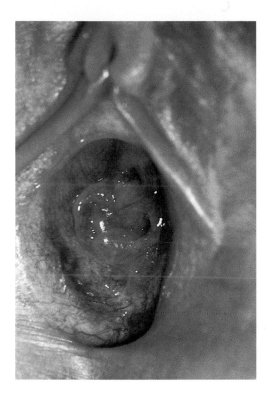

▲ **22.102 Female aged 7 years**
Distorted and partially obliterated hymen with laterally placed openings.

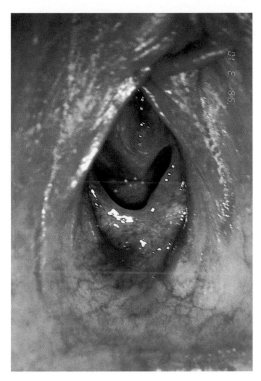

▲ **22.103 Female aged 8 years**
Asymmetric but crescentic hymen. Localized reddening at 7 o'clock.

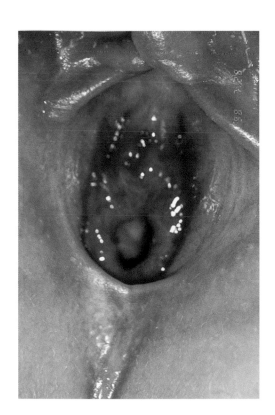

◀ **22.104 Female aged 12 months**
Markedly swollen but gaping hymen in an infant. Follow-up showed complete resolution of the signs.

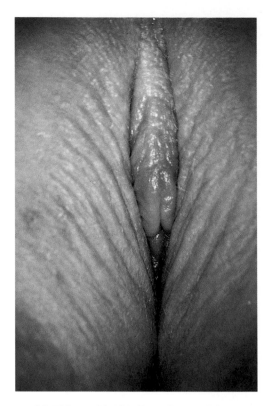

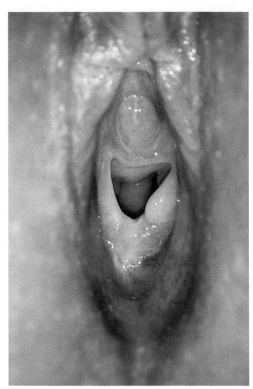

▲ **22.105,** ▲ **22.106 Female aged 9 years**
Marked wrinkling of the labia. Early oestrogen changes with asymmetrical hymenal opening and possible notch at 2 o'clock. Interpretation of signs more difficult with oestrogen present.

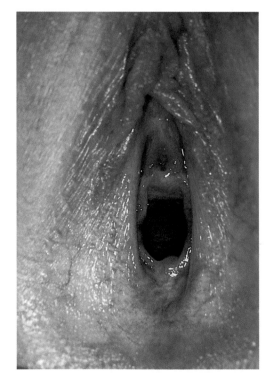

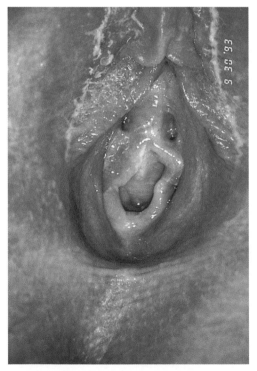

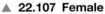

▲ **22.107 Female**
Widely gaping hymenal opening with little remaining hymen present. The edge is irregular, rolled, with several minor notches present, and note square appearance anteriorly. There are chronic skin changes, with thickened reddened skin.

▲ **22.108 Female aged 13 years**
An oestrogenized hymen with an irregular margin is seen. These are inconclusive findings.

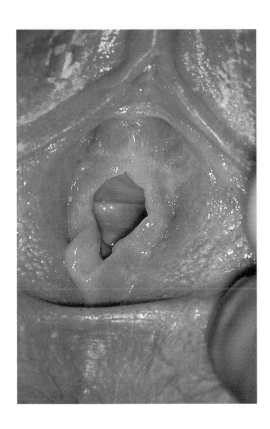

◀ 22.109 Female aged 10 years
Oestrogenized hymen is seen with a notched appearance at 6 o'clock; normal physiological discharge.

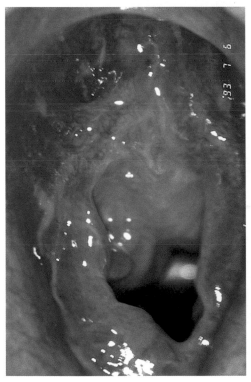

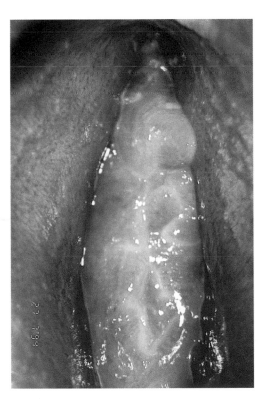

▲ 22.110, ▲ 22.111 Female aged 9 and 10 years
Figure 22.110 is a high-magnification view showing vulvitis and some early oestrogen change. The shape of the hymen is irregular posteriorly. Figure 22.111 taken 12 months later, shows a marked oestrogen effect with a physiological discharge. On this occasion the hymen was closed and appeared to be secondarily obliterated.

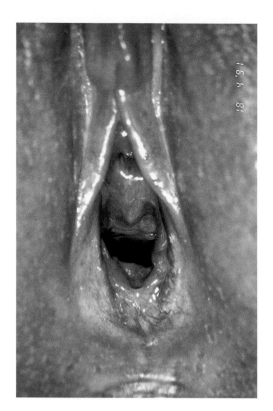

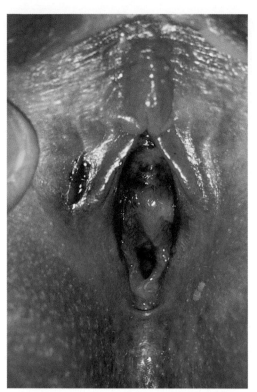

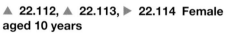

▲ 22.112, ▲ 22.113, ▶ 22.114 Female aged 10 years

Child seen after a straddle injury. Note the change in the shape of the hymen due to earlier abuse. There are abrasions periurethrally and on the labia minora. Early oestrogen changes are apparent. Note the dramatic effect that oestrogen has had on this hymen, which is now redundant, pale and appears to have a deep notch posteriorly still.

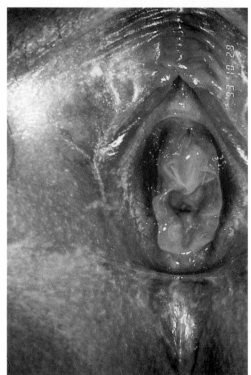

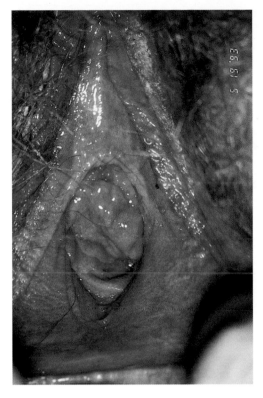

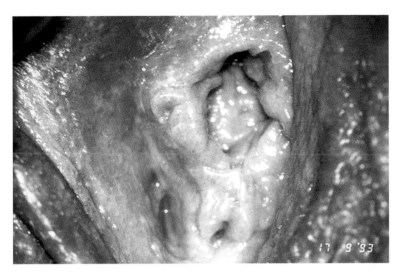

▲ **22.115 Female aged 15 years**
A redundant oestrogenized hymen is visible anteriorly but with little hymen persisting posteriorly. Vaginal examination admitted two fingers with ease, demonstrating the deceptive width of this hymen on inspection.

▲ **22.116 Female aged 15 years**
An oestrogenized hymen is seen, pale and thickened but very irregular and with only remnants persisting laterally and inferiorly. Vaginal examination admitted two fingers with ease.

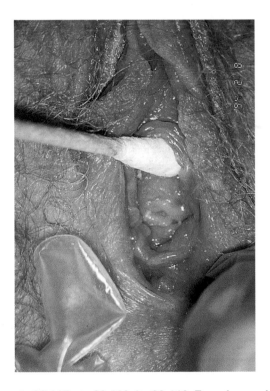

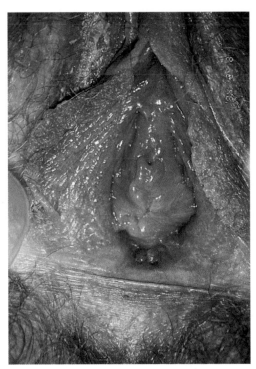

▲ **22.117,** ▲ **22.118,** ▶ **22.119 Female aged 14 years**
The photographs show an oestrogenized hymen with two warts visible inferiorly. The hymenal margin is demonstrated by use of a cotton wool bud and showing transection at 3 o'clock. The warts are well illustrated inferiorly.

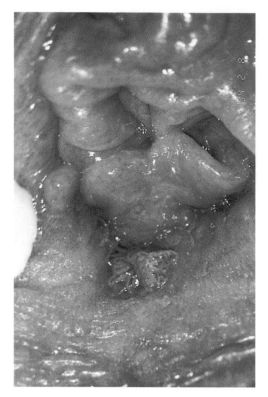

▲ **22.119**

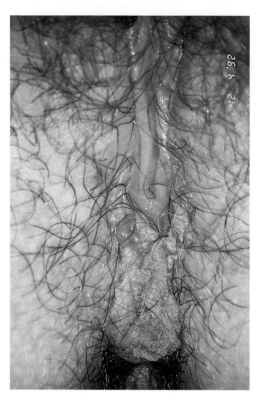

▲ **22.120 Female aged 15 years**
Thickened, redundant pigmented perineal skin
is seen.

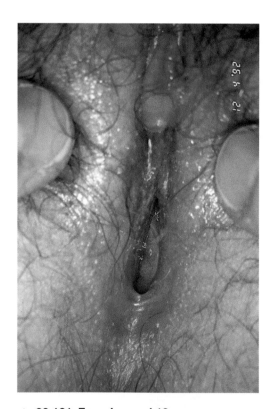

▲ **22.121 Female aged 13 years**
An oestrogenized hymen is seen associated
with labial fusion.

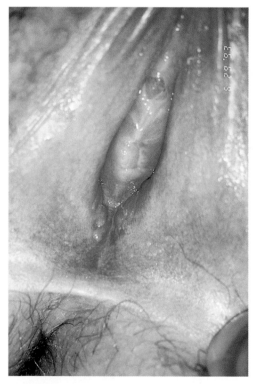

▲ **22.122 Female aged 10 years**
The oestrogenized hymen admitted the tip of
a little finger. There is an unusual nodular
appearance at the posterior fourchette.

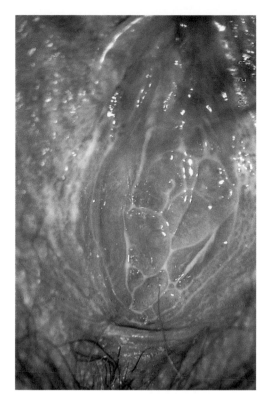

▲ **22.123 Female aged 16 years**
Note the oestrogenized appearance of the
hymen with physiological discharge. Note also
the appearance of the hymen in a consensually
sexually active teenager.

▲ **22.124 Female aged 14 years**
An oestrogenized but deficient hymen.

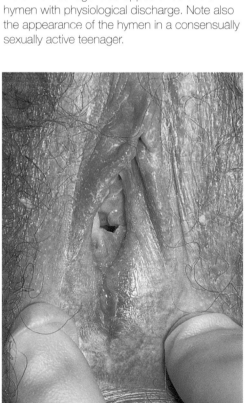

◀ **22.125 Female aged 15 years**
Pubertal girl. Well-healed scar extending from
the posterior fourchette across the perineum.
Note the deceptively small hymenal opening.
A medium-sized speculum was passed with
ease.

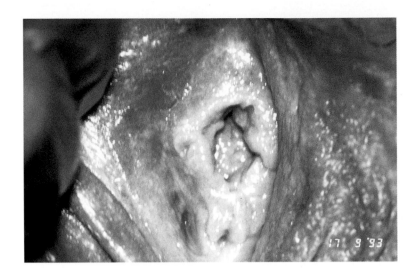

◀ **22.126 Female**
Postpubertal girl with redundant irregular hymen.

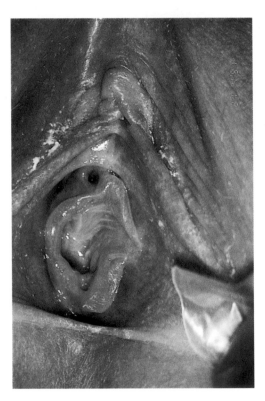

▲ **22.127 Female aged 14 years**
Postpubertal girl with deep transection at 3 o'clock and partial transection at 6 o'clock. The urethra is dilated.

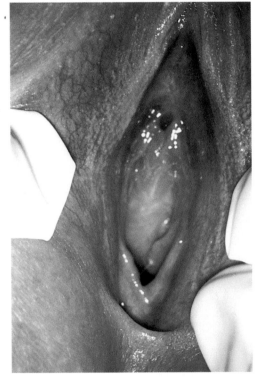

▲ **22.128 Female aged 10 years**
Early oestrogen changes in a child who had a previously damaged hymen.

Chapter 23

Anal Findings in Sexually Abused Children

Anal abuse is common but still denied by many in the UK and US. There is now better dialogue with girls in general about child sexual abuse (CSA) but neither girls or boys find it easy to talk about anal or oral sex. Healing is rapid and usually complete.

1. Perianal reddening is non-specific, i.e. it is associated with CSA, poor hygiene, diarrhoea, streptococcal infection. Scatches may be caused by the child with threadworms, eczema or an assailant grasping the child.

2. Swelling of the anal margin (the tyre sign) and anal verge haematoma are caused by forcible anal penetration.

3. A gaping anus is seen in the hours, possibly longer, after forcible penetration.

4. A lax anus is seen particularly in young children but also older children and teenagers who have been repeatedly buggered, also in neurogenic anus (e.g. spina bifda).

5. Reflex anal dilatation is a sign of anal penetration, which was used in the UK by police when homosexuality was illegal.

    The child is usually examined in the left lateral position, the buttocks are separated and the anus inspected over 30 seconds.

    A positive response occurs when the external anal sphincter dilates followed by the internal sphincter giving a view into the rectum. The sphincters repeatedly open and shut.

    Normal stool may be seen and does not invalidate the sign.

    Large, constipated stool protruding from the anal canal needs treating and the child re-examined later.

    There is disagreement about the relevance of various degrees of dilatation − 1−1.5 cm is usual, 2−2.5 cm may be occasionally seen.

    The sign is associated with CSA and appears to be a learned behaviour. The sign may be present for weeks to months.

6. The external sphincter relaxes after 10 seconds or rather longer and as usually the internal sphincter remains closed there is no view into the rectum. It is a normal phenomenon and has been called 'winking'.

7. Anal fissures cross the anal verge and may be single, multiple and 6 and 12 o'clock commonly, but may be at any site. Constipated young children in particular may have fissure but a good history of bowel dysfunction is required. Stretching of the anus as in buggery may cause similarly pain, bleeding and tear(s).

8. Dilated veins are associated with anal abuse and may present as a halo of flat veins, or dilated veins in an arc or encircling the anus.

    The veins, if any, should be described with the child in the left lateral position at less than 30 seconds.

9. In chronic anal abuse there may be skin changes perianally − thickening of the perianal skin, loss of skin folds and sometimes laxity. The anus may be deeply placed or funnelled − this sign is seen in teenagers.

10. Scars are seen in 10% or less and are linear or fan-shaped and may be associated with skin tags.

11. Sexually transmitted disease.

12. Bruises, burns and lacerations are sometimes inflicted.

13. It is important that it is recognized that there may be no signs of CSA, especially in teenagers, and if a lubricant is used.

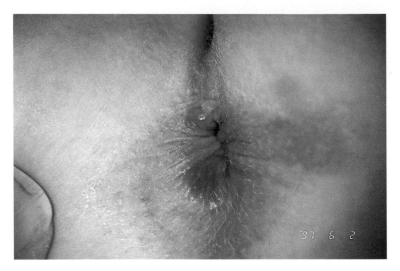

▲ **23.1 Female aged 7 years**
Perianal reddening with leases of veins and prominent skin fold at 12 o'clock.

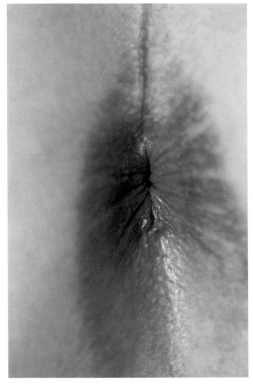

▲ **23.2 Male aged 9 years**
Perianal reddening is seen, and a dilated vein at 6 o'clock with some irregular skin folds at 7 o'clock and more irregular skin folds adjacent. This boy was handicapped, and therefore at greater risk of abuse of all types. Signs: reddening, irregular folds, veins.

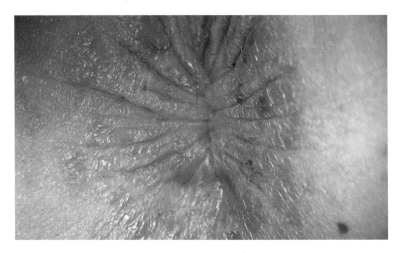

▲ **23.3 Male aged 3 years**
Perianal reddening is seen with superficial small abrasions. Signs: reddening, abrasions.

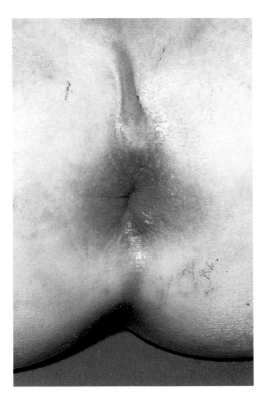

▶ **23.4 Male aged 3 years**
There is perianal reddening with swelling and scattered dilated veins and a deep fold at 9 o'clock. A reddened, prominent midline raphe is seen. Signs: reddening, veins, midline raphe, deep fold.

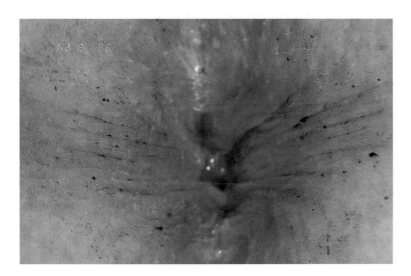

▲ **23.5**

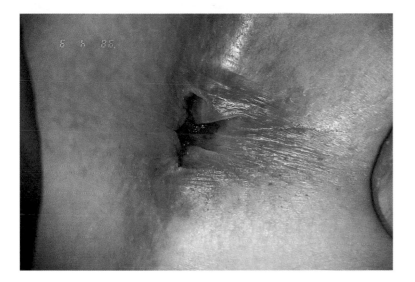

▲ **23.6**

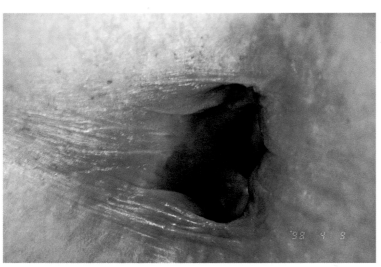

▲ **23.7**

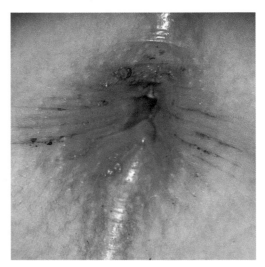

▲ **23.8**

◄ **23.5**, ◄ **23.6**, ◄ **23.7**, ▼ **23.8 Male aged 10 years**
Boy seen over 3 months. Figure 23.5: reddened, lax, acute fissure, dilated veins. Figures 23.6 and 23.7 (2 weeks later): laxity and gross reflex dilatation with swelling of the anal margin. Figure 23.8 (after removal and protection 3 months later): healing; no fissure, slight residual laxity and persistent soiling.

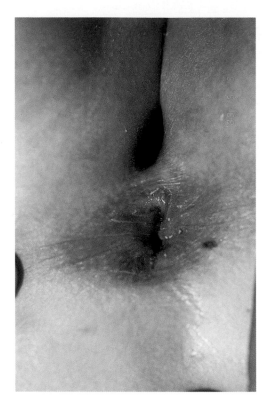
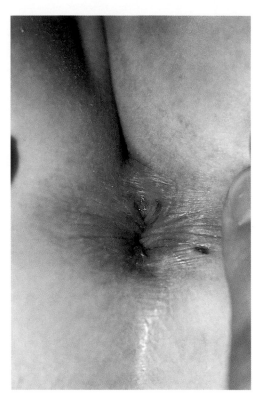

▲ 23.9, ▲ 23.10 **Female aged 5 years**

Figure 23.9 shows perianal reddening with a recent fissure at 12 o'clock extending across the anal margin. There is a possible healing fissure at 1 o'clock. Irregular skin folds are seen, with dilated veins in an arc. Figure 23.10 shows healing 1 month later – see anterior fissure. Signs: reddening, veins, acute fissure, healing fissure.

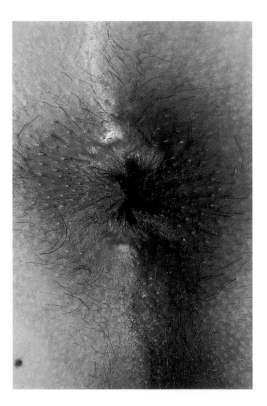

▶ 23.11 **Male aged 12 years**

Perianal reddening is seen with increased pigmentation. There are recent fissures at 1, 4, 6, 7 and 11 o'clock with scattered distended perianal veins at 5, 7, 8 and 10 o'clock and smooth areas at 6 and 12 o'clock. Signs: reddening, increased pigmentation, veins, acute fissures.

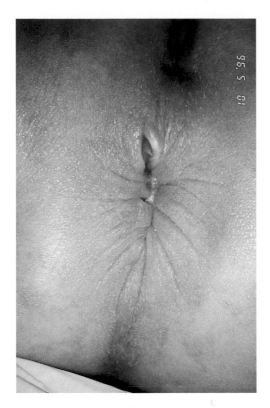

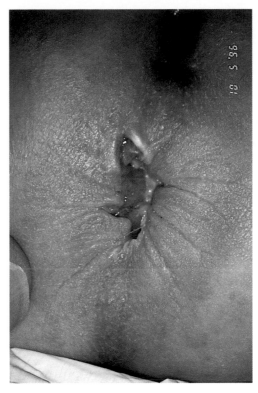

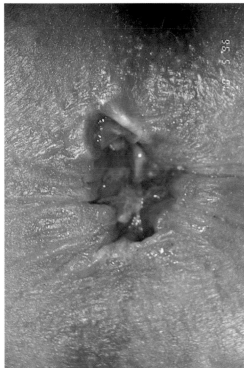

▲ **23.12,** ▲ **23.13,** ◀ **23.14 Female aged 6 months**
Series of views of an infant showing a substantial tear at 11 o'clock and with minimal traction, the anus reveals a complete loss of tone. This represents disruption of the anal sphincter.

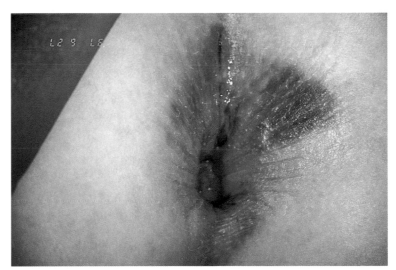

▲ **23.15 Female aged 5 years**
Girl with acute tear in the anus and perianal skin, with wedge-shaped areas of distended veins on both sides of the tear. Anus is lax with rectal mucosa prolapsing.

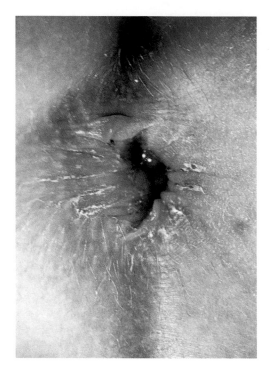

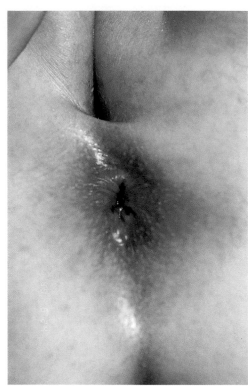

◄ 23.17 Female aged 15 months

Perianal reddening is seen with swelling and venous congestion. There is a disrupted fold pattern to the anus, and a healing fissure at 6 o'clock.

Signs: reddening and swelling, venous congestion, folds, fissure.

▲ 23.16 Female aged 2 years

There is perianal reddening with an anterior fissure at 12 o'clock running to a skin tag, a healing fissure at 7 o'clock and adjacent thickened fold/small tag. The anus is gaping and the rectal mucosa is visible.

Signs: reddening, tag, healing, fissures, gaping sphincter, visible mucosa.

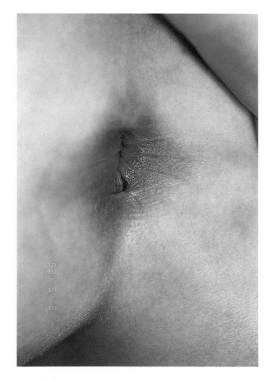

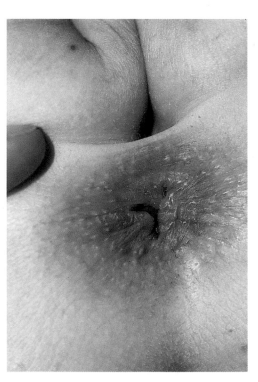

◄ 23.19 Female aged 3 years

There is some perianal reddening with scattered dilated veins and a recent fissure at 1 o'clock with a clear deficit in anal margin at 9 o'clock.

Signs: reddening, veins, fissure, deficit.

▲ 23.18 Male aged 3 years

There is some perianal reddening with an almost complete ring of dilated veins. A recent fissure is seen at 5 o'clock, along the fold.

Signs: reddening, veins, fissure.

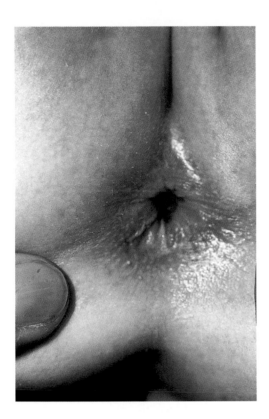

◀ 23.20 Female aged 2 years

Some perianal reddening is seen with scattered dilated veins. There is anal laxity and a healing fissure at 6 o'clock. Signs: reddening, veins, anal laxity, fissure.

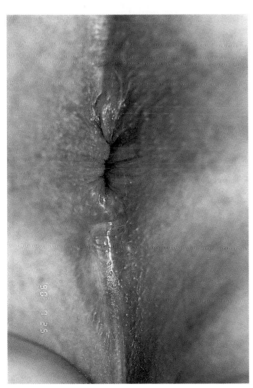

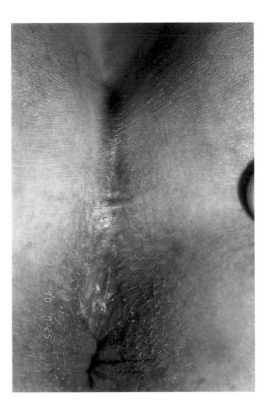

▲ 23.21, ▲ 23.22 Male aged 8 years

There is some perianal reddening with venous congestion. A skin tag is seen at 12 o'clock. There is a linear scar extending from just inferior to the anal margin anteriorly across the perineum, due to a previous knife wound. Signs: reddening, venous congestion, tag, scar.

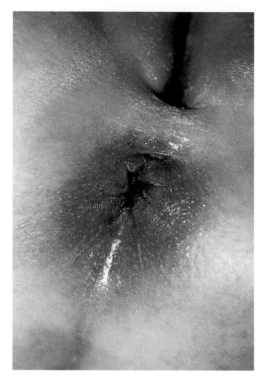

▲ **23.23 Female aged 12 months**
There is perianal reddening, with swelling and halo of veins, and recent stellate fissures. Signs: reddening and swelling, veins, acute fissures.

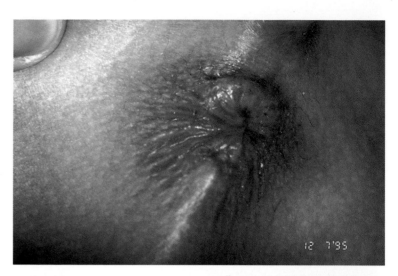

▲ **23.24, ▲ 23.25 Male aged 5 years**
Swelling of the anal margin (tyre sign) and small dilated veins. At follow-up 4 weeks later the swelling had settled but the veins remain. Veins may be the most persistent sign.

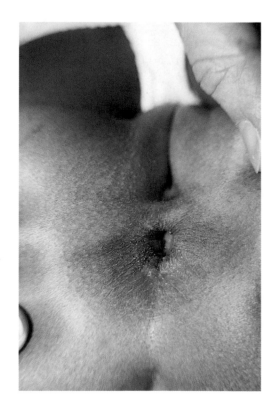

◄ **23.26 Female aged 2 years**
Tyre sign and lax dilating anus are seen. A dilated vein is visible at 7 o'clock. Signs: tyre sign, veins, laxity, dilating anus.

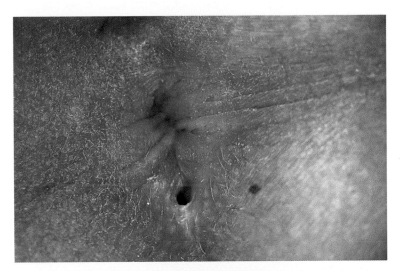

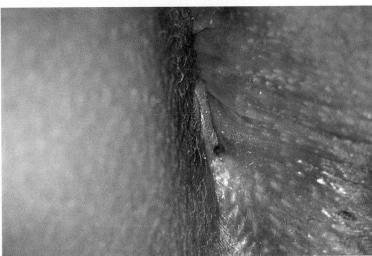

◀ **23.27,** ◀ **23.28 Female aged 2 years**
Figure 23.27 shows minimal perianal reddening, with irregular folds and an unhealed posterior fissure. The follow-up photograph after surgery (Fig. 23.28) shows a long posterior skin fold. The fissure has not completely healed distally. Signs: reddening, irregular folds, fissure, scar.

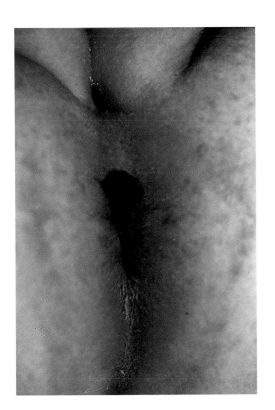

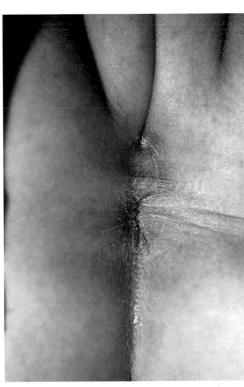

◀ **23.29,** ◀ **23.30 Female aged 18 months**
Some perianal reddening and a gaping anus are seen in Fig. 23.29. Healing has occurred 1 week later (Fig. 23.30). Signs: reddening, gaping, healing.

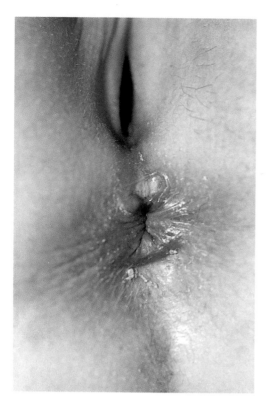 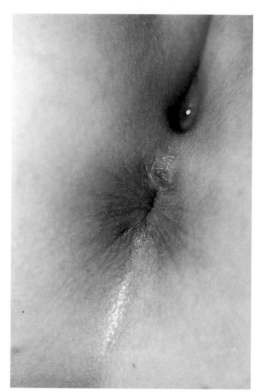

▲ **23.31,** ▲ **23.32 Female aged 8 years**
Minimal reddening is seen with an almost complete arc of dilated veins. There is a recent tear at 12 o'clock extending across the anal margin (Fig. 23.31). Healing is seen 3 months later with irregular folds anteriorly (Fig. 23.32). Signs: reddening, veins, recent fissure, healing.

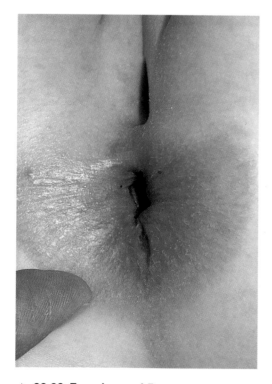 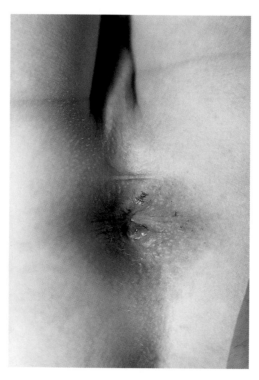

▲ **23.33 Female aged 5 years**
Perianal reddening is seen with a recent extensive fissure extending across the anal margin. The anus is gaping and stool is visible. Signs: reddening, gaping anus (not dilatation), acute fissure.

▲ **23.34 Male aged 9 years**
Minimal perianal reddening is seen and an anal verge haematoma at 5 o'clock.
Signs: reddening, anal verge haematoma.

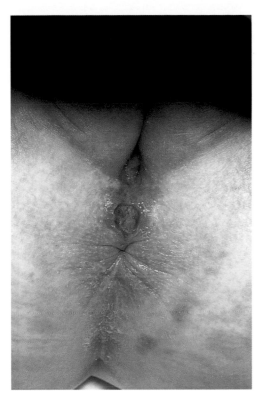

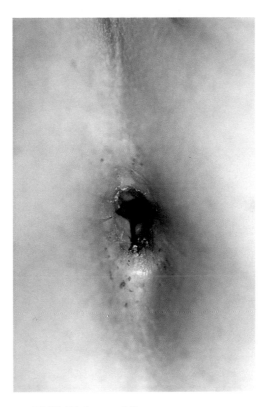

▲ **23.35 Female aged 15 months**
Some perianal reddening is visible, with an extensive tear anteriorly. Signs: reddening, acute fissure.

▲ **23.36 Male aged 9 years**
Smooth shiny perianal skin is seen and dilated veins are present. There is a gaping anus with a deep chronic posterior fissure. Signs: smooth shiny skin, veins, chronic fissure.

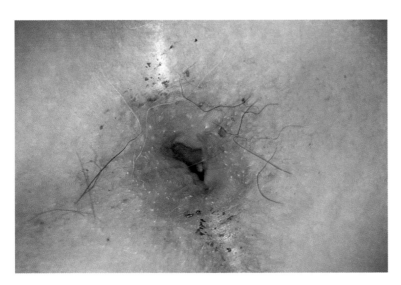

▲ **23.37 Male aged 11 years**
Lax, scattered veins, skin smooth. Irregular dilated opening.

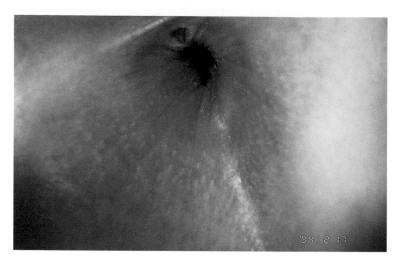

▲ **23.38 Female aged 4 years**
Pink, smooth skin is seen perianally with a healing fissure at 12 o'clock with a prominent fold. The anus is gaping. Signs: smooth shiny skin, fold, fissure, gaping.

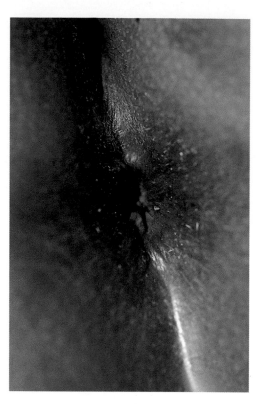

▲ **23.39 Female aged 9 years**
An irregular anal margin is shown with a pale scar at 1 o'clock and a skin tag at 7 o'clock with an adjacent dilated vein. The perianal skin is pigmented. Signs: pigmented skin, tag, vein, scar.

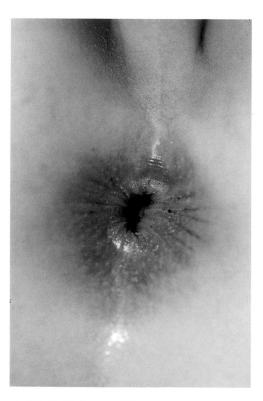

▲ **23.40 Male aged 7 years**
There is marked perianal reddening with a swollen anal verge, i.e. the tyre sign, and some laxity of the anus. Signs: reddening, swelling, laxity.

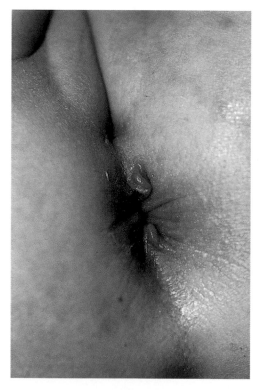

▲ **23.41 Female aged 5 years**
Large skin tags are seen at 6 and 12 o'clock. Signs: tags.

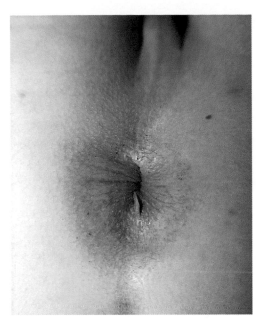

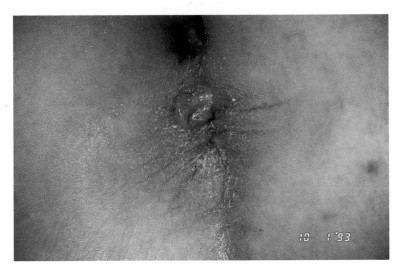

▲ **23.43 Female aged 5 years**
Irregular anal skin folds are seen with a large skin tag at 12 o'clock.
Signs: folds, tag.

▲ **23.42 Male aged 10 years**
There are dilated veins and a skin tag at
5 o'clock. Signs: veins, tag.

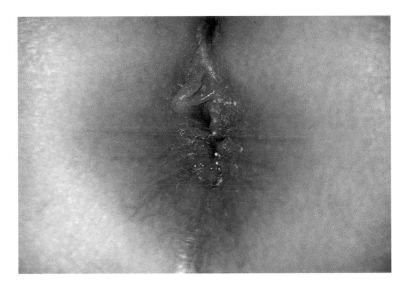

◀ **23.44 Female aged 2 years**
An irregular anal margin is seen with a skin tag
and linear scar extending anteriorly.
Signs: folds, tag, scar.

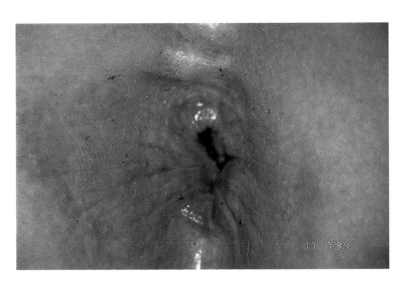

◀ **23.45 Male aged 8 years**
Scarred, disrupted and disorganized anus in a
deaf child.

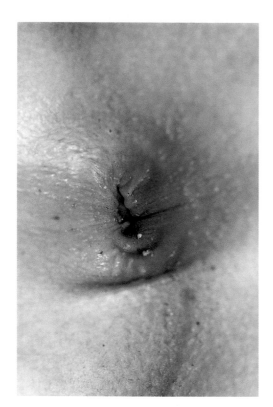

▲ **23.46 Male aged 9 years**
A funnelled anus is seen with a disorganized fold pattern and deficit with a prominent fold at 1 o'clock. The anus is lax. Signs: funnelled, folds, deficity, laxity.

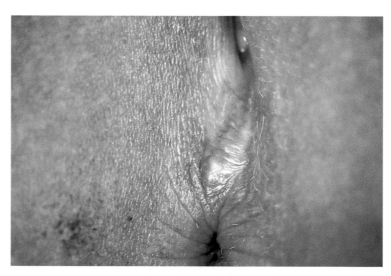

▲ **23.47 Female aged 6 years**
A distorted anal margin is visible with a large anterior scar. The anus is lax. Signs: scar, laxity.

▶ **23.48 Female aged 8 years**
There is a large vertical anterior scar extending from the anal margin across the perineum. Signs: scar.

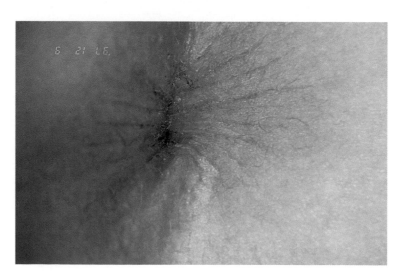

▶ **23.49 Male aged 5 years**
Fan-shaped scar radiating from the anus.

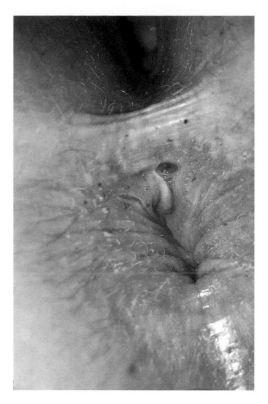

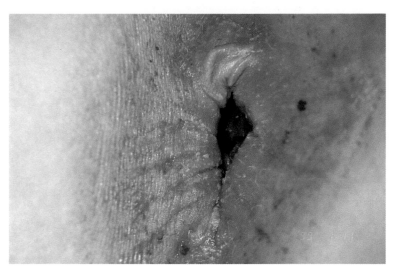

▲ **23.51 Female aged 4 years**
Skin reddened and abraded. Anus is dilated, lax and there is a large anterior skin tag.

▲ **23.50 Female aged 7 years**
A highly magnified view of the anal margin showing a linear scar at 12 o'clock extending across the anal margin. Signs: scar.

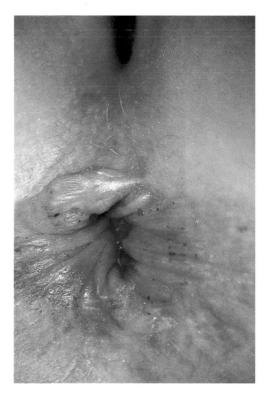

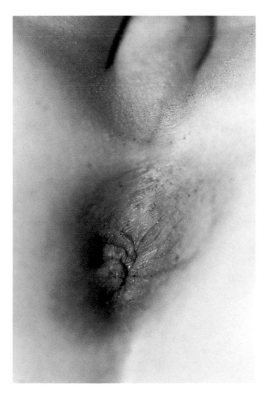

▲ **23.52 Female aged 7 years**
Perianal reddening is seen with a lax anus, irregular skin folds and a large anterior skin tag. Signs: reddening, folds, tag, laxity.

▲ **23.53 Male aged 12 years**
A funnelled anus is shown with swelling and irregular skin folds, and scattered veins. Signs: funnelling, folds, veins.

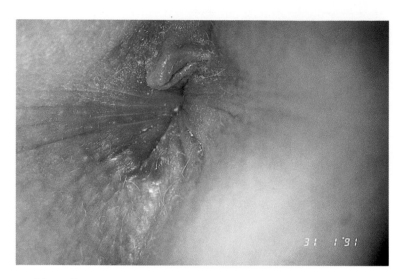

▲ **23.54 Female aged 3 years**
Perianal reddening is seen with a large anterior skin tag. Superficial fissures and venous congestion are seen at 5–6 o'clock.
Signs: reddening, tag, fissure, venous congestion.

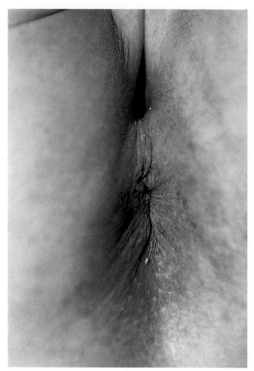

▲ **23.55 Female aged 4 years**
There is perianal reddening with dilated veins, and a very unusual and complex series of skin folds extending anteriorly and across the perineum. Sign: reddening, veins, folds.

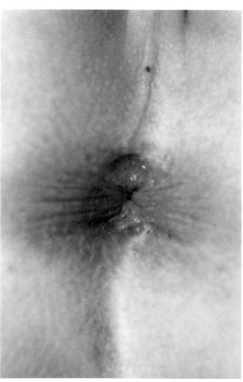

▶ **23.57 Male aged 3 years**
Perianal reddening is seen with an irregular anal margin and deficits at 3, 6 and 9 o'clock, with some laxity. There is a skin tag at 12 o'clock. A medium raphe is seen anteriorly. (This child coincidentally has dystrophia myotonica. Organic disease does not exclude the possibility of additional abuse. A normal sister had genital and anal signs consistent with sexual abuse.)
Signs: reddening, tag, raphe.

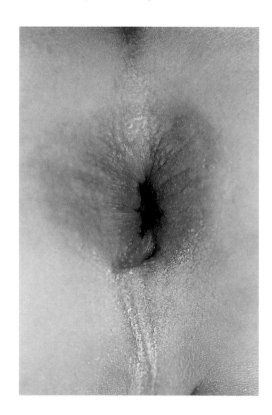

▲ **23.56 Male aged 7 years**
Some perianal reddening is seen with veins particularly marked between 6 and 9 o'clock. There is a normal raphe across the perineum.
Signs: reddening, veins, raphe.

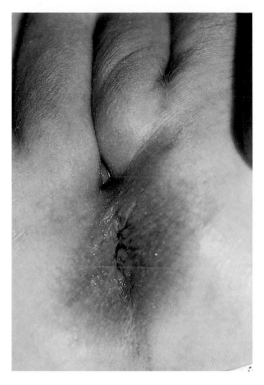

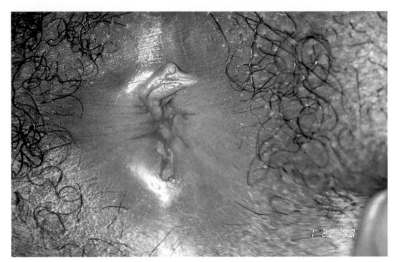

▲ 23.59 Female aged 12 years
A disorganized anal margin is seen with an unhealed fissure at 6 o'clock and a large skin tag anteriorly; in addition small skin tags are seen at 3 and 4 o'clock. Signs: fissure, tags.

▲ 23.58 Female aged 4 years
There is reddening perianally with dilated veins and a distorted anal margin. Signs: reddening, veins, distorted anal margin.

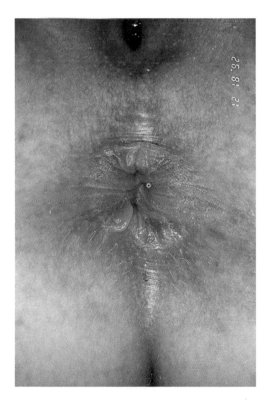

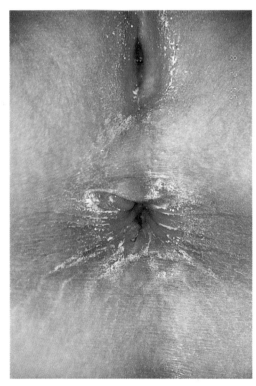

▲ 23.60 Female aged 18 months
Dilated veins are seen, with skin tags at 7, 11 and 12 o'clock, and an irregular margin. Signs: veins, tag, irregular margin.

▲ 23.61 Female aged 6 years
There is an irregular anal margin with some laxity and a large anterior skin tag. This child had Down's syndrome; anal laxity is not part of this syndrome. Signs: laxity, tag.

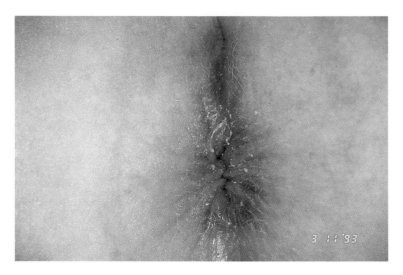

▲ **23.62 Female aged 3 years**
An almost complete ring of dilated veins is seen perianally and unusual skin folds at 7 and 11–12 o'clock. Signs: veins, folds.

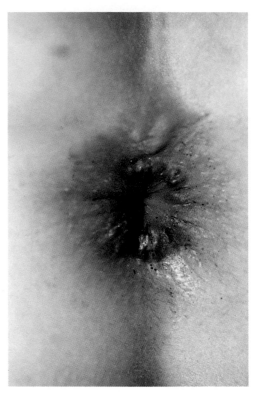

▲ **23.63 Male aged 5 years**
There is perianal reddening with a complete ring of markedly dilated veins and a scar anteriorly. Signs: reddening, veins, scar.

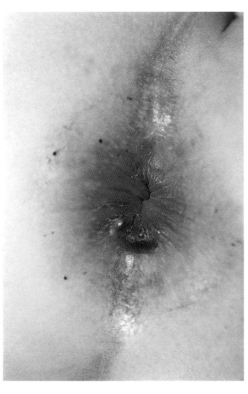

▲ **23.64 Male aged 8 years**
Perianal reddening is seen with an arc of dilated veins at 5–7 o'clock. Signs: reddening, veins.

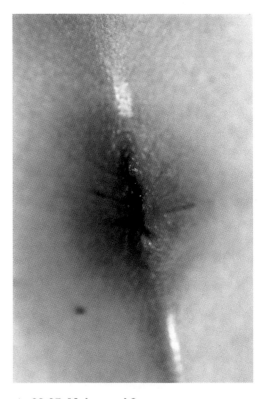

▲ **23.65 Male aged 8 years**
Increased perianal pigmentation is seen with a small dilated vein at 12 o'clock and a halo of venous congestion. Signs: pigmentation, veins.

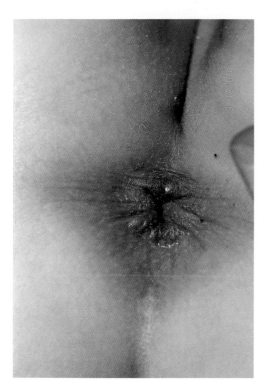

▲ **23.66 Female aged 3 years**
There is perianal reddening, a swollen margin
and a ring of dilated veins. Signs: reddening,
swollen, veins.

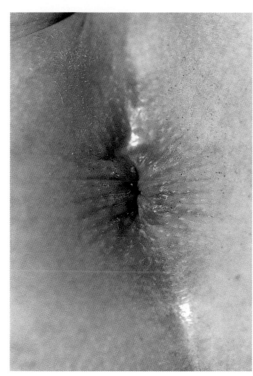

▲ **23.67 Male aged 8 years**
Perianal reddening is seen with swelling of the
anal margin giving an irregular appearance to
folds with dilated veins. There is a smooth area
at 12 o'clock. Signs: reddening, swollen, veins.

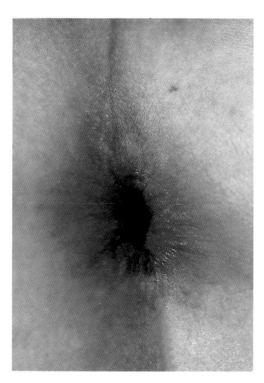

▲ **23.68 Male aged 5 years**
Perianal reddening is seen, with reflex anal
dilatation. There are dilated veins posteriorly
and deficits in the anal margin at 5 and
7 o'clock. (The child had a rectal polyp
diagnosed on proctoscopy.) Signs: reddening,
veins, reflex anal dilatation.

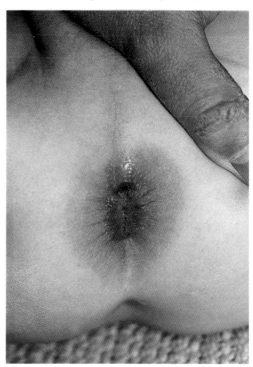

▲ **23.69 Male aged 4 years**
There is increased perianal pigmentation and a
complete ring of veins. Signs: pigmentation,
veins.

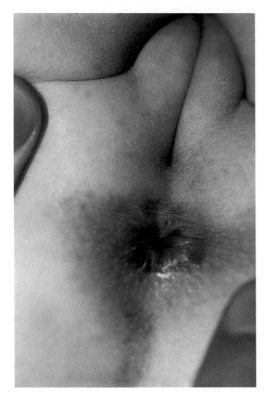

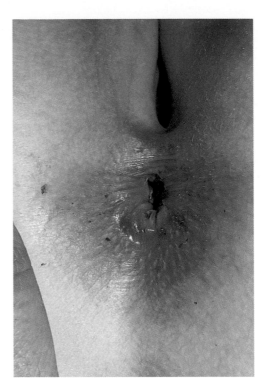

▲ **23.70 Female aged 2 years**
Perianal redness is seen, with perianal swelling.
There is an irregular anal margin with a skin tag
at 12 o'clock and a prominent fold at 7 o'clock,
and dilated veins anteriorly and posteriorly.
Signs: reddening, swollen, tag, veins.

▲ **23.71 Female aged 7 years**
Perianal reddening is seen with a halo of
dilated veins laterally and posteriorly. The anus
is gaping with heaped up skin folds posteriorly.
Signs: reddening, veins, folds, gaping.

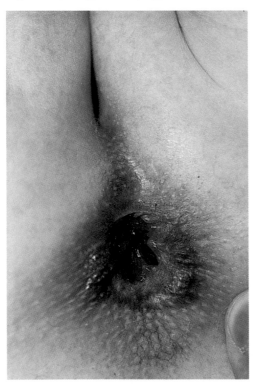

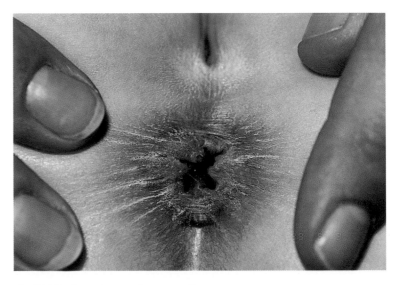

▲ **23.73 Female aged 12 months**
There is marked venous congestion and stellate appearance of the lax
anal sphincter with rectal mucosa visible. Signs: veins, laxity, rectal
mucosa.

▲ **23.72 Female aged 3 years**
Very congested perianal skin is seen with
prominent veins and a distorted anal margin.
The rectal mucosa is visible and the anus is lax.
Signs: veins, rectal mucosa, laxity.

▶ **23.74,** ▶ **23.75**
Male aged 10 years
Figure 23.74 shows perianal reddening with scattered dilated veins and irregular anal skin folds. The anus is dilated in Fig. 23.75 to show reflex anal dilatation and deficits in the anal margin at 5, 7 and 9 o'clock. Signs: reddening, veins, folds, deficits.

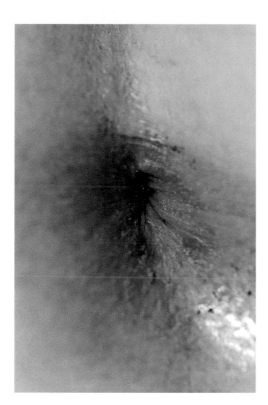

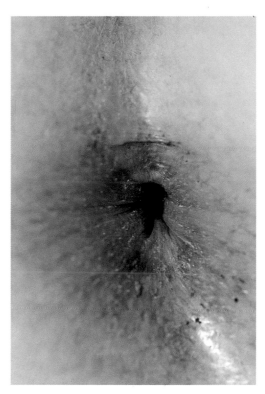

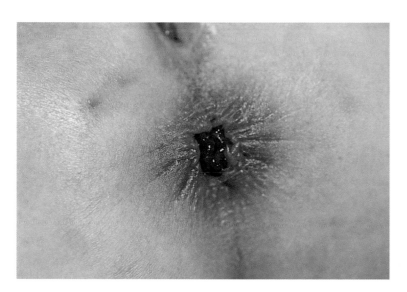

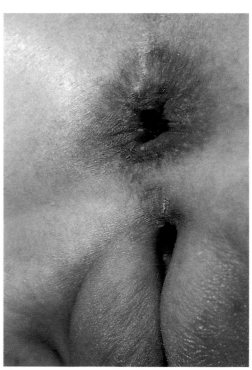

▲ **23.76 Female aged 15 months**
Perianal reddening is seen with dilated veins and the rectal mucosa prolapsing to a disorganized, lax anal sphincter. Signs: reddening, veins, laxity, rectal mucosa.

▲ **23.77 Female aged 2 years**
There is perianal reddening with venous congestion and swelling of the anal margin. The anal sphincter is lax and distorted with rectal mucosa visible. Signs: reddening, swollen, veins, laxity, irregular folds, rectal mucosa.

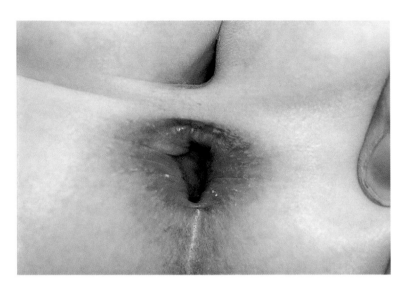

▲ **23.78 Female aged 4 years**
Perianal reddening is seen with a lax anal sphincter with visible rectal mucosa and dilated veins anteriorly. Signs: reddening, veins, laxity.

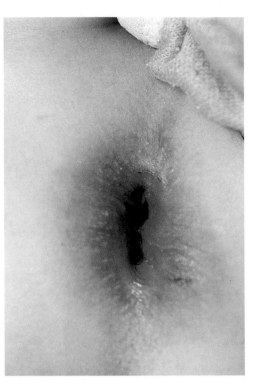

▲ **23.79 Male aged 3 years**
There is perianal reddening and smoothing of the skin perianally. Rectal mucosa is visible, and the sphincter is lax. Signs: reddening, smooth skin, laxity.

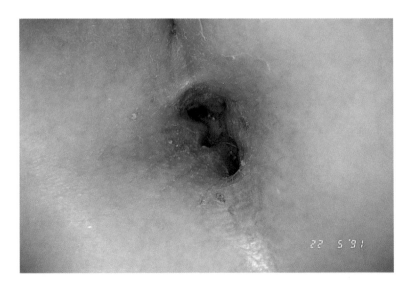

▲ **23.80 Female aged 4 years**
Roughened, thickened, perianal skin is seen with loss of skin folds. The anus is gaping with rectal mucosa visible. Signs: thickened skin, gaping, rectal mucosa.

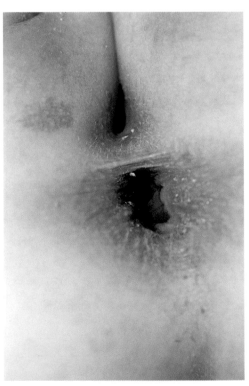

▲ **23.81 Female aged 3 years**
Perianal reddening is seen with scattered dilated veins, a reddened anal margin with loss of usual skin folds and anal dilatation. Signs: reddening, veins, anal dilatation.

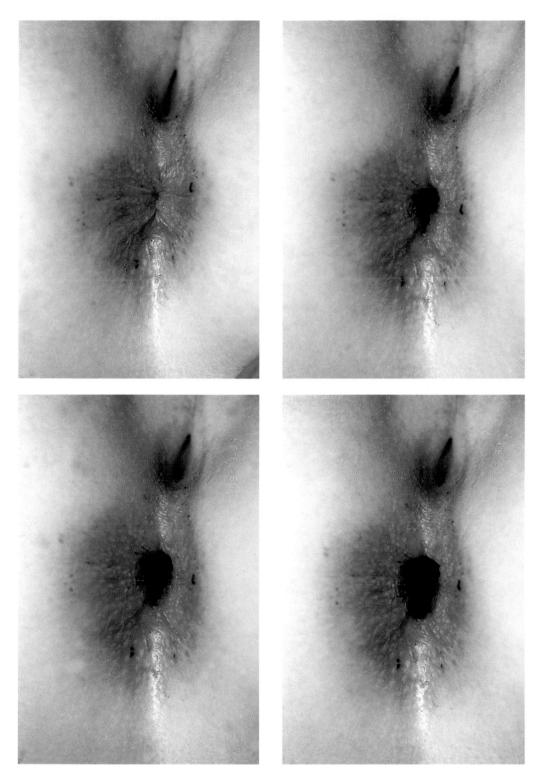

▲ **23.82,** ▲ **23.83,** ▲ **23.84,** ▲ **23.85 Female aged 5 years**
Perianal reddening with marked anal dilatation of increasing magnitude is shown across the four
photographs. There is an irregular margin with a few small veins visible.
Signs: reddening, veins, dilatation.

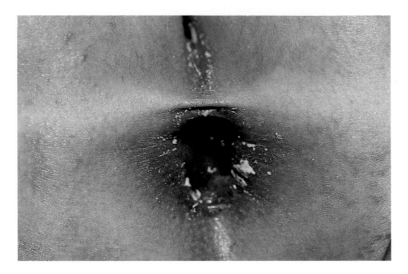

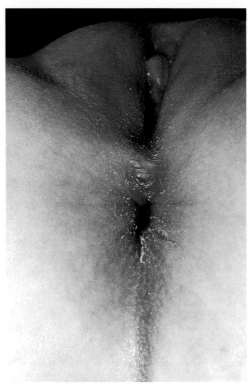

▲ 23.86, ▶ 23.87 **Female aged 2 years**
Some perianal reddening is seen in Fig. 23.86 with venous congestion. There is marked gaping/dilatation with a very thin irregular margin to the anal sphincter, and the rectal mucosa is prolapsing. Figure 23.87, taken 6 months later, shows healing. The anal margin is still irregular and appears thickened. There is an extensive scar anteriorly and a few small dilated veins. Signs: reddening, venous congestion, gaping, dilatation, rectal mucosa, scar.

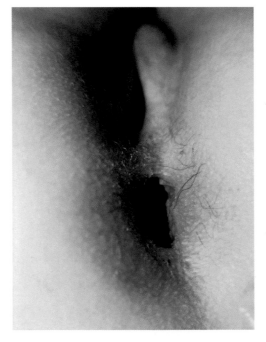

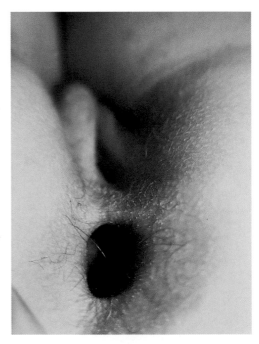

▲ 23.88, ▲ 23.89, ▶ 23.90, ▶ 23.91, ▶ 23.92, ▶ 23.93 **Female aged 12 years**
Figure 23.88 (above left) shows perianal reddening, thickened perianal skin and dilatation; in Fig. 23.89 (above right) there is stool clearly visible in the rectum. These two photographs were taken at the first examination. Figure 23.90 was taken 6 weeks later, Fig. 23.91 3 months after that, (Figure 23.92) 3 months later, and Fig. 23.93 3 months later. These show that over the next year the anal sphincter gradually developed increased tone. Signs: reddening, thickened skin, reflex anal dilatation.

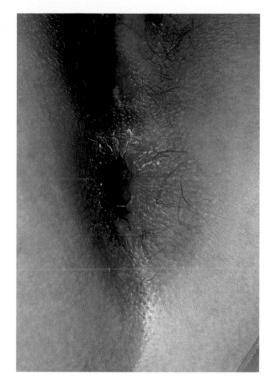

▲ 23.90

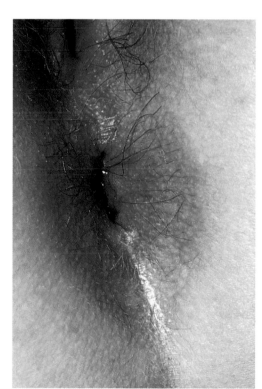

▲ 23.91

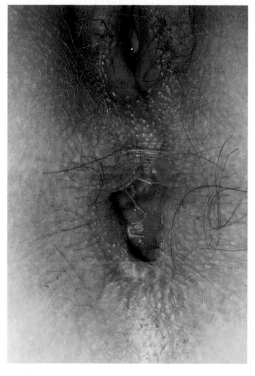

▲ 23.92

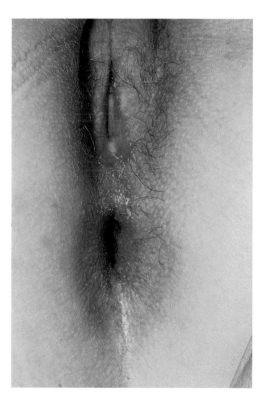

▲ 23.93

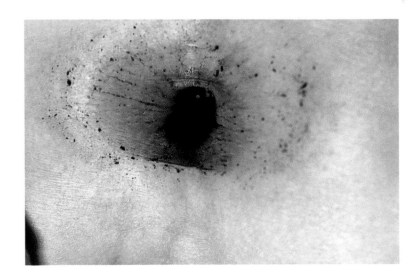

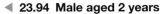

23.94 Male aged 2 years
There is marked perianal and anal reddening; the anus is widely gaping with rectal mucosa visible. The examination was carried out under sedation, the effect of which is not clearly established. Signs: reddening, gaping, rectal mucosa.

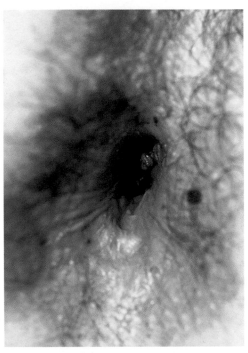

▶ **23.95 Male aged 17 years**
There is marked reflex anal dilatation. The posterior margin of the anus is very irregular and probably the site of previous fissures. Smooth perianal skin is seen, and stool is present in the rectum. (Note: if during the examination a child wishes to have his or her bowels opened it is better to re-examine the child again some time later. However, the presence of stool in the rectum does not invalidate the physical signs.)

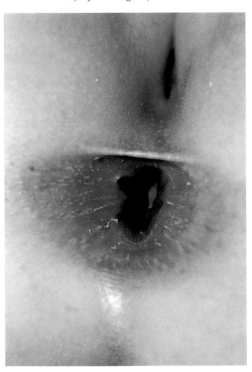

▲ **23.96 Female aged 4 years**
There is markedly red and swollen perianal skin with a lack of folds, marked anal dilatation with an irregular margin and stool present in the rectum. Signs: reddening, swollen, reflex anal dilatation.

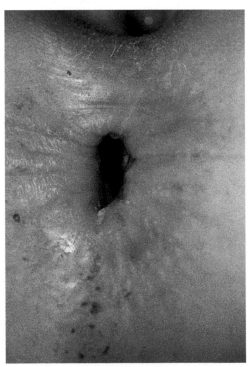

▲ **23.97 Female aged 6 years**
The perianal skin is smooth with new folds. Marked dilatation is seen with an irregular anal sphincter. Signs: smooth skin, reflex anal dilatation.

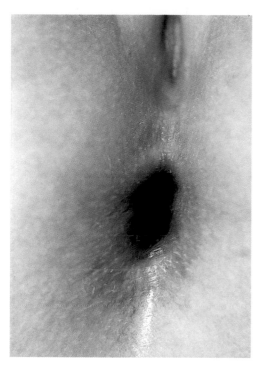

▲ **23.98 Female aged 5 years**
There is a marked perianal rim with reddening smooth skin, loss of anal folds and marked anal dilatation. Signs: reddening, smooth skin, reflex anal dilatation.

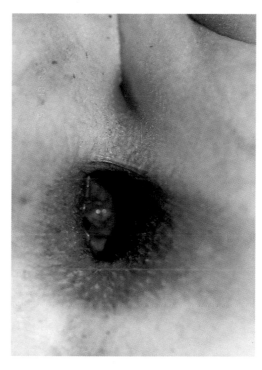

▲ **23.99 Female aged 5 years**
Perianal reddening is seen with loss of skin folds and marked anal dilatation. This child was markedly constipated and soiled. Her symptoms settled and the signs regressed as soon as she was admitted to foster care. She then disclosed sexual abuse within the family. This clinical picture demonstrates reflex anal dilatation, not the 'visibly relaxed' anus described in very severe chronic constipation where stools are protruding from the anus and the anal sphincter is therefore stretched about them.

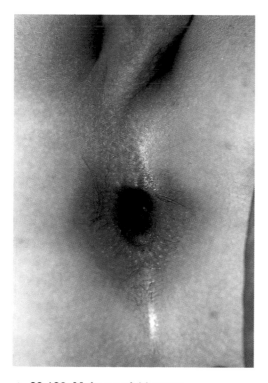

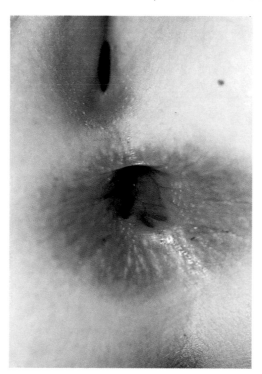

◀ **23.101 Female aged 5 years**
There is marked perianal reddening with some increased pigmentation, a markedly dilated anal sphincter with irregular margin and rectal mucosa prolapsing. The brother of this child had myotonic dystrophy.
Signs: reddening, pigmentation, reflex anal dilatation, mucosa prolapsing.

▲ **23.100 Male aged 11 years**
A dilating anus is seen with some smoothing of the skin and pigmentation with small scattered veins. Signs: pigmented skin, veins, smooth skin, reflex anal dilatation.

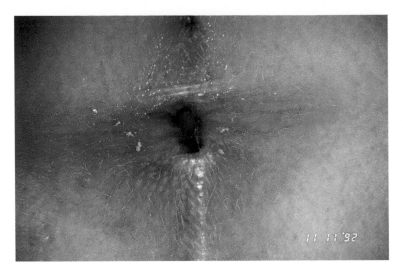

▲ **23.102 Female aged 5 years**
Thick and shiny perianal skin is seen with loss of skin folds, an irregular margin with a deficit at 10 o'clock and a lax anus. Signs: shiny skin, folds, deficit.

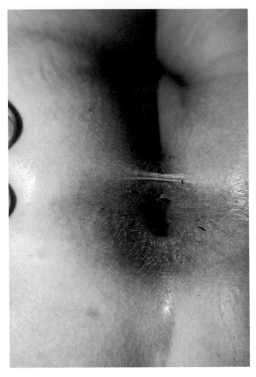

▲ **23.103 Female aged 4 years**
There is perianal reddening with an irregular anal margin and reflex anal dilatation. The perianal skin is thickened with loss of the usual skin folds, and rectal mucosa is visible. Signs: reddening, thickened skin, reflex anal dilatation, rectal mucosa prolapsing.

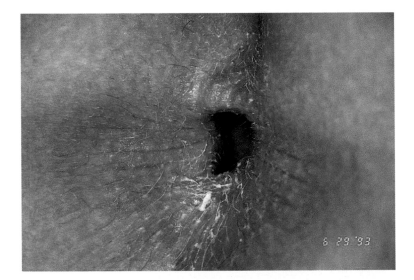

◀ **23.104 Female aged 13 years**
A thickened, smooth, pink anal verge is seen, with a dilated anus. Signs: skin changes, reflex anal dilatation.

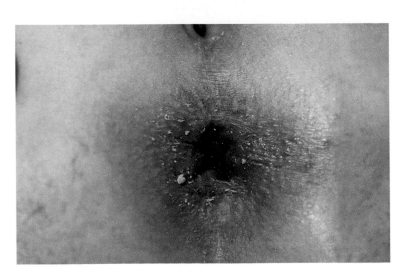

◀ **23.105 Female aged 9 months**
The perianal skin is red and swollen. There is an abraded anal canal and lax sphincter with visible mucosa. Signs: skin changes, laxity, abrasion anal canal.

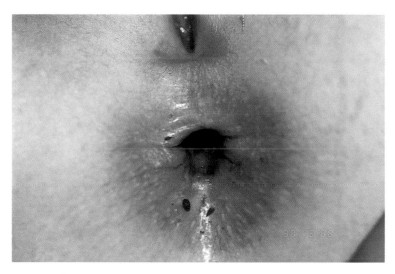

▲ **23.106 Female aged 4 years**
Thickened, smooth, red, shiny skin is seen, with swelling of the anal
verge. There is reflex anal dilatation, and the anus has deep folds at
2, 4, 8 and 10 o'clock. Signs: skin changes, reflex anal dilatation,
deep folds.

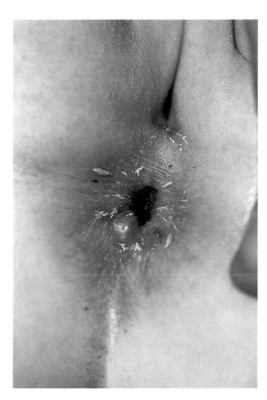

▲ **23.107 Female aged 3 years**
Perianal reddening is seen with a large dilated
vein at 6 o'clock and smaller veins at 4 and
5 o'clock. There is reflex anal dilatation with
rectal mucosa visible. Signs: reddening, veins,
reflex anal dilatation.

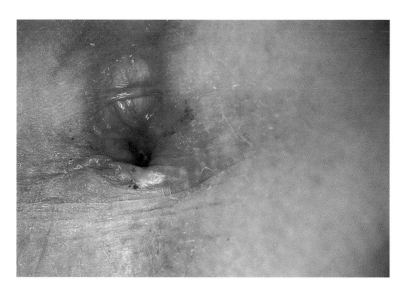

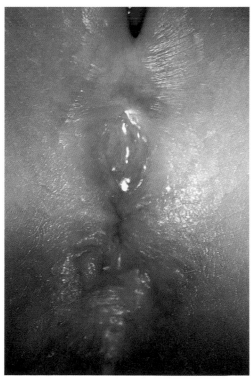

▲ **23.108,** ▶ **23.109 Female aged 10 years**
Red, swollen anal margin and wide anterior fissure, with reflex anal
dilatation and an unusual fold posteriorly. One month later (Fig. 23.109)
the anterior fissure has not healed. There is no anal dilatation. Skin tags
are seen posteriorly at 5, 6 and 7 o'clock, and unusual skin changes are
seen posteriorly. Signs: reddening, swollen, fissure, reflex anal dilatation,
tags.

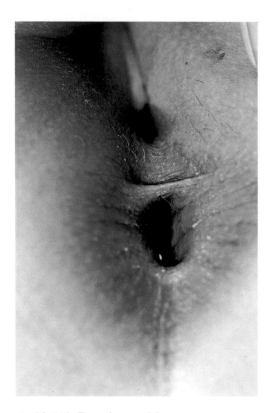

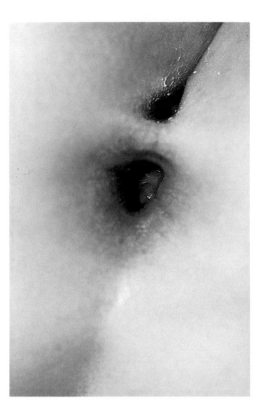

▲ **23.110 Female aged 9 years**
Perianal reddening and a gaping anus are
seen. The examination was carried out under
general anaesthetic, the effect of which is not
clear. Signs: reddening, gaping.

▲ **23.111 Female aged 3 years**
There is perianal reddening and the skin is shiny
and smooth. Venous congestion is seen, with
reflex anal dilatation and prolapsed mucosa.
Signs: reddening, venous congestion, skin
changes, rectal mucosa, reflex anal dilatation.

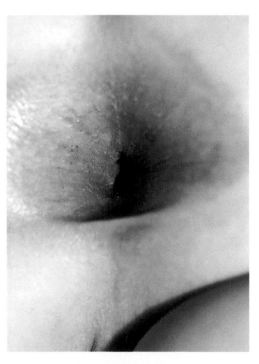

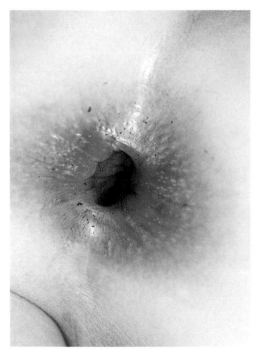

▲ **23.112 Male aged 10 years**
Perianal reddening, smooth skin and loss of
folds are seen, with reflex anal dilatation and
funnelled anus. Signs: reddening, skin
changes, reflex anal dilatation, funnelled.

▲ **23.113 Male aged 3 years**
Perianal reddening, smooth skin, dilating
sphincter with mucosa prolapsing and venous
congestion are seen. Signs: reddening, skin
changes, venous congestion, reflex anal
dilatation, rectal mucosa.

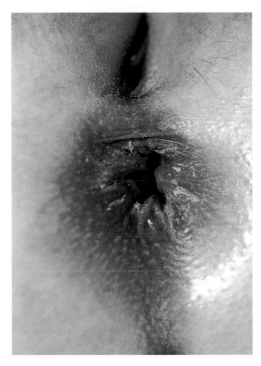

▲ **23.114 Female aged 3 years**
Perianal reddening, venous congestion, an
irregular margin and a lax sphincter are
seen. There are healing fissures at 5, 9 and
11 o'clock. Signs: perianal reddening, venous
congestion, laxity, fissures.

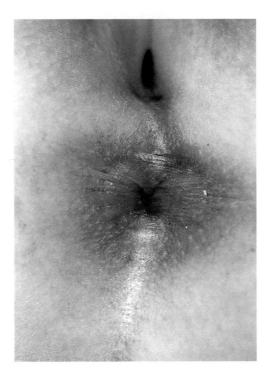

▲ **23.115 Female aged 5 years**
There is perianal reddening which continues
into the anal canal, swelling perianally, marked
venous congestion with a dilated arc of veins
anteriorly and a stellate line of anal closure.
Signs: reddening, venous congestion, dilated
veins, swelling, stellate line of closure.

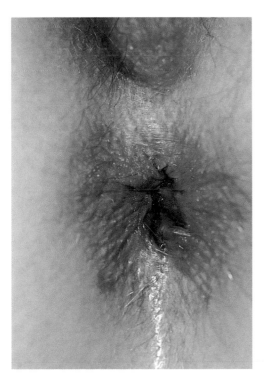

▲ **23.116 Female aged 11 years**
Perianal reddening is seen, with a disrupted
anal sphincter and an acute fissure at
6 o'clock. Rectal mucosa is visible, and there
is a tag at 5 o'clock. Signs: reddening, fissure,
disrupted anal sphincter, rectal mucosa.

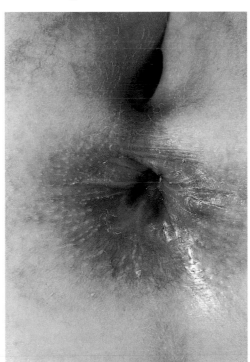

▲ **23.117 Female aged 6 years**
There is perianal reddening and swelling, with
venous congestion, laxity of the anal sphincter,
a superficial fissure at 2 o'clock and abrasions
at 5 o'clock. Signs: reddening, swollen, venous
congestion, laxity, fissure, abrasions.

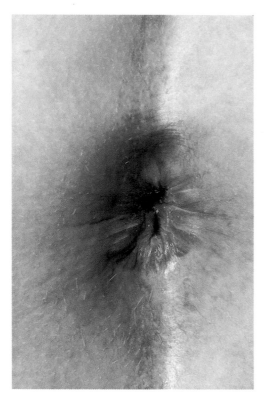

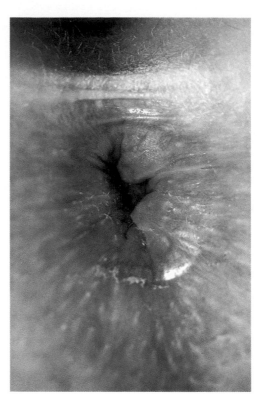

▲ **23.118 Male aged 10 years**
A distorted anal margin is visible with a definite scar posteriorly and possible scar anteriorly. There is venous congestion. Signs: distorted anal margin, scars, venous congestion.
Note: This photograph was taken 6 months after the photograph in Fig. 23.36 to show healing.

▲ **23.119 Female aged 4 years**
Perianal reddening is seen, with venous congestion, an anal verge deficit at 3 o'clock and a lax anal sphincter with rectal mucosa visible. Signs: perianal reddening, venous congestion, deficit in anal margin, laxity, rectal mucosa.

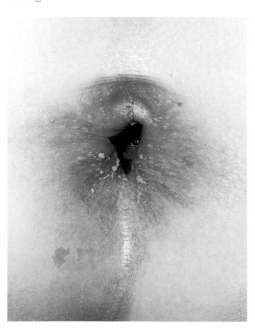

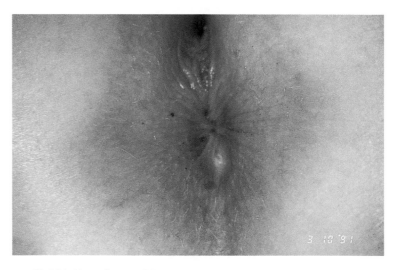

▲ **23.121 Female aged 5 years**
There is perianal pigmentation and a disorganized fold pattern. A scar is seen at 6 o'clock. There are irregular folds anteriorly. Signs: pigmentation, scar, folds.

▲ **23.120 Male aged 2 years**
There is perianal reddening, shiny, smooth skin, venous congestion and a gaping, lax sphincter with a deficit in the anal margin at 9 o'clock. Stool is visible. Signs: perianal reddening, skin changes, venous congestion, stool.

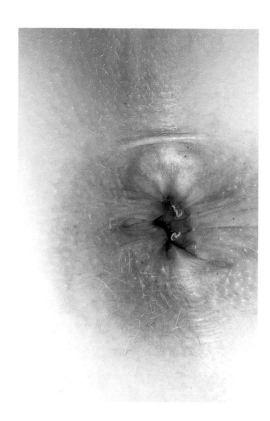

◀ **23.122 Male aged 5 years**
Perianal reddening is seen with thick and shiny skin. There is a fan-shaped anterior scar and probable posterior scar, an irregular anal margin, deficits at 5, 7 and 9 o'clock and a lax anus with threadworms visible. Signs: reddening, skin changes, deficits in anal margin, laxity, scars, threadworms.

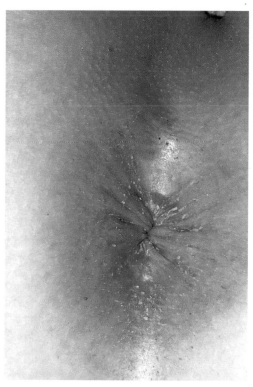

◀ **23.123**

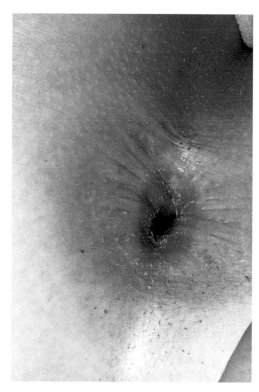

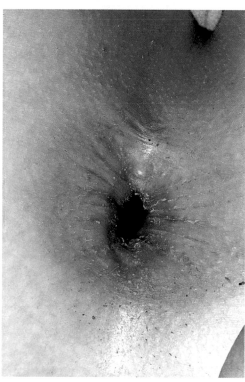

▶ **23.123,** ▲ **23.124,** ▶ **23.125 Male aged 8 years**
The perianal skin is red and smooth, with irregular folds. There is reflex anal dilatation in two phases. Signs: skin changes, folds, reflex anal dilatation.

◀ **23.125**

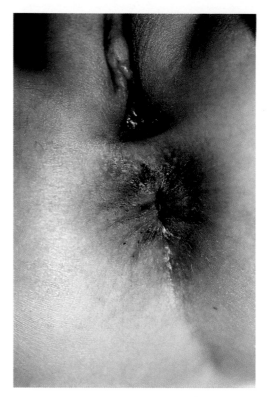

▲ **23.126 Female aged 2 years**
Marked perianal congestion is seen, with
swelling. (Note: there was a history of recurrent
rectal prolapse and anal abuse.) Signs: venous
congestion.

▲ **23.127 Male aged 7 years**
The perianal skin is red and smooth. There is
an irregular anal margin, and reflex anal
dilatation with stool visible in the rectum.

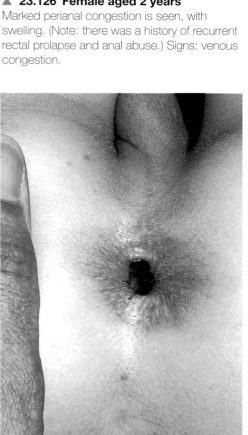

◄ **23.128 Male aged 9 years**
The perianal skin is red and smooth. There is
an irregular anal margin, and reflex anal
dilatation. Signs: skin changes, irregular margin,
reflex anal dilatation, stool. (Note: the boys in
Figs 23.127 and 23.128 were brothers and
both gave clear disclosures of anal abuse.
Stool in the rectum does not invalidate the
signs here.)

Chapter 24

Sexually Transmitted Diseases in Children and Adolescents

'Non-sexual transmission of STDs is rarely an issue in adults ... when STD occurs in children CSA must be suspected ...' (RCP 1991)

The risk of an STD in an abused child is in the order of 5% in young children to 25% in adolescents and the risk varies:

- depending on the age of the child, for example the acquisition of an STD neonatally may be from direct contact in the birth canal;
- the nature of the abuse, for example penetration is more likely to result in an acquired infection;
- sexual precocity of older children leading to multiple abusers;
- children who are symptomatic, for example who have a vaginal discharge;
- children who are asymptomatic are at a lower risk, but there remains the possibility of asymptomatic infection, particularly of *Chlamydia*.

STDs: There may be no symptoms early on

Symptoms of STDs:
- may be minimal;
- a vaginal or penile purulent discharge;
- pain, e.g. vulval or rectal;
- systemic illness.

STDs may lead to sterility if untreated

Screening for STDs
This might be the ideal for all children thought at risk of CSA but:

- Some children do not co-operate with the examination.
- Some children will co-operate with the exam but not swabs.
- Young children may tolerate 1 to 2 swabs, a 'minimal screen' has been evolved – a protocol is described below.

- Discussions with the local genito-urinary physician will inform as to local epidemiology and which investigations are indicated as well as suggesting therapy.
- It is good practice to have a teenage clinic, perhaps once a week, where a full examination can be undertaken. A GU nurse is an invaluable colleague both in skilled handling of the swabs but also in discussing sexual health with teenagers.
- STDs are important to recognize not only because of ill health in the short term but long-term sequelae such as pelvic inflammatory disease and the risk of infertility – it may therefore be necessary to give a general anaesthetic on occasion.
- A summary of necessary information is given in Table 24.1.
- Treatment is best discussed with local GU physicians and not advised in this paper.

STD may have no symptoms in early disease

Summary
- STDs are an uncommon complication of CSA in prepubertal girls but the prevalence rises rapidly in adolescents (both sexes).
- The sequelae should not be underestimated, for example pelvic inflammatory disease leading to sterility in girls.
- Proven STD is important forensically and ideally two swabs would be taken, for example to diagnose gonorrhoea. In addition, typing of the micro-organism would give further important information.
- If finding of an STD is to be used in court the microbiologist may be required to give evidence as to method and establish the 'chain of evidence'.
- It is to be remembered that STDs are transmitted sexually but a careful picture ('jigsaw') is needed to diagnose CSA.

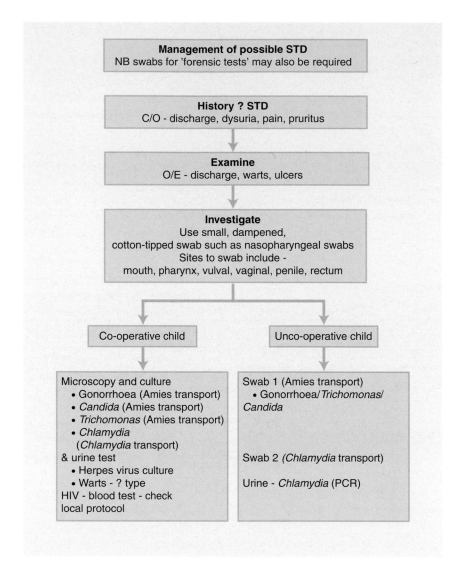

Management of possible STD
NB swabs for 'forensic tests' may also be required

History ? STD
C/O - discharge, dysuria, pain, pruritus

Examine
O/E - discharge, warts, ulcers

Investigate
Use small, dampened,
cotton-tipped swab such as nasopharyngeal swabs
Sites to swab include -
mouth, pharynx, vulval, vaginal, penile, rectum

Co-operative child

Unco-operative child

Microscopy and culture
• Gonorrhoea (Amies transport)
• *Candida* (Amies transport)
• *Trichomonas* (Amies transport)
• *Chlamydia*
  (*Chlamydia* transport)
& urine test
• Herpes virus culture
• Warts - ? type
HIV - blood test - check
local protocol

Swab 1 (Amies transport)
• Gonorrhoea/*Trichomonas*/
Candida

Swab 2 (*Chlamydia* transport)

Urine - *Chlamydia* (PCR)

Fig. 24.1

Table 24.1 Relevant information on common STDs (after RCP 1997)

	Incubation	Route of infection	Probability of CSA
Gonorrhoea	3–4 days	Birth canal Direct contact	*** ** if <2 years
Chlamydia	7–14 days	Birth canal Direct contact	*** ** if <3 years
Herpes	2–14 days	Birth canal Direct contact	**
Trichomonas	1–4 weeks	Birth canal Direct contact	*** if child >6 weeks
Warts	1 month – many months	*In utero* Birth canal Direct contact	*
Bacterial vaginosis	2–14 days	Direct contact	*
HIV	3 months	*In utero* Perinatal	*

Table 24.2 Timing of Forensic samples

Seminal fluid (SF)	Vaginal – 12–18 hours SF 6 days S	External swab taken before Internal
Spermatozoa (S)	Anus – 3 hours SF 3 days S Mouth – 12–14 hours S Clothing/bedding until washed S & SF	SF may be found on abdomen, thighs, anogenital area
Saliva	Mouth – 6–12 hours	Salivary DNA – bites, love-bites, anogenital area Semen – on saliva specimen or swab Drug/alcohol assay
Urine	As soon as possible	DNA Drug/alcohol/solvent
Blood		

Forensic sampling in possible child sexual abuse

General principles:

1. Forensic tests are based on Locard's principle that every contact leaves a trace.
2. Evidential trace material may be stains of blood, semen, vaginal fluid, faeces, saliva, lubricant or debris such as pubic hair and fibres.
3. The timing of the forensic sampling is critical for some investigations – see Table 24.2.
4. The method of sampling, labelling, storing and delivery of samples is important:
   - samples are usually given to a police officer with care as to the 'chain of evidence';
   - police forces will provide 'rape kits' but clinics should have equipment ready for the unexpected referral.
5. Plain swabs are used (non-albumen coated).
6. Moist material is collected with dry swabs and dry material with damp swabs – use a minimal amount of tap water.
7. Specimens are labelled immediately in a standard format, e.g. HS1, HS2 represent the first two specimens taken by Dr H Smith – and the site is recorded.
8. Control – unused dry and damp swabs are taken.
9. Other samples may be taken from furniture, clothing.
10. Table
    - bathing, urination, defaecation – all eliminate or dilute material;
    - NB drainage varies with age and mobility;
    - collect alien hairs;
    - pulled hairs are needed for DNA and not done routinely;
    - lubricant should be revealed on routine testing.
11. Adolescents and rape allegations – all investigations listed are indicated and usually a screen for STD, consider HIV testing. Requires follow-up medically. Is emergency contraception needed?

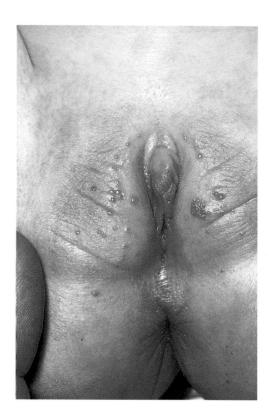

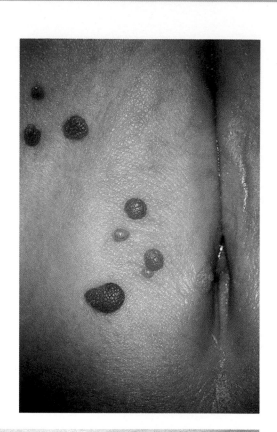

◀ **24.1 Female aged 13 months**
She presented to her doctor with unexplained lesions. Small scattered warts are seen across the flattened labia, and irregular skin is seen on the perineum. None of the carers of this child admitted to having a wart infection.
A 9-year-old uncle was known to have been involved in inappropriate sexual play. The diagnosis is an unexplained wart infection.

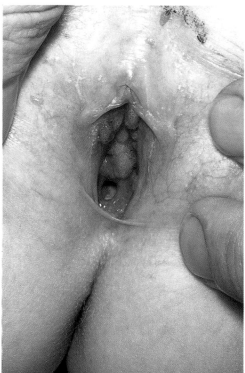

▲ **24.2, ▲ 24.3 Female aged 2 years**
Vulval warts in a child who presented with a hand burn.

▲ **24.4 Female aged 5 years**
The mother took her child to the doctor because of vaginal bleeding. The father was known to have penile warts. There are numerous vulval warts, mainly at the anterior introitus. A normal hymen is visible.

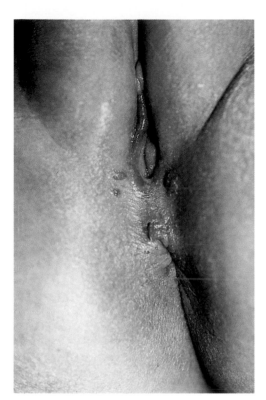

◄ 24.5 Female aged 3 years
She was taken to the doctor by her parents who were having difficulty in cleaning her bottom. There are unexplained perineal warts.

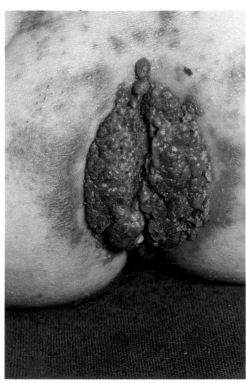

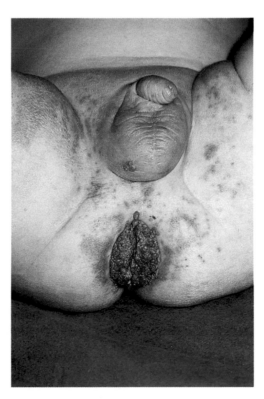

▲ 24.6, ▲ 24.7 Male aged 11 months
He was taken to the doctor for advice. Subsequently it was discovered that both of the separated parents had warts. Gross perianal warts are seen with a few seeded on the scrotum. The mode of transmission of these warts was uncertain.

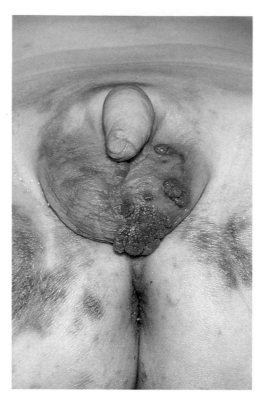

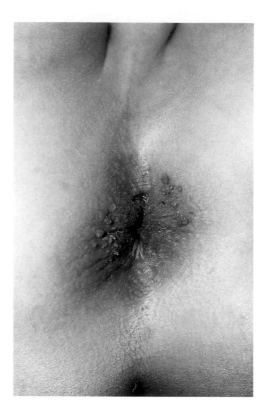

▲ **24.8 Male aged 18 months**
The mother asked the health visitor for advice. A large number of genital warts are seen, with co-existing nappy rash. The mode of transmission of these warts was uncertain

▲ **24.9 Male aged 6 years**
The mother took the child to the doctor for advice about the warts. Perianal warts are seen, with venous congestion and irregular folds with a posterior scar. This boy later alleged sexual abuse by his father.

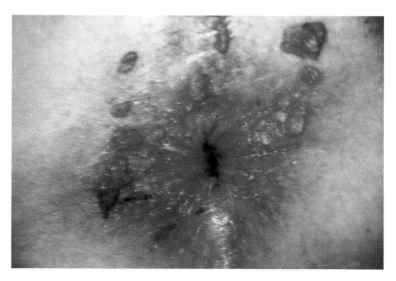

▲ **24.10 Male aged 7 years**
Boy with multiple perianal warts. There is some reddening and swelling of the anal verge.

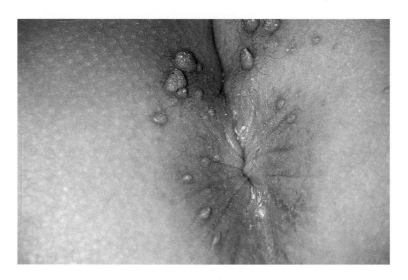

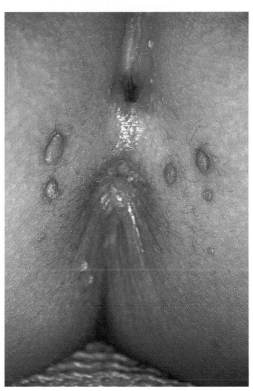

▲ 24.11, ▶ 24.12 Female aged 3 years

She was taken to the doctor by her mother for advice. Scattered perianal warts are visible, extending over the perineum. A friable posterior fourchette is show which bled on examination. The hymen was normal. The mother insisted that she had transmitted the warts from warts on her own hands but she had none. The mode of transmission of these warts was uncertain but was seen in association with signs consistent with intracrural intercourse.

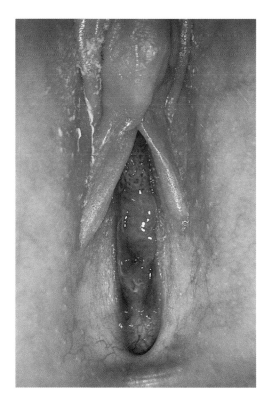

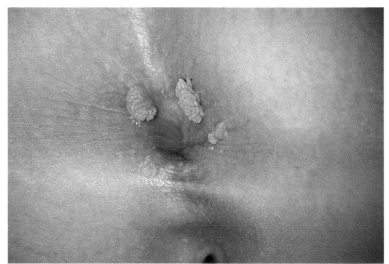

◀ 24.13, ▲ 24.14 Female aged 6 years

Girl's with introital and perianal warts.

▶ **24.15,** ▶ **24.16 Male twins aged 3 years**
They were taken to the doctor by their mother who was concerned about their warts. The warts developed within a day or two of each other. Perianal reddening is seen with swelling of the margin and venous congestion, and perianal warts. The father admitted to having penile warts but denied any abuse.

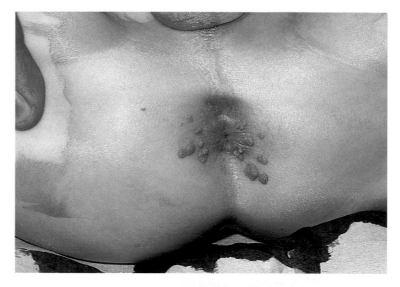

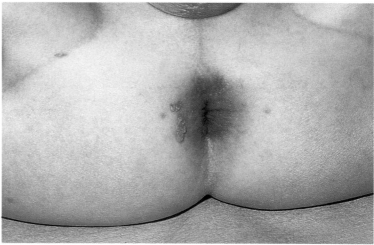

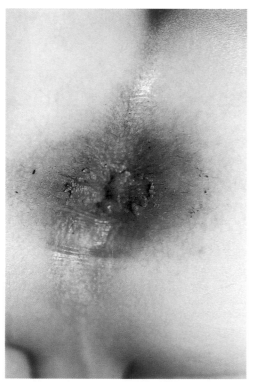

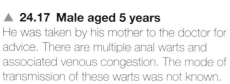

▲ **24.17 Male aged 5 years**
He was taken by his mother to the doctor for advice. There are multiple anal warts and associated venous congestion. The mode of transmission of these warts was not known.

▶ **24.18 Male aged 9 years**
One of five children all of whom had been seriously sexually abused. There is perianal reddening, dilated veins and irregular folds. Microbiological investigation showed the reddening to be due to *Candida* infection.

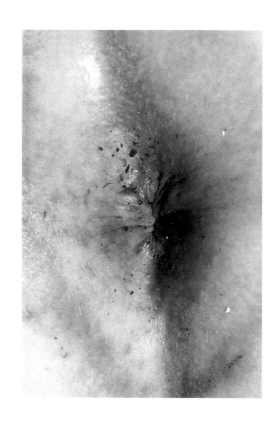

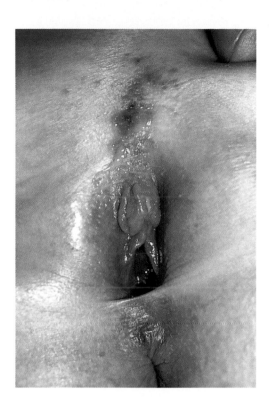

◄ 24.19 Female aged 5 years
She was referred by her doctor because of
purulent vaginal discharge. Marked vulvitis is
seen with purulent discharge. Microbiological
investigation was negative. Note the vascular
abnormality of the perineum.

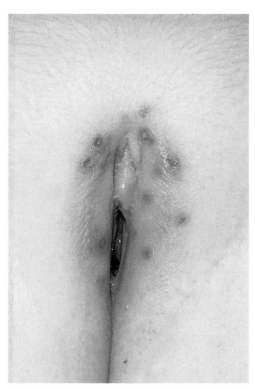

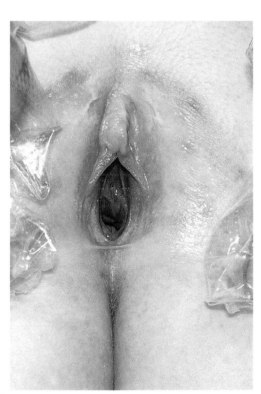

▲ 24.20, ▲ 24.21 Female aged 7 years
She was taken to the doctor by her mother because of a painful rash in the genital area. This child
and her siblings had been sexually abused by their father a year earlier, who had been convicted.
Multiple vesicles are seen on Fig. 24.20. Figure 24.21 was taken 3 days later and shows healing but
persisting discharge and gaping attenuated hymen. Microbiological investigation showed a herpes
type I infection.

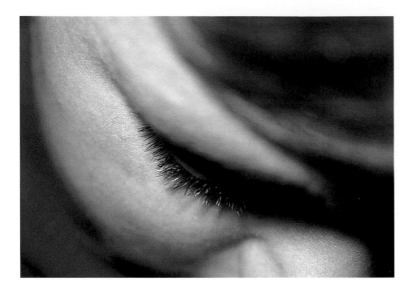

▲ **24.22 Female aged 3 years**

The child was referred to the paediatric department with an allegation of sexual abuse and was complaining of sore genitalia. Pubic lice are seen adherent to the eyelashes.

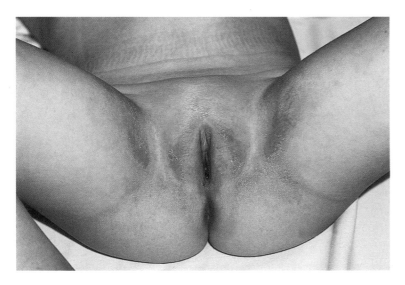

▲ **24.23 Female aged 3 years**

She was taken to the doctor complaining of soreness. Reddening of inner thighs and labia are seen. There was a purulent discharge. Microbiological investigation showed gonorrhoea. The child's father had gonorrhoea of the same type and was convicted.

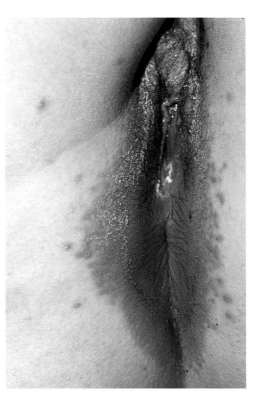

▲ **24.24 Female aged 14 years**

She went to her doctor complaining of soreness. There is a markedly inflamed vulva with satellite lesions. Microbiological investigation confirmed a candidal infection. This girl was sexually active and candidal infection is common in this group of teenagers.

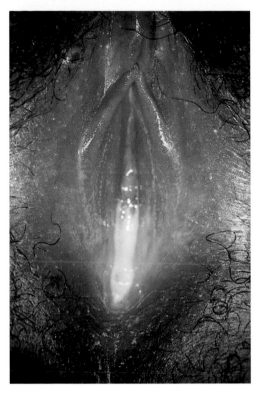

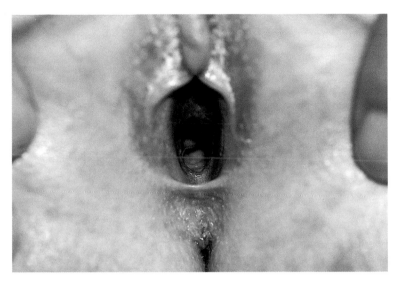

▲ **24.25 Female aged 11 years**
The child was taken by her grandmother to the
doctor because of purulent vaginal discharge
which had persisted over several months.
Vulvitis is seen with creamy coloured discharge.
There is a single small abraded area at
11 o'clock. Grossly abnormal anal findings
were also seen (see Fig. 23.59).
Microbiological investigation confirmed a
Trichomonas infection.

▲ **24.26 Female aged 8 years**
Social services referred the child because she
was living in a household with her brother who
was a convicted child abuser, and she was
known to have an offensive vaginal discharge.
There is marked vulvitis, and a gaping hymenal
opening with attenuation of the hymen and
a rolled edge. A vaginal ridge is seen at
9 o'clock. Microbiological investigation showed
a bacterial vaginosis.

Chapter 25

Differential Diagnosis of Sexual Abuse

The physical signs found in CSA are caused by trauma which may be complicated by infection or co-existent disorder, e.g. lichen sclerosis which itself may be precipitated by trauma.

Healing is often rapid in CSA and re-abuse frequent; both will change the signs.

The rate of healing depends on the degree of damage but scars are uncommon even in the very young.

The differential diagnosis of CSA is not extensive and the diagnosis more commonly is built up from the history, examination and other investigation (Tables 25.1–25.3). There are several clinical situations which are diagnostic, as listed:

◆ gonorrhoea, but repeat the swabs;

◆ pregnancy, remember to do DNA to confirm parentage;

◆ semen recovered from the child's body;

◆ physical findings:
  - tear in the posterior hymen;
  - attenuated hymen;
  - fissure crossing the anal margin, in the absence of bowel disease;
  - scarring – as a consequence of a vaginal or anal tear.

Symptoms such as bleeding, whilst highly correlated with CSA, have a differential diagnosis: trauma is the main cause in prepubertal girls and a careful assessment is needed – in straddle injury the child falls across a hard surface, trapping soft tissue – causing damage to the anterior tissues which may be asymmetrical; there is no penetration.

Female genital mutilation is against the law in the UK.

There is a growing debate in the UK on male circumcision – a general anaesthetic and analgesia is necessary if this ritual is thought necessary.

Table 25.1 Male genital injuries – differential diagnosis

History	Aetiology	Note
'Urethral bleeding'	Penetrative injury	CSA prepubertally ? in adolescence
	Forced retraction of foreskin	CSA prepubertally ? in adolescence
	Zip injury Bite – dog, horse	Usually seen still attached to zip May be difficult surgical repair
Unexplained injuries	Ligature, cut, 'nipped' Sucking injury Burn – cigarette, branding	Non-accidental injury – usually an adult abuser, male or female
Fell astride fence	Straddle injury	Careful history needed
Burn – girls too	Bullous impetigo	Small satellite lesions
Bruises – girls too	Grip marks, pressure Hand mark, strangulation	Check bleeding/clotting times

Table 25.2 Differential diagnosis

History	Aetiology	Note
Vaginal bleeding	Trauma – CSA – accidental Foreign body Vaginal tumour Precocious puberty Urethral prolapse	See* Straddle } Labial } not penetrative Rare, usually CSA Very rare Menarche < 8 years. Very rare
Vaginal discharge	An STD, e.g. *Trichomonas* Non-specific Minor trauma, e.g. rubbing Over-zealous washing by carer – may amount to CSA	Investigate as for CSA If recurrent? CSA ? CSA** Child may perceive as unpleasant and intrusive
Enlarged hymenal opening	Penetration	Tampon use does not damage – may be slight stretching – small tampons are about 1 cm
Vulvitis	Rubbing by abuser Infection as No.1	Masturbation does not cause symptoms unless it is obsessive/excessive
Labial fusion	Trauma – from nappy rash to forced penetration	In infancy a few cells are rubbed off giving a superficial short fusion; in rape the damage is in older girls, the fusion longer, thicker
Skin disorder/nappy rash	Lichen sclerosis Seborrhoeic dermatitis Psoriasis Eczema	May be related to trauma Looks like trauma Characteristic lesion
Vascular lesion	Congenital lesion, looks like a bruise	Labia minora Perineum

* No penetration.
** Harmful genital practices.

Table 25.3 The differential diagnosis of anal signs

History	Aetiology	Note
Increasing perianal inflammation	Streptococcal infection Candidiasis	Characteristic picture of cellulitis
Rash perianally/across perineum, labia	Eczema Seborrhoeic dermatitis Lichen sclerosis	Also nappy rash secondary to poor hygiene Steroid cream – may be secondary to trauma
Inflammatory bowel disease	Crohn's disease Haemolytic uraemic syndrome	Associated perianal disease, fissure, skin tags
Rectal bleeding	Rectal polyp Infection – Shigella Salmonella Fissure secondary to constipation	Diagnosed on proctoscopy Diagnosed microbiologically Diagnosed on history and examination
Congenital abnormality	Midline raphe Midline depressed shiny area at 6 & 12 o'clock	Distinguish from scars
Lax anus from birth	Neurogenic sphincters	Usually in association with neural tube defect
Swelling of sacral area	Rectal tumour	Rare
Accidental trauma	Sat on thorn plant	Environmental hazard

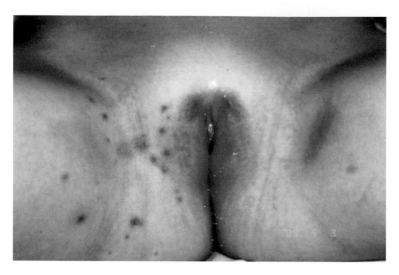

▲ **25.1 Female aged 4 years**
She was being sexually abused and developed secondary enuresis. Reddened labia are seen with satellite lesions. The signs are consistent with abuse and bed-wetting.

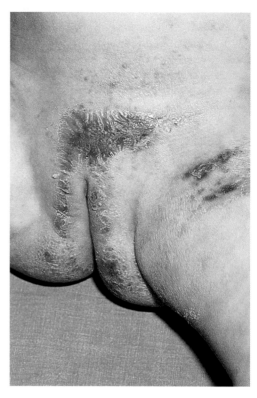

▲ **25.2 Female aged 3 years**
She was referred because the social worker was anxious about the possibility of a burn or sexual abuse. Blistering nappy rash is seen.

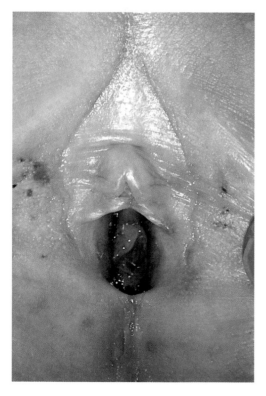

▲ **25.3 Female aged 4 years**
Girl with early lichen sclerosis. Notice the marked pallor and the scattered petechiae.

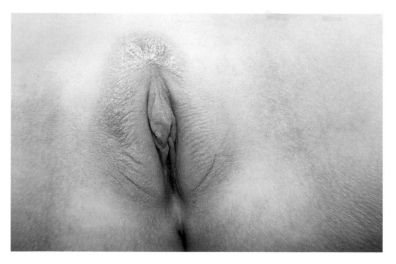

▲ **25.4 Female aged 6 years**
The child was referred because of sexualized behaviour, excessive mastubation and scratching. Thickened, dry, lichenified skin is seen across the mons pubis and labia majora, with wrinkled, flattened labia, and a scooped-out smooth posterior fourchette. Although initially it was felt that the physical signs were due to excessive scratching, it is more likely that this child was being sexually abused, i.e. intracrural intercourse.

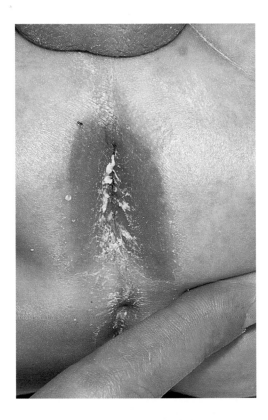

◀ 25.5 Male aged 3 months

His older sister had been sexually abused, and the referring doctor thought the baby had been abused also. There is marked perianal reddening. The diagnosis was nappy rash, which healed after being exposed for 24 hours.

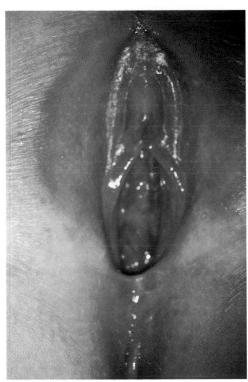

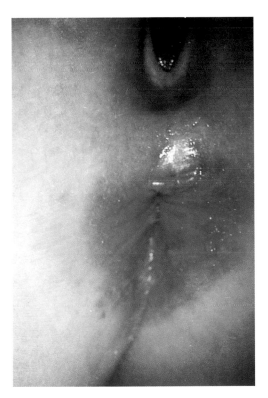

▲ 25.6, ▲ 25.7 Female aged 6 years

Girl with typical streptococcal infection with reddening and swelling both perianally and across the perineum. This girl should be re-examined when the infection with swelling has settled as it is not possible to have an opinion about the normality or otherwise of the genitalia and anus at this stage.

▶ **25.8 Male aged 6 years**
Referred by the doctor because of possible
sexual abuse. Reddened swollen perianal skin
is seen with superficial linear cracks. The signs
are consistent with a streptococcal infection,
which was proved microbiologically.

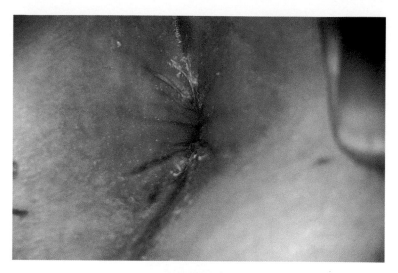

▶ **25.9 Male aged 10 months**
Referred because of a sore bottom and
possible fingernail scratches. Perianal
reddening is seen with small areas of skin loss.
The diagnosis was nappy rash associated with
diarrhoea.

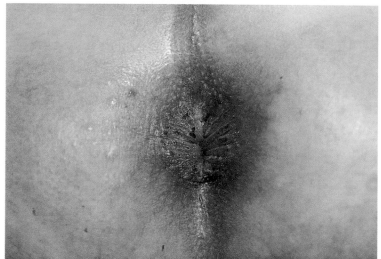

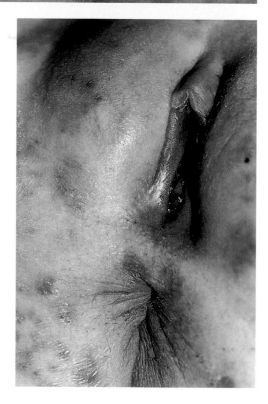

▶ **25.10 Female aged 18 months**
She was referred because of possible sexual
abuse. Marked nappy rash is seen. The child
also had signs of sexual abuse: congested
veins and a swollen red hymen are seen, which
are not features of nappy rash.

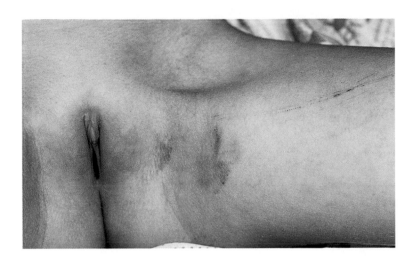

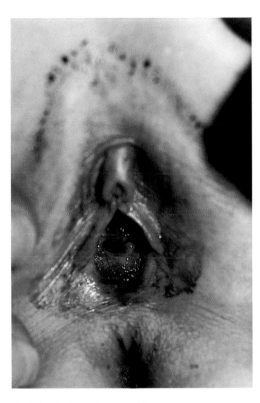

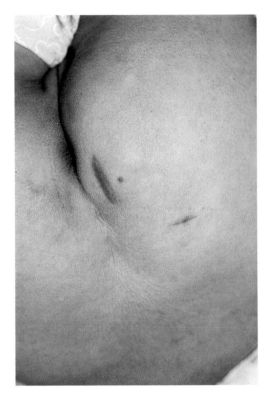

◀ **25.11 Female aged 6 years**
Child was referred to hospital after the school nurse noticed bruising on her legs. The child said this was caused by an accident on a home-made see-saw. A diffuse bruise is seen on the inner aspect of the left upper thigh with superficial abrasions. There was also bruising on the outer thighs, and signs of sexual abuse (the father was later convicted). The diagnosis was accidental injury.

▲ **25.12 Female aged 5 years**
She told her teacher she had fallen on the grass at school. She had grass marks on her dress and fresh blood in her pants. There is blood staining with a recent injury to the posterior fourchette. The hymen is red and swollen. This injury was not due to any ordinary accident. Injury of the posterior fourchette is usually specific for sexual assault or penetrating injury.

▲ **25.13 Female aged 4 years**
She was referred to the paediatrician because of possible sexual abuse. The history was that the child had had recurrent perianal soreness including abscess formation. The abscess had been surgically drained. The anus is normal; there is a surgical scar. The opinion was perianal abscess. There is no known association between sexual abuse and recurrent perianal abscesses in children.

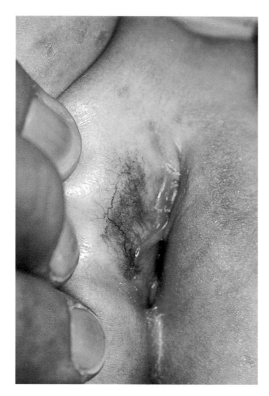

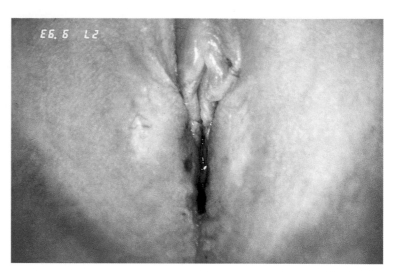

▲ **25.15**

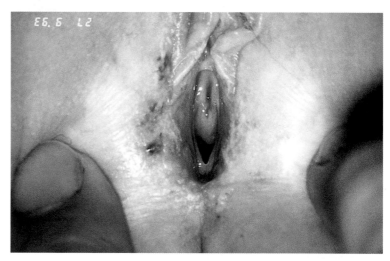

▲ **25.16**

▶ **25.17**

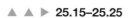

▲ **25.14 Female aged 2 years**
She was referred because of possible sexual abuse, after an older sibling was found to have been abused. There is unilateral haemangioma of the labia majora, due to a congenital vascular anomaly.

▲ ▲ ▶ **25.15–25.25**
This series of photographs shows lichen sclerosus et atrophicus. Note the depigmented area round the labia, perineum and anus, and telangiectasia which may bleed on contact. There is concern that lichen sclerosus may be associated or provoked by trauma as in sexual abuse. (Note: in several of these photographs there are genital or anal abnormalities which give rise to concern, and are not clearly the result of skin lesion.) (Sexual abuse of the child in Figs 25.19 and 25.20 was confirmed) (Figs 25.22 –25.24 by permission of Dr B. Priestley).

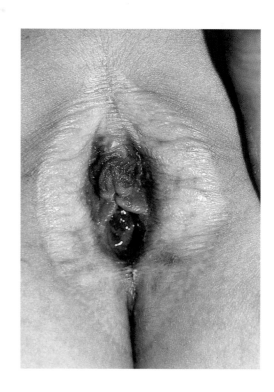

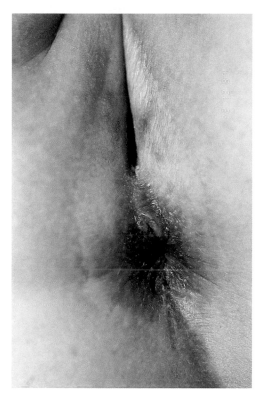

▲ 25.18

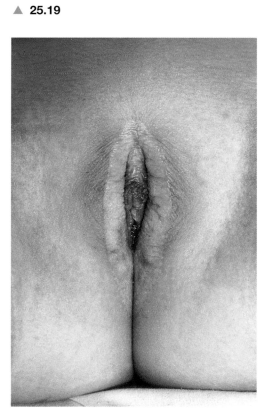

▲ 25.19

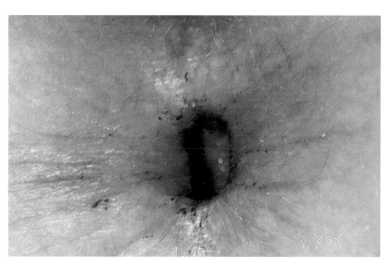

▲ 25.20

▲ 25.21 (continued overleaf)

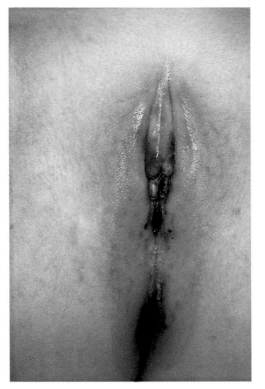

▲ 25.22

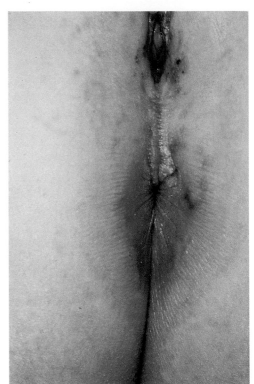

▲ 25.23

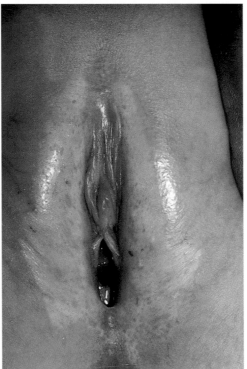

▲ 25.24

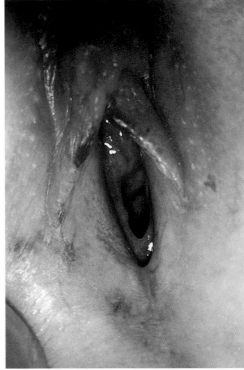

▲ 25.25

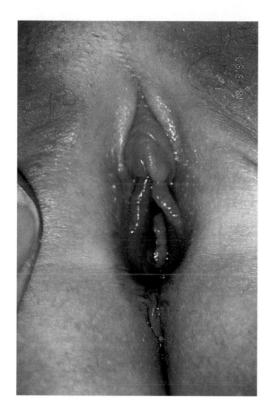

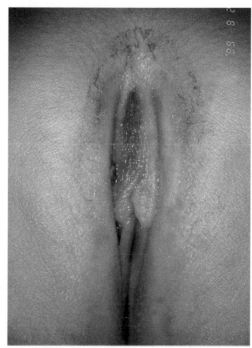

◄ 25.26 Female
Alleged straddle injury with markedly swollen
and reddened labia minora and bleeding.
The hymen is not clearly seen but looks
swollen. There is a prominent anterior anal fold.
Considerable doubt was expressed that this
was an accidental injury.

**◄ 25.27, ◄ 25.28
Female**
Girl with healing
straddle injury. Note
healing laceration on
inner aspect of the
labia majora
anteriorly.

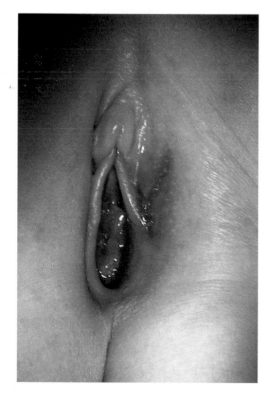

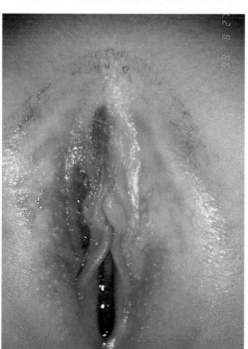

▲ 25.29 Female aged 4 years
She fell astride a climbing frame. Bruising to
labia majora and laceration lateral and anterior.
Hymen is swollen.

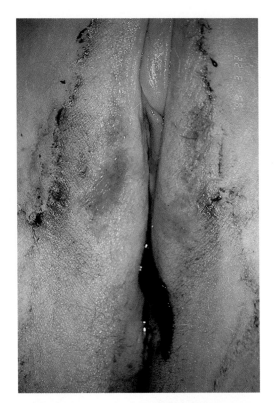

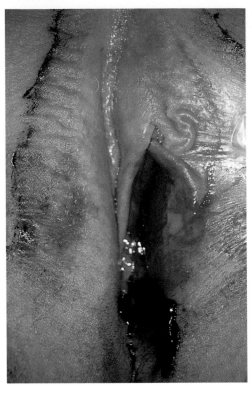

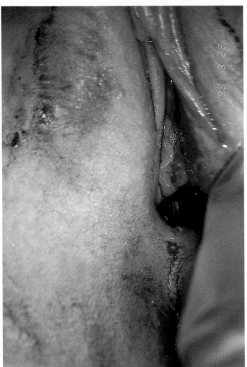

▲ ▲ ◄ 25.30–25.32 Female aged 6 years

She gave a clear history of falling on the corner of a drawer. Note bruising of the labia major and laceration of the inner aspect of the labia minora. Bleeding was quite extensive. The hymen looks normal.

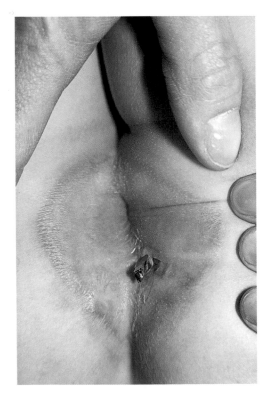

▶ 25.33 Male aged 4 years

He was referred because of a painful bottom. There was a history of falling on a milk bottle 2 years earlier. A shard of glass is seen protruding from the bottom. The diagnosis is accidental injury.

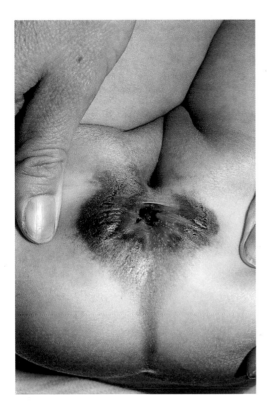
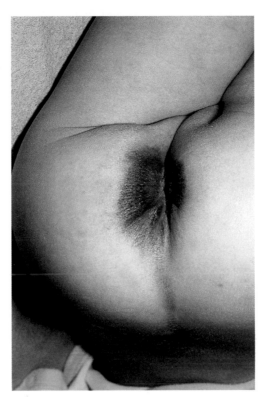

▲ **25.34, ▲ 25.35 Female infant**

She was referred because of rectal bleeding. There is marked venous congestion with perianal reddening and a gaping anus with prolapsing mucosa. The signs are due to a tumour. (Note the different nature of the venous congestion here as compared with venous congestion seen in sexual abuse.) (Figs 25.34 and 25.35 by permission of Dr M. Becker.)

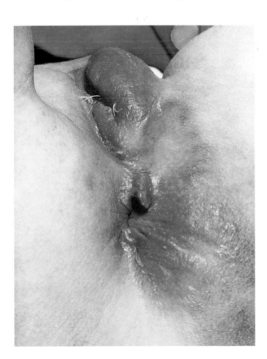

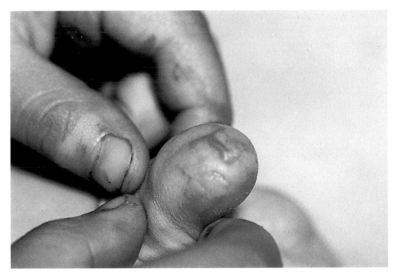

▲ **25.37 Male aged 5 years**

He was referred because his sibling had disclosed sexual abuse. There is a non-retractile foreskin, scarred, atrophic skin with prominent veins, and a displaced meatus. The diagnosis was xeroderma obliterans in a sexually abused boy.

▲ **25.36 Female aged 10 years**

She was referred by a gynaecologist who considered the possibility of sexual abuse. A grossly swollen left labia majorum is seen with perianal reddening and a large skin tag. The signs are consistent with Crohn's disease.